Cultural Diversity in Health & Illness

FIFTH EDITION

CulturalCare

There is something that transcends all of this
I am I . . . You are you
Yet. I and you
Do connect
Somehow, sometime.

To understand the "cultural" needs
Samenesses and differences of people
Needs an open being
See—Hear—Feel
With no judgment or interpretation
Reach out
Maybe with that physical touch
Or eyes, or aura
You exhibit your openness and willingness to
Listen and learn
And, you tell and share
In so doing—you share humanness
It is acknowledged and shared
Something happens—
Mutual understanding

—Rachel E. Spector

Cultural Diversity in Health & Illness

FIFTH EDITION

Rachel E. Spector, PhD, RN, CTN, FAAN

Associate Professor
Boston College School of Nursing
Chestnut Hill, Massachusetts

Prentice Hall Health
Upper Saddle River, New Jersey 07458

Library of Congress Cataloging-in-Publication Data

Spector, Rachel E.
   Cultural diversity in health & illness / Rachel E. Spector.—5th ed.
      p. ; cm.
   Includes bibliographical references and index.
   ISBN 0-8385-1536-3
     1. Transcultural medical care—United States. 2. Health attitudes—United States. 3. Transcultural nursing—United States. I. Title: Cultural diversity in health and illness.
II. Title.
    [DNLM: 1. Cultural Diversity—United States. 2. Attitude of Health Personnel—
United States. 3. Attitude to Health—United States. 4. Delivery of Health Care—
United States.
   WA 30 S741c 2000]
   RA418.5.T73 S64 2000
   362.1'0425—dc21

                                          99-046473

Publisher: *Julie Alexander*
Editor-in-Chief: *Cheryl Mehalik*
Acquisitions Editor: *Nancy Anselment*
Editorial Assistant: *Beth Ann Romph*
Director of Marketing: *Leslie Cavaliere*
Marketing Manager: *Kristin Walton*
Marketing Coordinator: *Cindy Frederick*
Director of Production and Manufacturing: *Bruce Johnson*
Managing Production Editor: *Patrick Walsh*
Production Liaison: *Cathy O'Connell*
Production Editor: *Karen Fortgang, bookworks*
Senior Production Manager: *Ilene Sanford*
Creative Director: *Marianne Frasco*
Cover Design: *Maria Guglielmo*
Cover Director: *Jayne Conte*
Composition: *Clarinda Company*
Presswork/Binding: *RR Donnelley and Sons, Harrisonburg*

Notice: The author and the publisher of this volume have taken care to make certain that the doses of drugs and schedules of treatment are correct and compatible with the standards generally accepted at the time of publication. Nevertheless, as new information becomes available, changes in treatment and in the use of drugs become necessary. The reader is advised to carefully consult the instruction and information material included in the package insert of each drug or therapeutic agent before administration. This advice is especially important when using new or infrequently used drugs. The publisher disclaims any liability, loss, injury, or damage incurred as a consequence, directly or indirectly, or the use and application of any of the contents of the volume.

Printed in the United States of America

10 9 8 7 6 5 4 3 2

ISBN 0-8385-1536-3

Prentice Hall International (UK) Limited, *London*
Prentice Hall of Australia Pty. Limited, *Sydney*
Prentice Hall Canada, Inc., *Toronto*
Prentice Hall Hispanoamericana, S.A., *Mexico*
Prentice Hall of India Private Limited, *New Delhi*
Prentice Hall of Japan, Inc., *Tokyo*
Simon & Schuster Asia Pte. Ltd., *Singapore*
Editora Prentice Hall do Brasil Ltda., *Rio de Janeiro*

I would like to dedicate this text to

My husband, Manny;
Sam, Hilary, Julia, and Emma;
Becky, Perry, and Naomi;
the memory of my parents, Joseph J. and Freda F. Needleman,
and my in-laws, Sam and Margaret Spector;
and the memory of my beloved mentor, Irving Kenneth Zola.

Contents

Preface

You don't need a masterpiece to get the idea.
                                                            —*Pablo Picasso*

In 1977 I wrote the first edition of *Cultural Diversity in Health and Illness* and have revised it several times since then; this is the fifth edition. The purpose of each edition has been to increase the reader's awareness of the dimensions and complexities involved in caring for people from diverse cultural backgrounds. I wished to share my personal experiences and thoughts concerning the introduction of cultural concepts into the education of health-care professionals. The books represented my answers to the questions:

- "How does one effectively expose a student to cultural diversity?"

and

- "How does one examine health-care issues and perceptions from a broad social viewpoint?"

As I had done in the classroom, I attempted to bring the reader into direct contact with the interaction between providers of care within the North American health-care system and the consumers of health care. The staggering issues of health care delivery are explored and contrasted with the choices that people may make in attempting to deal with health care issues.

It is now imperative, according to the most recent policies of the Joint Commission of Hospital Accreditation and the Health Care Financing Administration, that all health care providers be *culturally competent.* In this context, cultural competence implies that within the delivery of care the health care provider understands and attends to the total context of the client's situation; it is a complex combination of knowledge, attitudes, and skills. Yet,

- How do you really *inspire* people to *hear* the content?
- How do you *motivate* providers to *see* the world view and lived-experience of the patient? How do you assist providers to really bear witness to the living conditions and life ways of patients?
- How do you *liberate* providers from the burdens of *prejudice,* xenophobia, the "isms"—racism, ethnocentrism—and the "antis"?

Features

- **The HEALTH Traditions Quilt.** This edition of the book uses the no-tion of a "quilt" to present images and create the linkages from chap-ter to chapter. The HEALTH (HEALTH, when written this way, is defined as the balance of the person, both within one's being—physical, men-tal, spiritual—and in the outside world—natural, familial and commu-nal, metaphysical). The traditions quilt contains panels for each of the populations presented and several of the themes. This metaphor was selected because quilts are an old, creative art form that are invaluable objects in a home. Quilting, the creation of a quilt, is an art that is both absorbing and relaxing; the completed quilt provides protection, comfort, and warmth and often tells the stories of the person who cre-ated it. Quilts are invaluable treasures and heirlooms. In many ways the quilt is symbolic of and analogous to the concept of heritage and the traditions of a given people. This HEALTH Traditions Quilt is designed to awaken you to the richness of a given heritage and the symbolism, HEALTH beliefs, and practices inherent with many traditional cultures.

- **Three dimensions of health/illness issues.**
  1. **The worlds of the provider:** Health and illness from a personal perspective, from the background one carries from their immediate and historical families, and in the perspectives of the allopathic phi-losophy and health care delivery system.
  2. **The worlds of cultural differences:** Starting with background in-formation regarding culture and heritage and homeopathic philoso-phies that include HEALTH and healing traditions, both of natural and magico-religious dimensions.
  3. **The worlds of traditional HEALTH beliefs:** Examples of traditional HEALTH beliefs and practices among selected populations.
- **The Twentieth Century Time Line.** An overview of historic socio-cultural, public health and health policy events, and medical milestones from 1900–2000.

OVERVIEW

Unit I focuses on the provider's knowledge of his or her own culture.

- Chapter 1 explores the provider's knowledge of his or her own per-ceptions, needs, and understanding of health and illness.
- Chapter 2 explores family history and determines what methods were used to maintain, protect, and restore HEALTH in a given family.
- Chapter 3 focuses on the broad issues of health-care delivery, barriers, and alternatives.

Unit II develops the notion of choices in HEALTH care.

- Chapter 4 explores the concept of culture and the role it plays in one's perception of HEALTH and illness. This exploration is first outlined in general terms: What is culture? How is it transmitted? What is ethnicity? How does it affect a person?
- Chapter 5 describes the notions of HEALTH and HEALTH traditions are discussed. The HEALTH traditions model is explored as are natural methods of HEALTH restoration.
- Chapter 6 explores the concept of faith in the context of healing, or magico-religious, traditions. This is an increasingly important issue, which is evolving to a point where the professional must have some understanding of this phenomenon.
- Chapter 7 presents a discussion of the demographic backgrounds of each of the U.S. Census Bureau's categories of the population.

Once the study of each of these components has been completed, Unit III moves on to explore selected population groups in more detail.

These pages can neither do full justice to the richness of any one culture nor any one health-belief system. By presenting some of the beliefs and practices and suggesting background reading, however, the book can begin to inform and sensitize the reader to the needs of a given group of people.

The Epilogue is devoted to an overall analysis of the book's contents and how best to apply this knowledge in health planning, health education, and health-care delivery for both the patient and the health-care professional.

There is so much to be learned. Countless books and articles have now appeared that address these problems and issues. It is not easy to alter attitudes and beliefs or stereotypes and prejudices. Some social psychologists state that it is almost impossible to lose all of one's prejudices, yet alterations can be made. I believe the health-care provider must develop a sensitivity to personal fundamental values regarding health and illness. With acceptance of one's own values comes the framework and courage to accept the existence of differing values. This process of realization and acceptance can enable the health-care provider to be instrumental in meeting the needs of the consumer in a collaborative, safe, and professional manner.

The first edition of this book was the outcome of a *promesa*, a promise, I once made. The promise was made to a group of black and Hispanic students I taught in a medical sociology course in 1973. In this course, the students wound up being the teachers, and they taught me to see the world of health-care delivery through the eyes of the health-care consumer rather than through my own well-intentioned eyes. What I came to see, I did not always like. I did not realize how much I did not know; I believed I knew a lot. I have held on to the promise, and my experiences over the years have been incredible. I have met people and traveled. At all times I have held on to the idea and goal of attempting to help nurses and other providers be aware of and sensitive to the beliefs and needs of their patients.

I know that looking inside closed doors carries with it a risk. I know that people prefer to think that our society is a melting pot and that old beliefs and practices have vanished with an expected assimilation into mainstream North American life. Many people, however, have continued to carry on the traditional customs and culture from their native lands, and health and illness beliefs are deeply entwined within the cultural and social beliefs that people have. To understand health and illness beliefs and practices, it is necessary to see each person in his or her unique sociocultural world.

This book is written primarily for the student in basic allied health professional programs, nursing, medical, social work, and other health care provider disciplines. I believe it will be helpful also for providers in all areas of practice, especially community health, long-term oncology, chronic care settings, and hospice centers. I am attempting to write in a direct manner and to use language that is understandable by all. The material is sensitive, yet I believe that it is presented in a sensitive manner. At no point is my intent to create a vehicle for stereotyping. I know that one person will read this book and nod "Yes, this is how I see it," and someone else of the same background will say "No, this is not correct." This is the way it is meant to be. It is incomplete by intent. It is written in the spirit of open inquiry, so that an issue may be raised and so that clarification of any given point will be sought from the patient as health care is provided. The deeper I travel into this world of cultural diversity, the more I wonder at the variety. It is wonderfully exciting. By gaining insight into the traditional attitudes that people have toward health and health care, I find my own nursing practice is enhanced, and I am better able to understand the needs of patients and their families. It is thrilling to be able to meet, to know, and to provide care to people from all over the world. It is the excitement of nursing.

Acknowledgments

I have had a 25-year adventure of studying the forces of culture, ethnicity, and religion and their influence on health and illness beliefs and practices. Many, many people have contributed generously to the knowledge I have acquired over time as I have tried to serve as a voice for these beliefs and for the struggle to include this information not only in nursing education but in the educational content of all helping professions—including medicine and social work.

I deeply thank the people from the audiovisual Department of Boston College: Mary C. Binnell, Assistant Director, Graphics; Stephen Vedder, Assistant Director, Photography Production Service; Michal Hardoof-Raz, photographer, who painstakingly photographed many of the objects in my collection; Sarah Bastille, who was able to envision my notion of the quilt and able to "sew" each object or image into the panels—this quilt is a creation of love and the people who helped did so with that feeling; Wanda Anderson, Reference Librarian/Bibliographer, O'Neill Library, Boston College, led me to several of the texts used in developing the time line and offered helpful critiques during its development.

I particularly wish to thank the following people for their guidance and professional support over the years: Sally Barhydt, Elsie Basque, Dave Caroll, Julian Castillo, Leonel J. Castillo, Jenny Chan, Dr. P. K. Chan, Joe Colorado, Mary Crockett, Elizabeth J. Cucchiaro, Mary A. Dineen, Norine Dresser, Celeste Dye, Terry Fermino, Laverne Gallman, Elizabeth Garafalo, Omar Hendrix, Betty Koff, Orlando Isaza, Henry and Pandora Law, Barbara Ligouri, Hawk Littlejohn, Alfred Lui, Harold Lui, Patricia McArdle, Father Richard E. McCabe, S. Dale McLemore, Josie Morales, Virginia Swift, Sister Mary Nicholas Vincelli, Nora C. Wang, David Warner, Pat Wilson, and the late Irving Zola.

I also wish to thank my friends and family who have tolerated my absence at numerous social functions and the many people who have provided the numerous support services necessary for the completion of a project such as this.

A lot has happened in my life since the first edition of this book was published in 1979. My family has shrunk with the deaths of all four parents, and greatly expanded with a new daughter, Hilary, and a new son, Perry; and three granddaughters—Julia, Emma, and Naomi. The generations have gone, and come.

❁ *Credits for Quilt Panels*

Graphics

Mary C. Binell, Assistant Director, Graphics
Audiovisual Department
Boston College
Chestnut Hill, Mass.

Photography

Sarah Bastille
Michal Hardoof-Raz
Stephen E. Vedder, Assistant Director, Photography
Audiovisual Department
Boston College
Chestnut Hill, Mass.

Rachel E. Spector
Objects—Spector Collection

❁ *About the Author*

Dr. Rachel E. Spector has been a student of culturally diverse health and illness beliefs and practices for 25 years and has researched and taught courses on culture and health care for the same time span. Dr. Spector has had the opportunity to work in many different communities, including the American Indian and Hispanic communities in Boston, Massachusetts. Her studies in these culturals have taken her to many places, including much of the United States, Canada, Mexico, Cuba, Europe, Pakistan, Russia, Spain, Finland, Switzerland, France, and Israel. She was fortunate enough to collect traditional amulets and remedies from many of these diverse cultures and also to meet practitioners of traditional health care in those countries. She was instrumental in the creation and presentation of the exhibit "Immigrant Health Traditions" at the Ellis Island Immigration Museum, May 1994 through January 1995. She has exhibited health-related objects in several other settings.

Cultural Diversity in Health & Illness

FIFTH EDITION

Unit
I

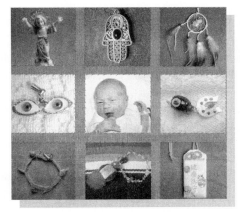

Provider
Self-Awareness

Unit 1 sets the stage for this book and enables you to become aware of health and illness beliefs, your and your family's historical health beliefs and practices in particular, and the health care delivery system in general. You are helped to

1. Understand health and illness and the sociocultural and historical phenomena that affect them.

2. Reexamine and redefine the concepts of health and illness.

3. Understand the multiple relationships between health and illness.

4. Associate the concepts of good and evil, and light and dark with health and illness.

5. Trace your family's practices in

   a. health maintenance;

   b. health protection; and

   c. health restoration.

6. Understand the interrelationships of sociocultural, public health, and medical events that have produced the crises in today's health-care system.

7. Trace the complex web of factors that

   a. contribute to the high cost of health care;

   b. determine payment for services;

   c. impede progress through the system;

   d. create barriers to utilization of the system.

Before you read Unit 1, please answer the following questions twice—first, as they relate directly to you and, second, as they relate to members of your family.

1. How do you define health?
2. What do you do to maintain your health?
3. What do you do to protect your health?
4. What do you do when you experience a noticeable change in your health?
5. Do you diagnose your own health problems?
6. From whom do you seek health care?
7. What do you do to restore your health? Give examples.
8. Do you use over-the-counter medications? Which ones and when?
9. How do you navigate the health-care system?
10. What are the barriers to your health care?

Chapter 1

Health and Illness

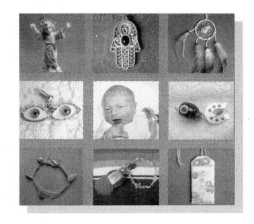

All things are connected. Whatever befalls the earth befalls the children of the earth.

—*Chief Seattle Suqwamish and Duwamish*

There are countless mirrors we can gaze into to ponder comprehensive notions of health and illness. How are they reflected throughout the contemporary dominant culture? In fact, we can begin our quest for a deeper understanding of the problems surrounding the delivery of adequate health care, by asking two fundamental questions: What is health? and What is illness? Once we find answers for these seemingly direct questions, we may then see the images of a comprehensive portrayal of health beliefs and cultural phenomena affecting health.

❋ *Health*

The answers to the first question, What is health? are not as readily articulated as you might assume. One response may be a flawless recitation of the World Health Organization (WHO) definition of health as a "state of complete physical, mental, and social well being and not merely the absence of disease." This answer may be recited with great assurance—a challenge is neither expected nor welcomed but may evoke an intense dispute in which the assumed right answer is completely torn apart. Answers such as "homeostasis," "kinetic energy in balance," "optimal functioning," and "freedom from pain" are open to discussion. Experienced health-care providers may be unable to give a comprehensive, acceptable answer to such a seemingly simple question. It is difficult to give a definition that makes sense without the use of some form of medical jargon. It is also challenging to define "health" in terms that a lay person can understand. (We lack skill in understanding "health" from the lay person's perspective.)

Figure 1–1 (From left to right, top to bottom) The Infant of Prague; Hand of God; dream catcher; "eyes of Saint Lucy"; identification bracelets; blue bead with horseshoe; red woven bracelet with jade amulets; beaded bracelet with the Virgin of Guadalupe, black jade, and a pom-pom; amulet. *(For more information on each picture see explanation at the end of chapter.*)*

One of the many definitions of health is in the *American Heritage Dictionary* (1976, paperback ed.):

> n. 1. The state of an organism with respect to functioning, disease, and abnormality at any given time. 2. The state of an organism functioning normally without disease or abnormality. 3. Optimal functioning with freedom from disease and abnormality. 4. Broadly, any state of optimal functioning, well being, or progress. 5. A wish for someone's good health, expressed as a toast.

Murray and Zentner (1975) have classically defined health as "a purposeful, adaptive response, physically, mentally, emotionally and socially, to internal and external stimuli in order to maintain stability and comfort."

These definitions—varying in scope and context—are essentially those that the student, practitioner, and educator within the health professions agree convey the meaning of "health." The most widely used and recognized definition is that of WHO. Within the socialization process of the health-care deliverer, the denotation of the word is that contained in the WHO definition. For other students, the meaning of the word "health" becomes clear through the educational experience.

In analyzing these definitions, we are able to discern subtle variations in denotation. If this occurs in the denotation of the word, what of the connotation? That is, are health-care providers as familiar with implicit meanings as with more explicit ones? Irwin M. Rosenstock (1966) commented that the health professions are becoming increasingly aware of the lack of clarity in the definition of health. Surely this is a contemporary and an accurate thought on the educational process, which is indeed deficient. He concludes that, "Whereas health itself is in reality an elusive concept, in much of research, the stages involved in seeking medical care are conceived as completely distinct."

The framework of both education and research in the health professions continues to rely on the more abstract definitions of the word *health*. When taken in a broader context, health can be regarded not only as the absence of disease but also as a reward for "good behavior." In fact, a state of health is regarded by many people as the reward one receives for "good" behavior, and illness as punishment for "bad" behavior. You may have heard something like "She is so good; no wonder she is so healthy," or a mother admonishing her child, "If you don't do such and such, you'll get sick." Situations and experiences may be avoided for the purpose of protecting and maintaining one's health. Conversely, some people seek out challenging, albeit dangerous, situations with the hope that they will experience the thrill of a challenge and still emerge in an intact state of health. One example of such behavior is driving at high speeds.

Health can also be viewed as the freedom from and the absence of evil. In this context, health is analogous to day, which equals good light. Conversely, illness is analogous to night, and evil, and dark. Illness, to some, is seen as a punishment for being bad or doing evil deeds; it is the work of vindictive evil spirits. In the modern education of health-care providers, these concepts of health and illness are rarely, if ever, discussed, yet if these concepts of health and illness are believed by some consumers of health-care services, understanding these varying ideas is important for the provider. Each of us enters the health-care community with our own culturally based concept of health. During the educational and socialization process in a health-care provider profession—nursing, medicine, or social work—we are expected to shed these beliefs and adopt the standard definitions. In addition to shedding these old beliefs, we learn, if only by unspoken example, to view as deviant those who do not accept the prevailing, institutional connotation of the word *health.*

The material that follows illustrates the complex process necessary to enable providers to return to and appreciate our former interpretations of health, to understand the vast number of meanings of the word *health*, and to be aware of the difficulties that exist with definitions such as that of the World Health Organization.

How Do You Define Health?

You have been requested to describe the term *health* in your own words. Many of you may initially respond by reciting the WHO definition. What does this definition really mean? The following is a representative sample of actual responses:

1. Being able to do what I want to do
2. Physical and psychological well-being, "physical" meaning that there are no abnormal functions with the body, all systems are without those abnormal functions that would cause a problem physically, and "psychological" meaning that one's mind is capable of a clear and logical thinking process and association
3. Being able to use all of your body parts in the way that you want to—to have energy and enthusiasm
4. Being able to perform your normal activities, such as working, without discomfort and at an optimal level
5. The state of wellness with no physical or mental illness
6. I would define health as an undefined term: it depends on the situations, individuals, and other things.

In the initial step of the unlocking process, it begins to become clear that no single definition fully conveys what health really is.* We can all agree on the WHO definition, but when asked, What does that mean? we are unable to clarify or to simplify that definition. As we begin to perceive a change in the connotation of the word, we may experience dismay, as that emotional

---

*The unlocking process includes those steps taken to help break down and understand the definitions of both terms—*health* and *illness*—in a living context. It consists of persistent questioning: What is health? No matter what the response, the question, What does that mean? is asked. Initially, this causes much confusion, but in classroom practice—as each term is written on the blackboard and analyzed—the air clears and the process begins to make sense.

response accompanies the breaking down of ideas. When this occurs, we begin to realize that as we were socialized into the provider culture by the educational process our understanding of health changed, and we moved a great distance from our older cultural understanding of the term. The following list includes the definitions of health given by students at various levels of education and experience. The students ranged in age from 19-year-old college juniors to adult nursing trainees and graduate students in both nursing and social work.

Junior Students
- A system involving all subsystems of one's body that constantly work on keeping one in good physical and mental condition

Senior Students
- Ability to function in activities of daily living to optimal capacity without requiring medical attention
- Mental and physical wellness
- The state of physical, mental, and emotional well-being

Adult Students
- Ability to cope with stressors; absence of pain—mental and physical
- State of optimal well-being, both physical and emotional

Graduate Students
- State of well-being that is free from physical and mental distress. I can also include in this social well-being, even though this may be idealistic.
- Not only the absence of disease but a state of balance or equilibrium of physical, emotional, and spiritual states of well-being

It appears that the definition becomes more abstract and technical as the student advances in the educational program. The terms explaining health take on a more abstract and scientific character with each year of removal from the lay mode of thinking. Can these layers of jargon be removed, and can we help ourselves once again to view health in a more tangible manner?

In further probing this question, let us think back to the way we perceived health before our entrance into the educational program. I believe that the farther back we can go in our memory of earlier concepts of health the better. Again, the question What is health? is asked over and over. Initially, the responses continue to include such terms and phrases as "homeostasis," "freedom from disease," or "frame of mind." Slowly, and with considerable prodding, we are able to recall earlier perceptions of health. Once again, health becomes a personal, experiential concept, and the relation of health to being returns. The fragility and instability of this concept also are recognized as health gradually acquires meaning in relation to the term *being*.

This process of unlocking a perception of a concept takes a considerable amount of time and patience. It also engenders dismay that briefly turns to anger and resentment. You may question why the definitions acquired and mastered in the learning process are now being challenged and torn apart. The feeling may be that of taking a giant step backward in a quest for new terminology and new knowledge.

With this unlocking process, however, we are able to perceive the concept of health in the way that a vast number of health-care consumers may perceive it. The following illustrates the transition that the concept passed through in an unlocking process from the WHO definition to the realm of the health-care consumer.

Initial Responses

- Feeling of well-being, no illness
- Homeostasis
- Complete physical, mental, and social well-being

Secondary Responses

- Frame of mind
- Subjective state of psychosocial well-being
- Activities of daily living can be performed

Experiential Responses

(Health becomes tangible; the description is illustrated by using qualities that can be seen, felt, or touched.)

- Shiny hair
- Warm, smooth, glossy skin
- Clear eyes
- Shiny teeth
- Being alert
- Being happy
- Freedom from pain
- Harmony between body and mind

Even this itemized description does not completely answer the question, What is health? The words are once again subjected to the question, What does that mean? and once again the terms are stripped down, and a paradox begins to emerge. For example, "shiny hair" may in fact be present in an ill person or in a person whose hair has not been washed for a long time, and a healthy person may not always have clean, well-groomed, lustrous hair. It becomes clear that no matter how much we go around in a circle in an attempt to define health, the terms and meanings attributed to the state can be challenged. As a result of this prolonged discussion, we never really come to an acceptable definition of health, yet by going through the intense unlocking process, we are able finally to understand the ambiguity that surrounds the word. We are, accordingly, less likely to view as deviant those people whose beliefs and practices concerning their own health and health care differ from ours.

Another health mirror reflects on the question, How do you keep yourself healthy? One method used to help answer this question is to use health diaries.

Health Diaries. Keeping a 30-day health diary is recommended to increase awareness of your own health status—physical, mental, and spiritual—and health practices. Comments will be most revealing! We recognize that, in spite of learning proper methods of health maintenance, we have poor nutritional and sleeping habits and rarely, if ever, seek medical help for what some of us consider "serious" bodily complaints. At best, we delay seeking care until we give up the idea that our symptoms will disappear. This diary has a very sobering effect. It also is used as an additional humanizing tool. The term *humanizing* is used here because just as we treat ourselves or delay in seeking help, we also ought not to judge people who, for various reasons, treat themselves or delay in seeking health care.

The following exercise is designed to help you tune in to your own daily health status:

> Keep a daily record of your health—physical, mental, and spiritual— status and behavior for 30 days. If an illness occurs, record what is done for it, why it is done, and what type of health-care services were used. Include in this record medications taken (prescription and nonprescription), eating, sleeping, exercise, recreational, and spiritual activities. When appropriate, note the reasons for your actions.
>
> The daily record, or diary, enables you to see how you react to the various stresses and strains of daily life. It reveals the intricacies of your daily lifestyle—the things you take for granted. For example: Do you eat three balanced meals a day? Do you get enough rest? Do you exercise? Many answers to the questions that initiated this unit will emerge in this diary!
>
> At the end of 30 days, reread this diary and analyze it in relation to recommended health practices.
>
> Typical entries for such a record follow.

Monday
- Overslept (went to bed at 3:00 A.M.)
- Skipped breakfast
- Dozed in class
- Cola drink and cheese crackers for lunch
- Two aspirins (headache)
- Hamburger and french fries for supper
- Crashed at 8:00 P.M.

Tuesday
- Up at 6:30 A.M. for clinical
- Milk and toast for breakfast
- Exercise—walk in hospital corridors
- Supper—lasagna, wine

- Headache—two aspirins
- Bed 8:00 P.M. (couldn't study)

Wednesday

- Up at 7:00 A.M. for 8:30 lecture
- Walked to hospital
- No breakfast (not hungry)
- Peanut butter and jelly for lunch
- Afternoon snack—milk and candy bar
- Study until 2:00 A.M.
- Two aspirins (headache)

Thursday

- Up at 6:30 A.M. for clinical
- Coffee and cheese sandwich for breakfast
- Walked to hospital (it rained)
- Almost slept on ward
- No lunch (out of funds, no time to cash check)
- Cola drink
- Walked in hospital corridors

The omission of any type of comments regarding spiritual health is note-worthy. I have collected health diaries for 25 years and have discovered that for the majority of contributors the mere mention of spirituality is taboo. Comments such as "spiritually—lack in health," "lacking spirituality," and "slacker," are the norm rather than an exception.

Preventive Care and Health Maintenance.   Health can be seen from many other viewpoints, and many areas of disagreement arise with respect to how this word can be defined. "Health is not merely an end in itself, but rather a means of attaining human well-being within the natural constraints in which man finds himself" (Hilleboe 1972).

The preparation of health-care workers tends to organize their education from a perspective of illness. Rarely (or superficially) does it include a study of the concept of health. The emphasis in health-care delivery has shifted from acute care to preventive care. The need for the provider of health services to comprehend this concept is therefore crucial. As this movement for preventive health care continues to take hold, become firmly entrenched, and thrive, multiple issues must be constantly addressed in answering the question, What is health? Unless the provider is able to understand health from the viewpoint of the patient, a barrier of misunderstanding is perpetuated. It is difficult to reexamine complex definitions dutifully memorized at an earlier time, yet an understanding of health from a patient's viewpoint is essential to the establishment of preventive health-care services because the perception of health is a complex psychological process. There tends to be no established pattern in what individuals and families see as their health needs and how they go about practicing their own health care.

Health maintenance and protection or the prevention of illness are by no means new concepts. As long as human beings have existed they have used a multitude of methods—ranging from magic and witchcraft to present-day immunization and lifestyle changes—in an ongoing effort to maintain good health and prevent debilitating illness. One traditional viewpoint regarding prevention was advanced by Richard Stark (1973): "Health maintenance has become our national obsession. Logic suggests that in order to maintain health we must prevent disease, and that is best accomplished by eating balanced meals, exercising regularly, and seeing the doctor once a year for a checkup." These words resonate today. The annual ritual of visiting a physician or nurse practitioner has been extensively promoted by the medical and nursing establishments and is viewed as effective by numerous lay people. A provider's statement often is required by a person seeking employment or life insurance. Furthermore, the annual physical examination has been advertised as the key to good health. A "clean bill of health" is considered essential for social, emotional, and even economic success. This clean bill of health is bestowed only by members of the health-care professions. The general public has been conditioned to believe that health is guaranteed if a disease that may be developing is discovered early and treated with the ever-increasing varieties of modern medical technology. Although many people believe in and practice the annual physical and screening for early detection of a disease, there are some—both within and outside the health-care professions—who do not subscribe to it. Preventive medicine grew out of clinical practice associated either with welfare medicine or with industrial or occupational medical practice. The approach of preventive medicine and health maintenance is the focus of health-care practice in the United States.

Box 1–1 *Healthy People 2010*

Just as *Healthy People 2000: National Health Promotion and Disease Prevention and Objectives* was a statement of national opportunities, *Healthy People 2010* was adjusted to continue in this trajectory. These prevention initiatives present a national strategy for significantly improving the health of the American people in the decade preceding the year 2000 and in the decades to follow. These documents recognize that lifestyle and environmental factors are major determinants in disease prevention and health promotion. They provide strategies for significantly reducing preventable death and disability, for enhancing quality of life, and for reducing disparities in health status among various population groups within our society.

Both *Healthy People 2000* and *2010* define two broad goals:

1. Increase the span of healthy life for all Americans.

   The first goal of *Healthy People 2000*, and now of *2010*, was to increase the quality as well as the years of healthy life. Here the emphasis is on the health status and nature of life, not just longevity.

   The life expectancy of Americans has steadily increased. In 1979, when the first *Healthy People: The Surgeon General's Report on Health Promotion and Disease Prevention* was published, the average life expectancy was 73.7 years. Based on current mortality experience, babies born in 1995 are expected to live 75.8 years. There is now increasing interest in other health goals such as preventing disability, improving functioning, and relieving pain and the distress caused by physical and emotional symptoms (www.health.gov/goal/).

2. Eliminate health disparities.

   This is a critical objective, as disparities are prominent between whites and the emerging majority. During the 1997 Healthy People progress reviews for Hispanics and Asian Americans and Pacific Islanders, a consensus emerged to do away with differential targets for racial and ethnic minority groups in *Healthy People 2010*. Subsequently, this recommendation was extended to people with low income, people with disabilities, women, and people in different age groups.

   The elimination of disparities is a bold step forward from the goal of *Healthy People 2000*, which was to reduce disparities in health status, health risks, and use of preventive interventions among population groups. *Healthy People 2000* special population targets were established for racial and ethnic minority groups, women, people with low incomes, people with disabilities, and specific age groups (i.e., children, adolescents, and the elderly). Targets were set, calling for greater improvements for each of these groups than for the total population. However, with the exception of service interventions, these targets rarely aimed at achieving equity by 2000. *Healthy People 2010*, in contrast, has set the goal of eliminating these disparities during the next decade.

   The elimination of disparities by the year 2010 requires new knowledge about the determinants of disease, and effective interventions for prevention and treatment. It also requires improved access for all to the resources that influence health. Research and a knowledge base dedicated to a better understanding of the relationships between health status and income, education, race and ethnicity, cultural influences, environment, and access to quality medical services is now imperative. The improvement of access to quality health care and the delivery of preventive and treatment requires working more closely with communities to identify culturally sensitive implementation strategies (www.health.gov/goal2).

Cultural competence, which is defined as a set of knowledge, skills, and attitudes that allows individuals, organizations, and systems to work effectively with diverse racial, ethnic, religious, and social groups, is an inherent component of this mandate (www.health.gov/goal2). It follows that CulturalCare is the mode of care that will develop within the scope of cultural competence.■

HEALTH STATUS AND DETERMINANTS

Health, United States, 1998, is the 22d report on the health status of the nation submitted by the secretary of health and human services to the president and Congress of the United States. It presents national trends in public health statistics. The following selected examples are relevant:

1. **Infant mortality** declined between 1983 and 1995 for infants of black and of white mothers at all educational levels.
2. Mothers with more education are more likely to have received **prenatal care** than less educated mothers.
3. **Overweight** was inversely related to family income among non-Hispanic white adolescents, but not among Mexican American or non-Hispanic black adolescents. **Sedentary lifestyle** was inversely related to family income among teenage girls and to a lesser extent among teenage boys.
4. **Life expectancy** is related to family income; people with lower family income tend to die at younger ages than those with higher income. In 1996 life expectancy at birth reached an all-time high of 76.1 years.
5. Less educated men and women have higher rates of **homicide** and **suicide** than those with more education.
6. Adults with low incomes are far more likely than those with higher incomes to report **fair or poor health status**.
7. Between 1988 and 1994 **hypertension** was more common among women of lower income than of higher income.

❀ *The Health Belief Model*

The health belief model (Figs. 1–2 a and b) is useful for transitioning from a discussion of health to that of illness. It illustrates the patient's perceptions of health and illness and can be modified to reflect the viewpoint of health-care providers. When implemented from the provider's viewpoint, the material provides a means of reinspecting the differences between professional and lay beliefs and expectations. Forging a link between the two helps one better understand how people perceive themselves in relation to illness and what motivates them to seek medical help and then follow that advice.

PERCEIVED SUSCEPTIBILITY

How susceptible to a certain condition do people consider themselves to be? For example, a woman whose family does not have a history of breast cancer is unlikely to consider herself susceptible to that disease. A woman whose mother and maternal aunt both died of breast cancer may well consider herself highly susceptible, however. In this case, the provider may concur with this perception of susceptibility on the basis of known risk factors.

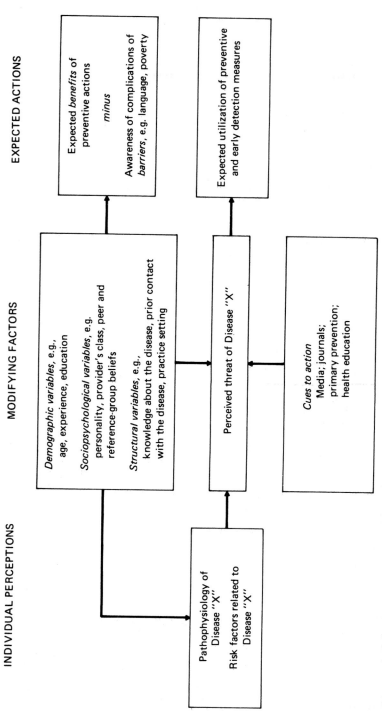

Figure 1–2.A Becker's "health belief model" as a predictor of preventive health behavior. (Reprinted with permission from M. H. Becker et al. "A New Approach to Explaining Sick Role Behavior in Low-Income Populations." *American Journal of Public Health* 64 (1974): 206).

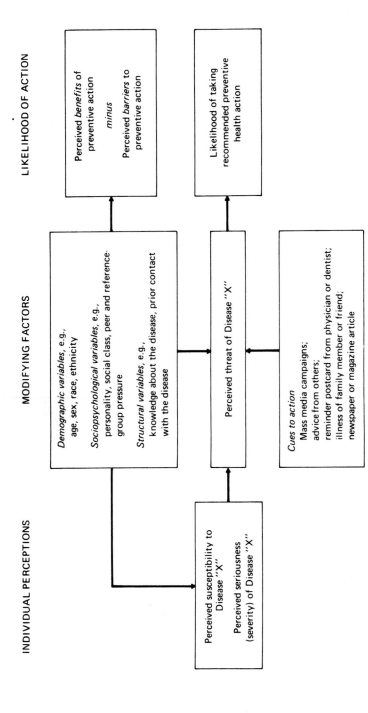

Figure 1–2B The health belief model from the patient's point of view.

PERCEIVED SERIOUSNESS

The perception of the degree of a problem's seriousness varies from one person to another. It is in some measure related to the amount of difficulty the patient believes the condition will cause. From a background in pathophysiology, the provider knows—within a certain range—how serious a problem is and may withhold information from the patient. The provider may resort to euphemisms in explaining a problem. The patient may experience fear and dread by just hearing the name of a problem, such as in the case of cancer.

PERCEIVED BENEFITS: TAKING ACTION

What kinds of actions do people take when they feel susceptible, and what are the barriers that prevent them from taking action? If the condition is seen as serious, they may seek help from a doctor or some other significant person, or they may vacillate and delay seeking and using help. Many factors enter into the decision-making process. Several factors that may act as barriers to care are cost, availability, and the time that will be missed from work.

From the provider's viewpoint, there is a protocol governing who should be consulted when a problem occurs, when during that problem's course help should be sought, and what therapy should be prescribed.

MODIFYING FACTORS

The modifying factors shown in Figures 1–2 a and b indicate the areas of conflict between patient and provider.

Demographic Variables: Race and Ethnicity.   The variables of race and ethnicity are cited most often as complex problem areas when the provider is white and middle class (or from one sociocultural economic class and the patient is from another) and the patient is a member of the emerging majority. The issues are complex and include overtones of personal and institutional racism. Such perceptions vary not only among groups but also among individuals.

Sociopsychological Variables.   Social class, peer group, and reference group pressures also vary between the provider and patient and among different ethnic groups. For example, if the patient's belief about the causes of illness is "traditional" and the provider's is "modern," an inevitable conflict arises between the two viewpoints. This conflict is even more evident when the provider is either unaware of the patient's traditional beliefs or is aware of the manifestation of traditional beliefs and practices and devalues them. Quite often, class differences exist between the patient and provider. The reference group of the provider may well be that of the "technological health system," whereas the reference group of the patient may well be that of the "traditional system" of health care and health-care deliverers.

Structural Variables.   Structural variables also differ when the provider and the patient see the problem from different angles. Often, each is seeing the same thing but is using different terms (or jargon) to explain it. Consequently, neither understands the other. Reference group problems also are manifested in this area, and the news and broadcast media are an important structural variable.

In summary, this section has attempted to deal solely with the concept of *health*. The multiple denotations and connotations of the word have been explored. A method for helping you to tune in to your health has been presented, a transitional discussion illustrating the plethora of issues to be raised later in the text has been included, and an overview of *Healthy People 2010* has set the tone for the remainder of the text.

❂ *Illness*

It is a paradox that the world of illness is the one that is most familiar to the providers of health care. It is in this world that the provider feels most comfortable and useful. Many questions about illness need to be answered:

- What determines illness?
- How do you know when you are ill?
- What provokes you to seek help from the health-care system?
- At what point does self-treatment seem no longer possible?
- Where do you go for help? And to whom?

We tend to regard illness as the absence of health, yet we demonstrated in the preceding discussion that health is at best an elusive term that defies a specific definition! Let us look at the present issue more closely. Is illness the opposite of health? Is it a permanent condition or a transient condition? How do you know if you are ill?

The *American Heritage Dictionary* defines *illness* as "Sickness of body or mind. b. sickness. 2. obsolete. Evil; wickedness." As with the word *health*, the word *illness* can be subjected to extensive analysis. What is illness? A generalized response, such as "abnormal functioning of a body's system or systems," evolves into more specific assessments of what we observe and believe to be wrong. Illness is a "sore throat," a "headache," or a "fever"—the latter determined not necessarily by the measurement on a thermometer, but by the flushed face, the warm-to-hot feeling of the forehead, back, and abdomen, and the overall malaise. The diagnosis of "intestinal obstruction" is described as pain in the stomach (abdomen), a greater pain than that caused by "gas," accompanied by severely upset stomach, nausea, vomiting, and marked constipation.

Essentially, we are being pulled back in the popular direction and encouraged to use lay terms. We initially resist this because we want to employ professional jargon. (Why use lay terms when our knowledge is so much greater?) It is crucial that we be called to task for using jargon. We must learn to be constantly conscious of the way in which the laity perceive illness and health care.

Another factor emerges as the word *illness* is stripped down to its barest essentials. Many of the characteristics attributed to health occur in illness, too. You may receive a rude awakening when you realize that a person perceived as healthy by clinical assessment may then—by a given set of symptoms—define himself as ill (or vice versa). For example, in summertime, one may see a person with a red face and assume that she has a sunburn. The person may, in fact, have a fever. A person recently discharged from the hospital, pale and barely able to walk, may be judged ill. That individual may consider himself well, however, because he is much better than when he entered the hospital—now he is able to walk! Thus perceptions are relative, and, in this instance, the eyes of the beholder have been clouded by inadequate information. Unfortunately, at the provider's level of practice, we do not always ask the patient, How do you view your state of health? Rather, we determine the patient's state of health by objective and observational data.

As is the case with the concept of health, we learn in nursing or medical school how to determine what illness is and how people are expected to behave when they are ill. Once these terms are separated and examined, the models that health-care providers have created tend to carry little weight. There is little agreement as to what, specifically, illness is, but we nonetheless have a high level of expectation as to what behavior should be demonstrated by both the client and provider when illness occurs. We discover that we have a vast amount of knowledge with respect to the acute illnesses and the services that ideally must be provided for the acutely ill person. When contradictions surface, however, it becomes apparent that our knowledge of the vast gray area is minimal, for example, whether someone is ill or becoming ill with what may later be an acute episode. Because of the ease with which we often identify cardinal symptoms, we find we are able to react to acute illness and may have negative attitudes toward those who do not seek help when the first symptom of an acute illness appears. The questions that then arise are, What is an acute illness, and how do we differentiate between it and some everyday indisposition that most people treat by themselves? When do we draw the line and admit that the disorder is out of the realm of adequate self-treatment?

These are certainly difficult questions to answer, especially when careful analysis shows that even the symptoms of an acute illness tend to vary from one person to another. In many acute illnesses the symptoms are so severe that the person experiencing them has little choice but to seek immediate medical care. Such is the case with a severe myocardial infarction, but what about the person who experiences mild discomfort in the epigastric region? Such a symptom could lead the person to conclude he or she has "indigestion" and to self-medicate with baking soda, an antacid, milk, or Alka-Seltzer. A person who experiences mild pain in the left arm may delay seeking care, believing the pain will disappear. Obviously, this person may be as ill as the person who seeks help during the onset of symptoms but will, like most people, minimize these small aches because of not wanting to assume the sick role.

THE SICK ROLE

The seminal work of Talcott Parsons (1966) helps explain the phenomenon of "the sick role." In our society, a person is expected to have the symptoms viewed as illness confirmed by a member of the health-care profession. In other words, the sick role must first be legitimately conferred on this person by the keepers of this privilege. You cannot legitimize your own illness and have your own diagnosis accepted by the society at large. There is a legitimate procedure for the definition and sanctioning of the adoption of the sick role and it is fundamental for both the social system and the sick individual. Thus, illness is not only a "condition" but also a social role. Parsons describes four main components that are inherent in the sick role.

1. "The sick person is exempted from the performance of certain of his/her normal social obligations." An example is a student or worker who has a severe sore throat and decides that she or he does not want to go to classes or work. For this person to be exempted from the day's activities, he or she must have this symptom validated by someone in the health-care system, a provider who is either a physician or a nurse practitioner. The claim of illness must be legitimized or socially defined and validated by a sanctioned provider of health-care services.

2. "The sick person is also exempted from a certain type of responsibility for his/her own state." For example, an ill person cannot be expected to control the situation or be spontaneously cured. The student or worker with the sore throat is expected to seek help and then to follow the advice of the attending physician or nurse in promoting recovery. The student or worker is not responsible for recovery except in a peripheral sense.

3. "The legitimization of the sick role is, however, only partial." When you are sick, you are in an undesirable state and should recover and leave this state as rapidly as possible. The student's or worker's sore throat is acceptable only for a while. Beyond a reasonable amount of time—as determined by the physician or nurse, peers, and the faculty or supervisors—legitimate absence from the classroom or work setting can no longer be claimed.

4. "Being sick, except in the mildest of cases, is being in need of help." Bona fide help, as defined by the majority of American society and other Western countries, is the exclusive realm of the physician or nurse practitioner. A person seeking the help of the provider now not only bears the sick role but in addition takes on the role of patient. Patienthood carries with it a certain prescribed set of responsibilities, some of which include compliance with a medical regimen, cooperation with the health-care provider, and following orders without asking too many questions, all of which leads to the illness experience.

THE ILLNESS EXPERIENCE

The experience of an illness is determined by what illness means to the sick person. Furthermore, illness refers to a specific status and role within a given society. Not only must illness be sanctioned by a physician for the sick person to assume the sick role, but it also must be sanctioned by the community or society structure of which the person is a member. Alksen (n.d.) divides this experience into four stages that are sufficiently general to apply to any society or culture.

Onset. Onset is the time when the person experiences the first symptoms of a given problem. This event can be slow and insidious or rapid and acute. When the onset is insidious, the patient may not be conscious of symptoms or may think that the discomfort will eventually go away. If, however, the onset is acute, the person is positive that illness has occurred and that immediate help must be sought. This stage is seen as the prelude to legitimization of illness. It is the time when the person in the preceding discussion may have experienced some fatigue, a raspy voice, or other vague symptoms.

Diagnosis. In the diagnostic stage of the illness experience the disease is identified or an effort is made to identify it. The person's role is now sanctioned, and the illness is socially recognized and identified. At this point the health-care providers make decisions pertaining to appropriate therapy. During the period of diagnosis the person experiences another phenomenon: dealing with the unknown, which includes fearing what the diagnosis will be.

For many people, going through a medical workup is an unfamiliar experience. It is made doubly difficult because they are asked and expected to relate to strange people who are doing unfamiliar and often painful things to their bodies and minds. To the lay person, the environment of the hospital or the provider's office is both strange and unfamiliar, and it is natural to fear these qualities. Quite often, the ailing individual is faced with an unfamiliar diagnosis. Nonetheless, the person is expected to follow closely a prescribed treatment plan that usually is detailed by the health-care providers but that, in all likelihood, may not accommodate a particular lifestyle. The situation is that of a horizontal–vertical relationship, the patient being figuratively and literally in the former position, the professional in the latter.

Patient Status. During the period of being a patient, the person adjusts to the social aspects of being ill and gives in to the demands of his or her physical condition. The sick role becomes that of patienthood, and the person is expected to shift into this role as society determines it should be enacted. The person must make any necessary lifestyle alterations, become dependent on others in some circumstances for the basic needs of daily life, and adapt to the demands of the physical condition as well as to treatment limitations and expectations. The environment of the patient is highly structured. The boundaries of the patient's world are determined by the providers of the health-care services, not by the patient. Herein lies the conflict.

Much has been written describing the environment of the hospital and the roles that people in such an institution play. As previously stated, the hospital is typically unfamiliar to the patient, who, nevertheless, is expected to conform to a predetermined set of rules and behaviors, many of which are unwritten and undefined *for* the patient—let alone *by* the patient.

Recovery. The final stage—recovery—is generally characterized by the re-linquishing of patient status and the assumption of prepatient roles and activities. There is often a change in the roles a person is able to play and the activities able to be performed once recovery takes place. Often, recovery is not complete. The person may be left with an undesirable or unexpected change in body image or in the ability to perform expected or routine every-day activities. One example might be that of a woman who enters the hospital with a small lump in her breast and who, after surgery, returns home with only one breast. Another example is that of a man who is a laborer and enters the hospital with a backache and returns home after a laminectomy. When he returns to work, he cannot resume his job as a loader. Obviously, an entire lifestyle must be altered to accommodate such newly imposed changes.

From the viewpoint of the provider, this person has recovered. Her or his body no longer has the symptoms of the acute illness that made surgical treatment necessary. In the eyes of the former patient, illness persists because of the inability to perform as in the past. So many changes have been wrought that it should come as no surprise if the person seems perplexed and uncooperative. Here, too, there is certainly conflict between society's expectations and the person's expectation. Society releases the person from the sick role at a time when, subjectively, the person may not be ready to relinquish it.

Table 1–1 is a tool designed for the assessment of the patient during the four stages of illness. Originally designed as a sociological measuring tool, the material has been altered here to meet the needs of the health-care provider in achieving a better understanding of patient behavior and expectations. If the provider is able to obtain answers from the patient to all the questions raised in Table 1–1, understanding the patient's behavior and perspective and subsequent attempts to provide safe, effective care become easier.

Another method of dividing the illness experience into stages was developed by the late Dr. Edward A. Suchman (1965). He described the five components that follow.

1. *The Symptom Experience Stage*—The person is physically and cognitively aware that something is wrong and responds emotionally.

2. *The Assumption of the Sick Role Stage*—The person seeks help and shares the problem with family and friends. After moving through the lay referral system, seeking advice, reassurance, and validation, the person is temporarily excused from such responsibilities as work, school, and other activities of daily living as the condition dictates.

3. *The Medical Care Contact Stage*—The person then seeks out the "scientific" rather than the "lay" diagnosis, wanting to know: Am I really sick? What is wrong with me? What does it mean? At this point, the sick person needs some knowledge of the health-care system, what the system offers, and how it functions. This knowledge assists in selecting resources and in interpreting the information received.

Table 1-1 A Tool for the Assessment of the Patient During the Four Stages of Illness

Onset	Diagnosis	Patient Status	Recovery
A. The Meaning of the Illness			
1. What symptoms does this patient complain of?	1. Does he or she understand the diagnosis?	1. Has his or her perception of the illness changed?	1. What are signs of recovery?
2. How does he or she judge the extent and kind of disease?	2. How does he or she interpret the illness?	2. What are the changes in his or her life as a consequence of it?	2. Can he or she resume prepatient role and functions?
3. How does this illness fit with his or her image of health? Himself, Herself?	3. How can he or she adapt to the illness?	3. What is his or her goal in recovery—the same level of health as before the illness, attainment of a maximal level of wellness, or perfect health?	3. Has his or her self-image been changed?
4. How does the disease threaten him or her?	4. How does he or she think others feel about it?	4. How does he or she relate to medical professionals?	4. How does he or she see present state of health—as more vulnerable or resistant?
5. Why does he or she seek medical help?		5. What are his or her social pressures leading to recovery?	
		6. What is motivating him or her to recover?	
B. Behavior in Response to Illness			
1. How does he or she control anxiety?	1. What treatment agents were used?	1. How does he or she handle the patient role?	1. Are there any permanent aftereffects from this illness?
2. How are affective responses to concerns expressed?		2. How does he or she relate to the medical personnel?	2. How does he or she resume old roles?
3. Did he or she seek some form of health care before he or she sought medical care?			

From: Alksen, L., Wellin, E., Suchman, E., et al. A Conceptual Framework for the Analysis of Cultural Variations on the Behavior of the Ill. Unpublished report. (New York City Department of Health, n.d.) Reprinted with permission.

4. *The Dependent-Patient Role Stage*—The patient is now under the control of the physician and is expected to accept and comply with the prescribed treatments. The person may be quite ambivalent about this role, and certain factors (physical, administrative, social, or psychological) may create barriers that eventually will interfere with treatment and the willingness to comply.

5. *The Recovery or Rehabilitation Stage*—The role of patient is given up at the recovery stage, and the person resumes—as much as possible—his or her former roles.

THE ILLNESS TRAJECTORY

Yet another way of explaining illness is to follow the trajectory of a given illness that a given person may experience. The term *trajectory* is applied to the following phases as they summarize the social science approaches that have

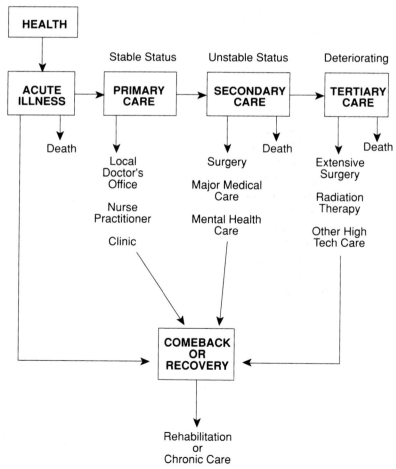

Figure 1–3 The illness trajectory.

been discussed to answer our second fundamental question, What is illness? and begin to shift our focus to the responses and experiences people have to and with illness. The focus now begins to move to the active role the patient plays in shaping and experiencing the course of a given illness. For example, the person with an illness may experience the following trajectory: acute illness, comeback or recovery, stable status, unstable status, deterioration, and death. The acute phase most often is treated in the acute care hospital, and the early phases of comeback and rehabilitation occur in this setting. The management of the chronic phase, except for acute episodes, is performed at home or in an institution that is either a rehabilitation facility or a long-term care institution (see Fig. 1–3). The illness profoundly affects the lives of the ill and their families—financially, emotionally, and spiritually. Further consideration of this phenomenon is found in later chapters.

MORBIDITY AND MORTALITY

There are countless indicators of the prevalence of diseases in the general population. As one example, the data presented in Table 1–2 illustrate the changes in age-adjusted death rates from 1970 to 1996 per 100,000 resident population.

As you can see, there have been countless explanatory words and models developed over time to define health and illness. Each of these is valid, each of these is time-tested, each of these is relevant as we go forward into the new century and into the millennium.

In summary, this chapter has introduced the dominant culture's perception of health and illness through countless lenses. The writings of a number

Table 1–2 | **Age-adjusted Deaths from Selected Causes of Death: United States, 1970–1996 Per 100,000 Resident Population**

Cause of Death	1970	1980	1990	1996
All Causes	714.3	585.8	520.2	491.6
1. Diseases of the heart	253.6	202.0	152.0	134.5
2. Malignant neoplasms	129.8	132.8	135.0	127.9
3. Cerebrovascular diseases	66.3	40.8	27.7	26.4
4. Chronic obstructive pulmonary diseases	123.3	15.9	19.7	21.0
5. Motor vehicle accidents	27.4	22.9	18.5	16.2
6. Pneumonia and influenza	22.1	12.9	14.0	12.8
7. Diabetes mellitus	14.1	10.1	11.7	13.6
8. Human immunodeficiency virus infection			9.8	11.1
9. Suicide	11.8	11.4	11.5	10.8
10. Homicide	9.1	10.8	10.2	8.5

From: National Center for Health Statistics. Health, United States, 1998, with Socioeconomic Status and Health Chartbook. (Hyattsville, Md., 1998), p. 203.

of sociologists have been examined in terms of applicability to health-care delivery. Material related to mortality has been included to further illustrate the phenomenon of illness.

❧ *References*

Alksen, L., et al. n.d. *A Conceptual Framework for the Analysis of Cultural Variations in the Behavior of the Ill.* Unpublished report. New York City Department of Health, 2.

Becker, M. H., Drachman, R. H., and Kirscht, J. P. 1974. *The Health Belief Model and Personal Health Behavior.* Thorofare, N.J.: B. Slack.

Hilleboe, H. E. 1972. Preventing Future Shock: Health Developments in the 1960s and Imperative for the 1970s: The Eleventh Brontman Lecture. *American Journal of Public Health* (February): 139.

Mechanic, D. 1968. *Medical Sociology.* New York: Free Press of Glencoe, 80.

Murray, R., and Zentner, J. 1975. *Nursing Concepts for Health Promotion.* Englewood Cliffs, N.J.: Prentice-Hall.

National Center for Health Statistics. *Health, United States, 1998, with Socioeconomic Status and Health Chartbook.* Hyattsville, Md.

Parsons, T. 1966. Illness and the Role of the Physician: A Sociological Perspective. In *Medical Care: Readings in the Sociology of Medical Institutions,* edited by W. R. Scott and E. H. Volkart. New York: Wiley, 275.

Rosenstock, I. M. 1966. Why People Use Health Services. *Millbank Memorial Fund Quarterly* 44(3) (July): 94–127. Discussion of article.

Stark, R. 1976. The Case Against Regular Physicals. *New York Times Magazine* (25 July): 10.

Suchman, E. A. 1965. Stages of Illness and Medical Care. *Journal of Health and Human Behavior* 6(3) (Fall): 114.

INTERNET SOURCES

http://www.health.gov/healthypeople/2010Draft/scripts/feframes.cfm?secname=goal1

http://www.health.gov/healthypeople/2010Draft/scripts/feframes.cfm?secname=goal2

http://www.health.gov/healthypeople/2010Draft/scripts/term.cfm?/Chapname=mental

*Figure 1-1 from page 1
From left to right—top to bottom: A baby is born—a new life begins. Many folk methods may be used to "create" this baby and safeguard it once born. The chapter-opening quilt panel of birth-related images depicts objects families may use to aid conception or to protect, maintain, and/or restore the health of a baby, mother, or young child. **The Infant of Prague**—was purchased from a Santera in a Botanica in the metropolitan Boston area, who suggested that this statue be placed in the room of a couple desiring to conceive. She told of several women who had used it and that it was most successful. **The Hand of God**—was purchased in Jerusalem and may be worn by women from many religious backgrounds for protection from the "evil eye." The blue bead in the center is said to add greater protection. **The Dream Catcher**—is from the American Indian Ojibway Nation. It is believed that dreams have magical qualities. The dream catcher is placed on an infant's cradle

board or hung in its room. When hung, the dream catcher captures dreams as they go by—good dreams drift gently with the help of the feathers, to the sleeping baby; bad dreams are captured in the web. The crystal is hung in the center to enhance the dreams. The **"Eyes of Saint Lucy,"** of Italian origin, may be worn or pinned on a baby to prevent blindness. The newborn baby wears identification bracelets. The one on her right wrist is marked with a red ribbon, as the baby was born to an Rh negative mother. In folk traditions the red string has several other meanings—one being protection from the evil eye. **The Blue bead with horseshoe**—is an amulet from a Palestinian community in Northern Israel, and it may be hung on the baby's crib or placed in the car for protection from the evil eye and good luck. A red woven bracelet with jade amulets may be placed on the wrist of a Chinese baby to protect it from evil spirits. A **beaded bracelet** with the Virgin of Guadalupe, black jade, and a red pom-pom may be placed on the wrist of a Mexican baby to protect it from the evil eye. An **amulet** may be pinned on the clothing of a Japanese baby for protection.

Chapter 2

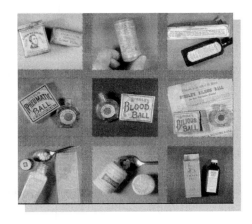

Familial Folk Remedies

As modern medicine becomes more impersonal, people are recalling with some wistfulness old country cures administered by parents and grandparents over the generations.
      —*F. Kennet,* Folk Medicine—Fact and Fiction

Given the difficulty of defining health and illness, it can be assumed that you may have little or no working knowledge of personally practiced "folk medicine" or traditional medicine within your own family. In addition to exploring the already described questions regarding the definitions of health and illness, it is beneficial to your understanding to describe how you maintain, protect, and restore your health. A common form of self-medication and treatment is the use of aspirin for headaches and colds, or occasional diet supplements with vitamins. Initially, one may admit to using tea, honey, and lemon and hot or cold compresses for headaches and minor aches and pains. For the most part, however, we tend to look to the health-care system for the treatment of minor illness.

There is an extremely rich tradition in the United States related to self-care. This includes the early use of patent medicines. Throughout most of their history, patent medicines enjoyed a free existence and were most popular with the people of the times. Some of the most popular medicines of the early twentieth century contained alcohol; others contained opium and cocaine. This served to increase their popularity, and the practice continued until passage of the Food, Drug, and Cosmetic Act of 1938 (Armstrong and Armstrong 1991).

The chapter-opening quilt panel, "American Traditions," of patent remedies portrays images of the time when families, perhaps yours, used popular patent medicines to protect, maintain, and/or restore their overall health.

Figure 2–1 (From left to right, top to bottom) Dr. M. Simmon's Liver Medicine and Dixon's Liver Pills, Piso's Tablets, Cardui, Steel's Rheumatic Ball, Steele's Blood Ball, Steele's Bilious Ball, Alka-Zane, Mac Laren's Mustard Cerate, Swamp Root. (*For more information on each picture see explanation at the end of the chapter.**)

As you can see in the concluding legend, these medicines served a wide variety of needs, and the manufacturers were quite flamboyant in their claims.

Folk medicine today is related to other types of medicine that are practiced in our society. It has coexisted, with increasing tensions, alongside modern medicine and was derived from academic medicine of earlier generations. There is ample evidence that the folk practices of ancient times have been abandoned only in part by modern health-care belief systems, for many of these beliefs and practices continue to be observed today. Today's popular medicine is, in a sense, commercial folk medicine. Yoder (1972) describes two varieties of folk medicine.

1. Natural folk medicine—or rational folk medicine—represents one of humans' earliest uses of the natural environment and utilizes herbs, plants, minerals, and animal substances to prevent and treat illnesses.
2. Magicoreligious folk medicine—or occult folk medicine—represents the use of charms, holy words, and holy actions to prevent and cure illnesses.

❧ *Natural Folk Medicine*

Natural folk medicine has been and still is widely practiced in the United States and throughout the world. In general, this form of prevention and treatment is found in old-fashioned remedies and household medicines. These remedies have been passed down for generations, and many are in common use today. Much folk medicine is herbal in nature, and the customs and rituals related to the use of these herbs vary among ethnic groups. Specific knowledge and usages are addressed throughout this text. Commonly, across cultures, these herbs are found in nature and are used by humans as a source of therapy, although how these medicines are gathered and specific modes of use may vary from group to group and place to place. In general, folk medical traditions prescribed the time of year in which the herb was to be picked; how it was to be dried; how it was to be prepared; the method, amount, and frequency of taking, and so forth. Chapter 5 explores this system in more detail.

MAGICORELIGIOUS FOLK MEDICINE

The magicoreligious form of folk medicine, too, has existed for as long as humans have sought to protect and restore their health. It has now come to be labeled by some as "superstition," yet for believers, it may take the form of religious practices related to health protection and healing. Chapter 6 addresses this belief system in more detail. One example is a form of unofficial religious healing that is not connected to churches, known as "powwowing," "charming," or "conjuring." In these practices, charms, amulets, and physical manipulations are used in the attempt to cure an illness.

Were you ever ill? What did your mother or grandmother do to take care of you? From whom did they seek advice first? Did they consult someone in your own ethnic or religious community to find out what was wrong? What remedies did they use? Do you know the health and illness beliefs and practices that were or are a part of your heritage? The following procedure is useful for making you aware of the overall history and health belief–related folklore* knowledge of your family.

Because the folk history of each family is unique, you may want to discover more than health beliefs and practices with this interview. Ask questions about your family surname, traditional first names, family stories, the history of family "characters" or notorious family members, how historical events affected your family in past generations, and so forth. Then, in interviewing your maternal† grandmother or great-aunt and your mother, obtain answers to the following questions.

1. What is the family's ethnic background? Country of origin? Religion?
2. What did they do to maintain health? What did their mothers do?
3. What did they do to protect health? What did their mothers do?
4. What home remedies did they use to restore health? What did their mothers use?

There are two reasons for exploring your familial past. First, it draws your attention to your ethnic heritage and belief system. Many of your daily habits relate to early socialization practices that are passed on by parents or additional significant others. Many behaviors are both subconscious and habitual, and much of what you believe and practice is passed on in this manner. By digging into the past, remote and recent, you can recall some of the rituals you observed either your parents or grandparents perform. You are then better able to realize their origin and significance. There are many beliefs and practices that are ethnically similar, and socialization patterns tend to be similar among ethnic groups as well. Religion also plays a role in the perception of, interpretation of, and behavior in health and illness.

The maternal side is selected for the interview because in today's society of interethnic and interreligious marriages, it is assumed that the ethnic beliefs and practices related to health and illness of the family are more in tune with the mother's family than with the father's. By and large, nurturance has been the domain of women in most cultures and societies. The mother tends to be the person within a family who cares for family members when illness occurs. She also tends to be the prime mover in preventing illness and seeking health care. It is the mother who tells the child what and how much to eat and drink, when to go to bed, and how to dress in inclement weather. She shares her knowledge and experience with her offspring, but usually the daughter is singled out for such experiential sharing.

A second reason for this examination of familial health practices is to sensitize you to the role your ethnic heritage has played. You must reanalyze the concepts of health and illness and, once again, view your own definitions from

*Folklore: the body of skills and knowledge passed on from one person to another for specific reasons.
†An explanation for choosing the maternal side follows in the text.

another perspective. If your familial background is presented in a class or other group setting, the peer group is able to see the people in a different light. A group observes similarities and differences among its members. You discover peer beliefs and practices that you originally had no idea existed. You may then be able to identify the "why" behind many daily health habits, practices, and beliefs.

Quite often, you may be amazed to discover the origins of these health practices. The "mysterious" behavior of a roommate or friend may be explained by reflecting on its origin. It is interesting to discover cross-ethnic practices within one's own group, as some people believe that a given practice is an "original," practiced only by their family. Many religious customs, such as the blessing of the throat, are now conceptualized in terms of health and illness behavior. Table 2–1 lists a sample of responses to the questions that students obtained from members of the maternal side of their families.

Table 2–1 | Family Health Histories Obtained from Students of Various Ethnic Backgrounds and Religions

Austrian (United States), Jewish

Health Maintenance
Eat wholesome foods, homegrown fruits and vegetables
Bake own bread

Health Protection
Camphor around the neck (in the winter) in a small cloth bag to prevent measles and scarlet fever

Health Restoration
Sore throat: Go to the village store, find a salted herring, wrap it in a towel, put it around the neck, and let it stay there overnight; gargle with salt water
Boils: Fry chopped onions, make a compress, and apply to the infections

Black and Native American, Baptist

Health Maintenance
Eat balanced meals three times a day
Dress right for the weather

Health Protection
Keep everything clean and sterile
Stay away from people who are sick
Regular checkups
Blackstrap molasses

Health Restoration
Bloody nose: Place keys on a chain around neck to stop
Sore throat: Suck yolks out of eggshell; honey and lemon; baking soda, salt, warm water; onions around the neck; salt water to gargle

| Table 2–1 | —Continued

Black African (Ethiopia), Orthodox Christian

Health Maintenance
Keep the area clean
Pray every morning when getting up from bed

Health Protection
Eat hot food, such as pepper, fresh garlic, lemon

Health Restoration
Eat hot and sour foods, such as lemons, fresh garlic, hot mustard, red pepper
Make a kind of medicine from leaves and roots of plants mixed together
Colds: Hot boiled milk with honey
Evil eye: They put some kind of plant root on fire and make the man who has the evil eye smile and the man talks about his illness

Canadian, Catholic

Health Maintenance
Cleanliness
Food: People should eat well (fat people used to be considered healthy)
Prayer: Health was always mentioned in prayer

Health Protection
Sleep
Lots of good food
Elixirs containing herbs and brewed, given as a vitamin tonic
Wear camphor around the neck to ward off any evil spirit; use Father John's medicine November to May

Health Restoration
Kidney problems: Herbal teas
Colds: Hot lemons
Infected wounds: Raw onions placed on wounds
Cough: Shot of whiskey
Sinuses: Camphor placed in a pouch and pinned to the shirt
Fever: Lots of blankets and heat make you sweat out a fever
Headache: Lie down and rest in complete darkness
Aches and pains: Hot Epsom salt baths
Eye infections: Potatoes are rubbed on them or a gold wedding ring is placed on them and the sign of the cross is made three times

Eastern Europe (United States), Jewish

Health Maintenance
Go to doctor when sick (mother)
Health care for others, not self (mother)
Reluctantly sought medical help (grandmother)
Health for self not a priority (grandmother)
Physician twice a year (mother)
Doctor only when pregnant (grandmother)

(continued)

| Table 2–1 | —Continued |

Eastern Europe (United States), Jewish—Continued

Health Protection

Observe precautions, such as dressing warmly, not going out with wet hair, getting enough rest, staying in bed if not feeling well (mother)

Not much to prevent illness—very ill today with chronic diseases (grandmother)

Vitamins and water pills

Health Restoration

Colds: Fluids, aspirin, rest

Stomach upset: Eat light and bland foods

Muscle aches: Massage with alcohol

Sore throat: Gargle with salt water, tea with lemon and honey

Insomnia: Glass of wine

Chicken soup used by mother and grandmother

English, Baptist

Health Maintenance

Eat well; daily walks; read; keep warm

Health Restoration

Earache: Honey and tea, warm cod-liver oil in ear; stay in bed

Cold: Heat glass and put on back

English, Catholic

Health Maintenance

Lots of exercise, proper sleep; lots of walking; no drinking or smoking; hard work

Bedroom window open at night

Take baths

Never wear dirty clothing

Good housekeeping

Immediate cleanup after meals; wash pan before meals

Rest

Health Protection

Maintain a good diet; fresh vegetables; vitamins; little meat; lots of fish; no fried foods; lots of sleep

Strict enforcement of lifestyle

Keep kitchen at 90°F in winter and house will be warm

Health Restoration

Cuts: Wet tobacco

Colds: Chicken soup; herb tea made from roots; alcohol concoctions; Vicks and hot towels on chest; lots of fluids, rest; Vicks, sulfur and molasses

Sore throat: Four onions and sugar steeped to heal and soothe the throat

Rashes: Burned linen and cornstarch

English, Episcopal

Health Maintenance

Thorough diet, vitamins

Enough sleep

Cod-liver oil

| Table 2-1 |

English, Episcopal—Continued

Health Restoration
Colds and sore throats: Camphor on chest and red scarves around chest

French (France), Catholic

Health Maintenance
Proper food; rest; proper clothing; cod-liver oil daily

Health Protection
Every spring give sulfur and molasses for 3 days as a laxative to get rid of worms

Health Restoration
Colds: Rub chest with Vicks; honey

French Canadian, Catholic

Health Maintenance
Wear rubbers in the rain and dress warmly; take part in sports; active body; lots of sleep

Health Protection
Sulfur and molasses in spring to clear the system
Cod-liver oil in orange juice
No "junk foods"; play outside; walk; daily use of Geritol; camphor on clothes; balanced meals

Health Restoration
Colds: Brandy with warm milk; honey and lemon juice; hot poultice on the chest; tea, whiskey, and lemon
Back pain: Mustard packs
Rashes: Oatmeal baths
Sore throat: Wrap raw potatoes in sack and tie around neck; soap and water enemas
Warts: Rub potato on wart, run outside and throw it over left shoulder

German (United States), Catholic

Health Maintenance
Wear rubbers; never go barefoot; long underwear and stockings
Wash before meals; change clothes often
Take shots
Take aspirin
Good diet

Health Protection
No sweets at meals
Drink glass of water at meals
Cod-liver oil
Plenty of milk
Exercise
Spring tonic; sulfured molasses

Health Restoration
Coughs: Honey and vinegar
Earache: Few drops of warm milk in the ear; laxatives when needed
Swollen glands or mumps: Put pepper on salt pork and tie around the neck
Constipation: Ivory soap suppositories

(continued)

Table 2-1 —Continued

German (United States), Catholic—Continued

Sore throat: Saltwater gargle
Sore back: Hot mustard plaster
Stye: Cold tea-leaf compress
Cramps: Ginger tea
Coughs: Honey and lemon; hot water and Vicks; boiled onion water, honey and lemon
Fever: Mix whiskey, water, and lemon juice and drink before bed—causes person to perspire and break fever
Headache: Boil a beef bone and break up toast in the broth and drink
Recovery diet: Boil milk and shredded wheat and add a dropped egg—first thing eaten after an illness

Iran (United States), Islam

Health Maintenance
Cleanliness
Diet

Health Protection
Dress properly for the season and weather; keep feet from getting wet in the rain
Inoculations

Health Restoration
Sore throat: Gargle with vinegar and water
Cough: Honey and lemon
Indigestion: Baking soda and water
Sore muscles: Alcohol and water
Rashes: Apply cornstarch

Irish (United States), Catholic

Health Maintenance
Good food, balanced diet
Vitamins
Blessing of the throat
Wear holy medals, green scapular
Dress warmly
Plenty of rest
Avoid "fast foods"
Attitudes were important: "Good living habits and good thinking": "Eat breakfast—if late for school, eat a good breakfast and be a little late"; "Don't be afraid to spend on groceries—you won't spend on the doctor later."
Keep clean
Keep feet warm and dry
Outdoor exercise, enjoy fresh air and sunshine
Brush teeth; if out of toothpaste use table salt, or Ivory soap, or Dr. Lyon's Tooth Powder
Be clean, wear clean clothes
Early to bed ("Rest is the best medicine.")

Health Protection
Clean out bowels with senna for 8 days
Every spring, drink a mixture of sulfur and molasses to clean blood

Table 2–1

Irish (United States), Catholic—Continued

Avoid sick people
Onions under the bed to keep nasal passages clear
During flu season, tie a bag of camphor around the neck
Never go to bed with wet hair
Eat lots of oily foods
Take Father John's Medicine every so often
Prevent evil spirits: Don't look in mirror at night and close closet doors
Drink senna tea at every vacation—cleans out the system
Maintain a strong family with lots of love
Be goal-oriented
Nurture a strong religious faith

Health Restoration
See doctor only in emergency
Fever: Spirits of niter on a dry sugar cube or mix with water; cold baths; alcohol rubdowns
Earache: Heat salt, put in stocking behind the ear
Colds: Tea and toast; chest rub; vaporizer; hot lemonade and a tablespoon of whiskey; mustard plasters; Vicks on chest; whiskey; Vicks in nostrils; hot milk with butter, soups, honey, hot toddies, lemon juice and egg whites; ipecac ("cruel but good medicine"); whiskey with hot water and sugar; soak feet in hot water and sip hot lemonade
Coughs: Cough syrup (available on stove all winter) made from honey and whiskey; Vicks on chest; mustard plaster on chest; onion-syrup cough medicine; steam treatment; swallow Vicks; linseed poultice on chest; flaxseed poultice on back, red flannel cloth soaked in hot water and placed on chest all night
Menstrual cramps: Hot milk sprinkled with ginger; shot of whiskey, glass of warm wine; warm teas; hot-water bottle on stomach
Splinters: Flaxseed poultice
Sunburn: Apply vinegar; put milk on cloth and apply to burn; a cold, wet tea bag on small areas such as eyelids
Nausea and other stomach ailments: Hot teas; castor oil; hot ginger ale; bay leaf; cup of hot boiled water; potato for upset stomach; baking soda; gruel
Sore throat: Paint throat with iodine, honey and lemon, Karo syrup; paint with kerosene oil internally with a rag and then tie a sock around the neck; paint with iodine or Mercurochrome and gargle with salt and water, honey, melted Vicks
Insect bites: Vaseline or boric acid
Boils: Oatmeal poultice
Cuts: Boric acid
Headaches: Hot poultice on forehead; hot facecloth; cold, damp cloth to forehead; in general, stay in bed, get plenty of rest and sleep, a glass of juice about once an hour, aspirin, and lots of food to get back strength
Stye: Hot tea bag to area

Italian (United States), Catholic
Health Maintenance
Hearty and varied nutritional intake; lots of fruit, pasta, wine (even for children), cheese, homegrown vegetables, and salads; exercise in form of physical labor; molasses on a piece of bread, or oil and sugar on bread; hard bread (good for the teeth)

(continued)

Table 2–1	—Continued

Italian (United States), Catholic—Continued

Pregnancy: Two weeks early: girl
  Two weeks late: boy
  Heartburn: baby with lots of hair
Eat (solved emotional and physical problems); fruit at end of meal cleans teeth; early to bed and early to rise

Health Protection
Garlic cloves strung on a piece of string around the neck of infants and children to prevent colds and "evil" stares from other people, which they believed could cause headaches and a pain or stiffness in the back or neck (a piece of red ribbon or cloth on an infant served the same purpose)
Keep warm in cold weather
Keep feet warm
Eat properly
Never wash hair or bathe during period
Never wash hair before going outdoors or at night
Stay out of drafts
To prevent "evil" in the newborn, a scissor was kept open under the mattress of the crib
To prevent bowlegs and keep ankles straight, up to the age of 6 to 8 months a bandage was wrapped around the baby from the waist to the feet
If infants got their nights and days mixed up, they were tied upside down and turned all the way around

Health Restoration
Chicken soup for everything from colds to having a baby
Boils: Cooked oatmeal wrapped in a cloth (steaming hot) applied to drain pus
Headache: Fill a soup bowl with cold water and put some olive oil in a large spoon; hold the spoon over the bowl in front of the person with the headache; while doing this, recite words in Italian and place index finger in the oil in the spoon; drop three drops of oil from the finger into the bowl; by the diameter of the circle the oil makes when it spreads in the water the severity of the headache can be determined (larger = more severe); after this is done three times the headache is gone
  Kerchief with ice in it is wrapped around the head; mint tea
Upset stomach: Herb tea made with herbs sent from Italy
Sore throat: Honey; apply Vicks on throat at bedtime and wrap up the throat
Sprains: Beat eggs whites, apply to part, wrap part
Fever: Cover with blankets to sweat it out
Cramps: Creme de menthe
Poison ivy: Yellow soap suds
Colic: Warm oil on stomach
Acne: Apply baby's urine
Sucking thumb: Apply hot pepper to thumb
High blood pressure: In Italy for high blood pressure, colonies of blood suckers were kept in clay, where they were born; the person with high blood pressure would have a blood sucker put on his fanny, where it would suck blood; it was thought that this would lower his blood pressure; the blood suckers would then be thrown in ashes and would then throw up the blood they had sucked from the person. If the blood sucker died, it alerted the person to see a doctor because it sometimes meant that there was something wrong with the person's blood
Stomachache: Camilla and maloa (herbs) added to boiled water

| Table 2-1 |

Italian (United States), Catholic—Continued

Colds: Boiled wines; coffee with anisette

Pimples: To draw contents, apply hot flaxseed

Toothache: Whiskey applied topically

Backache: Apply hot oatmeal in a sock; place a silver dollar on the sore area, light a match to it; while the match is burning put a glass over the silver dollar and then slightly lift the glass, and this causes a suction, which is said to lift the pain out

To build up blood: Eggnog with brandy; marsala wine and milk

Muscle pain: Heat up carbon leaves (herb) and bundle in a hot cloth to make a pack (soothes any discomfort)

Norwegian (Norway), Lutheran

Health Maintenance
Cod-liver oil
Cleanliness
Rest

Health Protection
Immunizations

Health Restoration
Colds and sore throat: Hot peppermint drink and Vicks

Nova Scotian, Catholic

Health Maintenance
Sleep; proper foods

Health Protection
Cut up some onions and put them on back of stove to cook; feed them to all

Health Restoration
Colds: Boil carrots until jellied, add honey; as expectorant boil onions, add honey

Sore throat: Coat a tablespoon of molasses with black pepper

Earache: Put few drops of heated camphorated oil in ear; melt chicken fat and sugar, put in ear

Psoriasis: Hang a piece of lead around the neck

Earache with infection: To drain the infection, cut a piece of salt pork about 2 inches long and 3/4 inch thick and insert it into the infected ear and leave for a few days

Cold in the back: Alcohol was put in a small metal container, a piece of cotton on a stick was placed in the alcohol, ignited, and put in a *banky* (a type of glass resembling a whiskey glass); this was put on the back where the cold was and left for half an hour and a hickeylike rash would develop; it was believed that the rash would drain the cold

Skin ulcer and infection: A sharp blade was sterilized and used to make a small incision in the skin, and live blood suckers were placed in the opening, they would drain the infection out; when the blood sucker was full, it would fall to a piece of paper, be bled, placed in alcohol, and reused

Polish (United States), Catholic

Health Maintenance
Use of physician
Eating good, nutritious foods
Plenty of rest
Cod-liver oil

(continued)

Table 2–1	—Continued

Polish (United States), Catholic—Continued

Health Protection
Exercise; good diet; eat fresh homegrown foods; work; good personal hygiene

Health Restoration
Headache: Take aspirin, hot liquids
Sore muscles: Heating pads and hot compresses
Colds: Drink hot liquids, chicken soup, honey

Swedish (United States), Protestant

Health Maintenance
Eat well-balanced meals
A lot of walking
Routine medical examinations
Cod-liver oil

Health Protection
Eat an apple a day
"I don't do a blooming thing"; eat well
Eat sorghum molasses for general all-round good health
Dress appropriately for weather
Blessing of the throat on St. Blaise Day

Health Restoration
Cough: Warm milk and butter
Rundown and tired: Eat a whole head of lettuce
Sick: Lots of juices and decarbonated ginger ale; lots of rest
Upset stomach: Baking soda
Sore throat: Gargle with salt and take honey in milk; herringbone wrapped in flannel around
   the neck
Anemia: Cod-liver oil
Bee stings: Poultice
Lumbago: Drink a yeast mixture
Black eye: Leeches
Earache: Warm oil
Congestion: Steamy bathroom
Fever: Blankets to sweat it out

❧ *Consciousness Raising*

RECOGNIZING SIMILARITIES

In my experience, as the group discussion continues, people realize that many personal beliefs and practices do in fact differ from what they are being taught in nursing or medical education to accept as the right way of doing things. Participants begin to admit that they do not seek medical care when the first symptoms of illness appear. On the contrary, they usually delay seeking care and often elect to self-treat at home. They also recognize that there are many preventive and health-maintenance acts learned in school with which they choose not to comply. Sometimes they discover that they are following an entire self-imposed regimen for health-related problems and are not seeking any outside intervention.

Another facet of a group discussion is the participants' exposure to the similarities that exist among them in terms of protection and health maintenance. To their surprise and delight, they find that many of their daily acts—routines that are taken for granted—directly relate to methods of maintaining and protecting health.

As is common in most large groups, students seem to be shy at the beginning of this exploration. As more and more members of the group are willing to share their experiences, however, other students feel more comfortable and share more readily. A classroom tactic I have used to break the ice is to reveal an experience I had on the birth of my first child. My mother-in-law, an immigrant from Eastern Europe, drew a circle around the child's crib with her fingers and spat on the baby three times to prevent the evil spirits from harming him. Once such an anecdote is shared, other participants have less difficulty in remembering similar events that may have taken place in their own homes.

Students have a variety of feelings about the self-care practices of their families. One feeling discussed by many students is shame. A number of students express conflict in their attitudes: They cannot decide whether to believe these old ways or to drop them and adopt the more modern ones they are learning in school. (This is an example of cognitive dissonance.) Many admit that this is the first time they have disclosed these beliefs and practices in public, and they are relieved and amazed to discover similarities with other students. The acts may have different names or be performed in a slightly different manner, but the uniting thread among them is to prevent evil (illness) and to maintain good (health).

TRANSFERENCE TO PATIENTS

The effects of such a verbal catharsis are long remembered and often quoted or referred to throughout the remainder of a course. The awareness we gain helps us understand the behavior and beliefs of our patients better. Given this understanding, we are comfortable enough to ask patients how they interpret a symptom and how they think it ought to be treated. We begin to be more sensitive to people who delay in seeking health care or fail to comply with preventive measures and treatment regimens. We come to recognize that we do the same thing. I believe that the increased familiarity with home health practices and remedies helps us project this awareness and understanding to the patients who are served.

Analyzed from a "scientific" perspective, the majority of these practices do have a sound basis. In the area of health maintenance (see Table 2–1), one notes an almost universal adherence to activities that include rest, balanced diet, and exercise.

In the area of health protection various differences arise, ranging from visiting a physician to wearing a clove of garlic around the neck. Although the purpose of wearing garlic around the neck is "to keep the evil spirit away," the act also forces people to stay away: What better way to cut down exposure to wintertime colds than to avoid close contact with people?

One person remembered that during her childhood her mother forced her to wear garlic around her neck. Like most children, she did not like to be different from the rest of her schoolmates. As time went on, she began to have frequent colds, and her mother could not understand why this was happening. The mother followed her child to school some weeks later and discovered that she removed the garlic on her way to school, hiding it under a rock and then replacing it on the way home. There was quite a battle between the mother and daughter! The youngster did not like this method of protection because her peers mocked her.

A discussion of home remedies is of further interest when each of the methods presented is analyzed for its possible "medical" analogy and also for its prevalence among various religious and ethnic groups. Many of the practices and remedies, to the surprise and relief of students, tend to run throughout groups but have different names or contain different ingredients. Table 2–1 illustrates examples of this information.

In this day of computers and sophisticated medicine, including transplants and intricate surgery, the most prevalent need expressed by people who practice folk medicine is to protect a given person and prevent "evil" from harming this person or to remove the "evil" that may be the cause of the health problem. As students, we analyze and discuss a problem and its folk treatments and we begin to see how evil continues to be considered the cause of illness and how often the treatment is then designed to remove it.

Each person testifies to the efficacy of a given remedy. Many state that when their grandmothers and mothers shared these remedies with them, they experienced great feelings of nostalgia for the good old days, when things seemed so simple. Some people may express a desire to return to these practices of yesteryear, whereas others openly confess that they continue to use such measures—sometimes in addition to what a health-care provider tells them to use or often without even bothering to consult a provider.

The goal of this kind of consciousness-raising session is to reawaken the participant to the types of health practices within her or his own family. The other purpose of the sharing is to make known the similarities and differences that exist as part of a cross-ethnic phenomenon. We are intrigued to discover the wide range of beliefs that exist among our peers' families. We had assumed that these people thought and believed as we did. For the first time, we individually and collectively realize that we all practice a certain amount of folk medicine, that we all have ethnically specific ways of treating illness, and that we, too, often delay in seeking professional health care. We learn that most people prefer to treat themselves at home and that they have their own ways of treating a particular set of symptoms—with or without a prescribed medical regimen. The previously held notion that "everybody does it this way" is shattered.

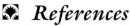 References

Armstrong, D., and Armstrong, E. M. 1991. *The Great American Medicine Show.* New York: Prentice Hall.

Kennet, F. 1976. *Folk Medicine—Fact and Fiction: Age-Old Cures, Alternative Medicine, Natural Remedies.* New York: Crescent Books, 9.

Yoder, D. 1972. Folk Medicine. In *Folklore and Folklife,* edited by R. H. Dorson Chicago: University of Chicago Press, 191–193.

❧ *Publishing Houses with Listings Related to Folk Medicine*

The following list is but a sample of the vast number of presses that publish materials related to folk life and medicine.

- *Illinois*
  University of Illinois Press
  54 East Gregory Drive
  Champaign, IL 61820

- *Kentucky*
  University Press of Kentucky
  663 South Limestone Street
  Lexington, KY 40506-0336

- *Michigan*
  Michigan State University Press
  1405 South Harrison Road
  Suite 25
  Manly Miles Bldg.
  East Lansing, MI 48823-5202

- *New Mexico*
  The University of New Mexico Press
  Albuquerque, NM 87131

- *Pennsylvania*
  University of Pennsylvania Press
  Blockley Hall, 13th floor
  Philadelphia, PA 19104-6261

- *North Carolina*
  The University of North Carolina Press
  Post Office Box 2288
  Chapel Hill, NC 27515-2288

- *Tennessee*
  AASLH Press
  172 Second Ave., North
  Nashville, TN 37201

  The University of Tennessee Press
  293 Communications Building
  Knoxville, TN 37996-0325

❀ *Folklife Centers*

The following is a listing of selected folklife centers in the United States. From these centers, one may obtain films and literature related to folklife and medicine.

- *California*
  Center for the Study of Comparative Folklore and Mythology
  University of California, Los Angeles
  Los Angeles, CA 90024

  California Folklore Society
  421 Baughman Ave.
  Claremont, CA 91711
  They Publish *Western Folklore*

- *Kentucky*
  Appalshop
  P.O. Box 743A
  Whitesburg, KY 41858

- *Missouri*
  Missouri Cultural Heritage Center
  Conley House
  Conley and Sanford Streets
  Columbia, MO 65211

- *Nevada*
  Folk Arts Program
  Nevada State Council of the Arts
  329 Flint Street
  Reno, NV 89501

- *Tennessee*
  Center for Southern Folklore
  1216 Peabody Avenue
  Memphis, TN 38104

- *Washington, DC*
  Within the federal government, resources for folklore and folklife endeavors in Washington, DC, are concentrated in four agencies.

  1. The Library of Congress
  2. The Smithsonian Institution
  3. The National Endowment for the Arts
  4. The National Endowment for the Humanities

  Although their programs are complementary, each operates under separate guidelines, supporting and coordinating activities that differ in purpose and scope.

AMERICAN FOLKLIFE CENTER

- The Library of Congress
  Washington, DC 2054
  (202) 287-6590
  Folkline (202) 287-2000: A telephone information service
  Folklife Sourcebook: A resource guide to relevant organizations

This center was created by Congress in 1976 to "preserve and present" American folklife. It is an educational and research program.

ARCHIVE OF FOLK CULTURE

- The Library of Congress
  Washington, DC 20540
  (202) 287-5510

This is the public reference and archival arm of the American Folklife Center.

OFFICE OF FOLKLIFE PROGRAMS

- Smithsonian Institution
  955 L'Enfant Plaza, Suite 2600
  Washington, DC 20560
  (202) 287-3424

This office, created in 1977, is the coordinative office for folklife activities within the Smithsonian Institution.

NATIONAL COUNCIL FOR THE TRADITIONAL ARTS

- 806 15th Street, NW, Suite 400
  Washington, DC 20005
  (202) 639-8370

This is a private, nonprofit organization that presents the National Folk Festival each year, organizes folk culture tours in this country and abroad, develops publications and radio programs, and offers consultant assistance.

THE AMERICAN FOLKLORE SOCIETY

- 1703 New Hampshire Avenue, NW
  Washington, DC 20009

Membership in this society, founded in 1888, is open to all persons interested in folklore. It serves as a forum for the preservation of folklore.

ANCESTRY

- P.O. Box 476
  Salt Lake City, UT 84110

This organization sells several publications that may be useful in developing your family history.

*Figure 2-1 from page 27
Dr. M. Simmon's Liver Medicine and Dixon's Liver Pills were popular forms of veg-etable medicines used to "treat a sick headache, sour stomach, colic, indigestion, biliousness, and diseases arising from torpidity of the liver." Simmon's powder was dissolved in boiling water and allowed to stand for 12 hours. The liquid was then strained through a clean cloth and taken in measured doses. It could also be ingested dry by "taking a large pinch of the powder on the tongue and washing it down with a swallow of water." Dixon's pills were used as needed. Each preparation sold for 25¢; each held a patent. **Piso's Tablets** were a healing and astringent tonic from 1913. They were used to treat such maladies as ulcers, sores, and afflictions of the skin and mucous membranes. This package sold for 60¢. **Cardui** was a vegetable tonic produced by McElree in Chattanooga, Tennessee. The thick liquid con-tained 19% alcohol, which was used as a solvent and preservative of the active medicinal in-gredients. One use was as an antispasmodic for painful periods. This particular bottle sold for $1.00; the medicine was patented. **Steel's Rheumatic Ball** was said to be a concen-trated vegetable compound reduced to a pill that cured acute and inflammatory rheuma-tism, sciatica, neuralgia, gout, and lumbago. These pills were manufactured in New York by the Ball Medicine Company, and the package sold for $1.00. **Steele's Blood Ball** was a med-ication that claimed to enrich and purify the blood, clear the complexion, and infuse rich blood through the system. It was said to cure scrofula, jaundice, blood poisoning, pimples, blotch, and mercurial diseases. These pills were manufactured in New York by the Ball Med-icine Company, and the package sold for 50¢. **Steele's Bilious Ball** was a medication used to treat all disorders of the liver. The instruction pamphlet claimed that "Biliousness is the Germ of all Disease." "This medicine is the cure." It was a household remedy for young and old and claimed to cure all disorders of the liver, including fever, torpid liver, indiges-tion, and headache. These pills were manufactured in New York by the Ball Medicine Com-pany, and the package sold for 25¢. **Alka-Zane** was an effervescent compound and patent medicine used to reduce excess acidity of the urine and to promote diuresis. It contained no lactate, sulfate, tartrate, or sodium chloride. Thus it could be used in conditions where a salt-free diet was important and diuresis desired. **Mac Laren's Mustard Cerate** was an ointment rubbed on the chest for coughs and colds, pneumonia, bronchitis, and croup, and on the body to treat headache, sore joints and muscles, and neuralgia. Inscribed on the top is the saying: "I'm the little doctor." It held a patent. **Swamp Root** is a liquid preparation used, even today, to flush the kidneys and bladder, thereby aiding in their work of eliminat-ing waste matter. It contains 10.5% alcohol and various herbs such as peppermint, cape aloes, oil of juniper, and buchu leaves incorporated into a syrup. The alcohol was used to preserve the ingredients.

Chapter 3

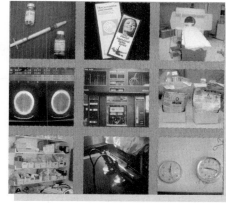

Health-Care Delivery: Issues, Barriers, and Alternatives

The health-care system of this nation is in crisis, and the visionary words and observations of Dr. John Knowles in 1970 ring true today:

> American medicine, the pride of the nation for many years, stands on the brink of chaos. To be sure, our medical practitioners have their great moments of drama and triumph. But, much of U.S. medical care, particularly the everyday business of preventing and treating illness, is inferior in quality, wastefully dispensed, and inequitably financed. Medical manpower and facilities are so maldistributed that large segments of the population, especially the urban poor and those in rural areas, get virtually no care at all, even though their illnesses are most numerous and, in a medical sense, often easy to cure.

We are now living in the 21st century, the third millennium; the problems of health-care delivery have grown exponentially, and solutions are more elusive than ever. Doctors in the United States administer the world's most expensive medical (illness) care system. The costs of U.S. health care soared from $4 billion in 1940 to the 1996 figure of $1.035 trillion—an enterprise that exceeds all the goods and services produced by half the states in the country. Health has become this country's biggest business, and it accounts for 13.6% of our gross domestic product, as shown in Table 3–1 and Figure 3–2. In fact, nearly $3708 was spent in 1996 on health care for every man,

Figure 3–1 (From left to right, top to bottom) Syringe and vials, health education brochures, X-ray equipment, CT scan, laboratory equipment, blood for transfusions, emergency room equipment, paddles, clocks. *(For more information on each picture see explanation at the end of chapter.*)*

Table 3-1 **Gross Domestic Product and National Health Expenditures: 1960–1996**

	Gross Domestic Product in Billions of Dollars	National Health Expenditures in Billions of Dollars	Percentage of GDP in Health Expenditures
1960	526.6	26.9	5.1
1970	1,035.6	73.2	7.1
1980	2,784.3	247.3	8.9
1990	5,743.8	699.5	12.2
1996	7,636.4	1,035.0	13.6

Note: Gross domestic product (GDP) is the market value of the goods and services produced by labor and property located in the United States.
From: National Center for Health Statistics. *Health, United States, 1998, with Socioeconomic Status and Health Chartbook.* (Hyattsville, Md., 1998), p. 341.

woman, child, and fetus. (Rodwin 1999, 135) Table 3–2 compares, over time, the amount of money paid per capita both in the United States and several other nations.

The health-care system is both a source of national pride—for if one has the money, it certainly is possible to get the finest medical care in the world—and a source of deep embarrassment, for those who are poor or uninsured may well be wanting for care; in fact, one out of six Americans do not have health insurance. Negative changes in the delivery of care since the early 1990s include the following:

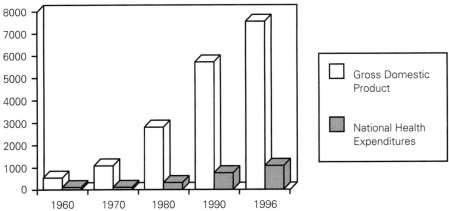

Figure 3-2 Gross domestic product and national health expenditures, 1960–1996. Gross domestic product (GDP) is the market value of the goods and services produced by labor and property located in the United States. [*From:* National Center for Health Statistics. *Health, United States, 1998, with Socioeconomic Status and Health Chartbook.* (Hyattsville, Md., 1998), p. 341.]

Table 3–2 Per Capita Health Expenditures Adjusted to U. S. Dollars in Selected Countries: 1960, 1980, 1995, and 1996

Country	1960	1980	1995	1996
United States	$141	$1052	$3633	$3708
Switzerland	93	850	2412	2412
Luxembourg	***	617	2206	***
Germany	91	860	2134	2222
Canada	105	729	2069	2002
Greece	16	190	703	748
Korea	***	71	666	***
Hungary	***	***	562	***
Mexico	***	***	386	384
Turkey	***	77	272 (1994)	***

***—data not available

From: National Center for Health Statistics. *Health, United States, 1998, with Socioeconomic Status and Health Chartbook.* (Hyattsville, Md., 1998), p. 342 and Rodwin, V. G. "Comparative Analysis of Health Systems: An International Perspective," in *Health Care Delivery in the United States,* ed. S. Jonas and A. R. Kovner. (New York: Springer, 1999), p. 135. © 1999 Springer Publishing Company, Inc., New York 10012. Used by permission.

- Limits on access to quality health care, and the erosion of care;
- Profits made by health-care organizations that drain resources from patient care; for-profit health maintenance organizations (HMOs) constitute over 65% of the market;
- The distortion of clinical decision making because of financial considerations within the scope of managed care that leads to inappropriate discharges and the lack of follow-up care (Ad Hoc Committee to Defend Health Care 1997).

Despite this high expenditure and the large numbers of hospital beds, we were not healthier in 1996 than people from other nations. In fact, 22 other nations had lower infant mortality rates, and 26 had lower death rates from cardiovascular diseases (see Table 3–3). The following clinical examples serve to illustrate the former situation:

- *Limits on access to quality health care, and the erosion of care.*
  A young mother in Brooklyn, who had been arrested for starving her baby, whom she was breast-feeding, was found to have visited an outpatient clinic in New York Methodist Hospital. She was turned away for lack of a Medicaid card and the money—$25.00—to cover the fee for service for a scheduled checkup for her baby (Bernstein 1998, 3).
- *Profits made by health-care organizations that drain resources from patient care.*
  Resources of enormous worth, such as nonprofit hospitals, visiting nurse agencies, even hospices, are being taken over by for-profit companies. The profits include $100 per patient per day in for-profit

Table 3–3 | **Health Care Expenditures and Health Status: 1994–1995**

Country	Health Expenditure as % of GDP	Life Expectancy at Birth		Infant Mortality/1000 Live Births
		Females	Males	
Canada	9.2	81.3	75.3	6
France	9.6	81.9	73.9	5
Germany	10.5	79.5	73	5.3
Italy	7.6	80.8	74.4	6.2
Japan	7.2	82.8	76.4	4.3
Spain	7.6	81.2	73.2	5.5
United Kingdom	6.9	79.7	74.3	6
United States	14.2	79.2	72.5	8

From: Rodwin, V. G. "Comparative Analysis of Health Systems: An International Perspective," in *Health Care Delivery in the United States,* ed. S. Jonas and A. R. Kovner. (New York: Springer, 1999), p. 144. © 1999 Springer Publishing Company, Inc., New York 10012. Used by permission.

hospitals, large salaries for executives, and large overheads (Ad Hoc Committee to Defend Health Care 1997).

- *The distortion of clinical decision making because of financial considerations within the scope of managed care that leads to inappropriate discharges and the lack of follow-up care.*

A 91-year-old frail woman in acute congestive heart failure was admitted to a secondary-level community hospital. She was treated and discharged on the third day after admission without adequate concern for long-term care and rehabilitation. Her bed was stripped even before she was able to leave the room. The family did not want her discharged without an adequate long-term care plan and placement and offered to cover the $800 daily charges. The offer was refused. The major concern of the hospital was to stay within the managed-care protocol, and the requests for adequate long-term care planning were ignored.

In addition, despite innumerable efforts to make health care safer for patients, the error count is on the rise. In Massachusetts alone, the number of errors rose from 30 in 1994 to 123 in 1998. Such errors included the following:

- *Medication errors*—For example, a patient was given twice the dose of a medication that was ordered, and a child was given three doses of chemotherapy instead of one.
- *Surgical errors*—For example, a patient died in surgery after receiving the wrong anesthetic, and surgery was done on a person's healthy limb.

Table 3–4 | **National Health Expenditures as Percentage of Total Health-Care Expenditure: 1960, 1980, and 1996**

	1960	1980	1996
Total expenditure in billions of dollars	$26.9	$247.3	$1,035.1
Hospital care	34.5%	41.5%	34.6%
Physician services	19.7	18.3	19.5
Dentist services	7.3	5.4	4.6
Nursing home care	3.2	7.1	7.6
Home health care	0.2	1	2.9
Drugs and medical nondurables	15.8	8.7	8.8
Other products and services	7.3	5.8	9.7
Public health activities	1.4	2.7	3.4
Administration	4.3	4.8	5.9
Research and construction	6.3	4.7	3

Source: National Center for Health Statistics, *Health, United States, 1998, with Socioeconomic Status and Health Chartbook.* (Hyattsville, Md., 1998), p. 346.

- *Quality of care errors*—For example, a patient did not receive oxygen as ordered.
- *Emergency-room treatment errors*—For example, patients were not tended to in an appropriate way.
- *Dumping*—Patients were shifted from one setting to another. A 27-year-old pregnant woman in labor was transferred to another hospital and the ambulance driver got lost. The baby died (Tye 1999).

How did we get to this critical situation? What factors converged to bring us to this dramatic breaking point? Whereas, because of the unprecedented growth of biomedical technology, we have witnessed the tremendous advancement in medical science and in its ability to perform an astounding variety of lifesaving procedures, now, not only can we no longer afford to finance these long-dreamed-of miracles, but the dream has become a nightmare. Table 3–4 and Figure 3–3 illustrate the changing distribution of dollars spent for health care.

This chapter briefly traces the history of events and developments from 1850 to the present that have led us to this destination. Then, a time line with more details of events, begins in 1900 and delineates sociocultural, public health, and allopathic health-care milestones through the twentieth century. In addition, the common problems we all experience when we seek health care, the pathways we follow when we experience a health problem, the view of medicine as a means of social control, and an introduction to health-care alternatives are presented. You are strongly encouraged to probe more deeply into each of these areas.

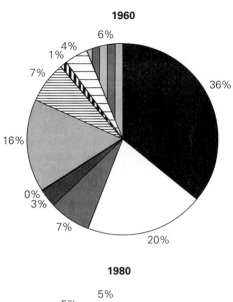

1960

6%
4%
1%
7%
16%
0%
3%
7%
36%
20%

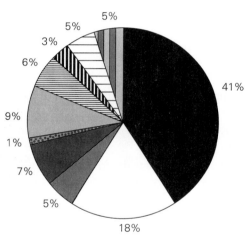

1980

5%
5%
3%
6%
9%
1%
7%
5%
41%
18%

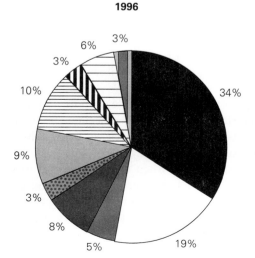

1996

6%
3%
3%
10%
9%
3%
8%
5%
34%
19%

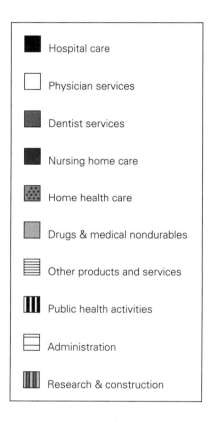

■ Hospital care

☐ Physician services

▦ Dentist services

■ Nursing home care

▥ Home health care

▨ Drugs & medical nondurables

▤ Other products and services

▥ Public health activities

☐ Administration

▥ Research & construction

Figure 3–3 Health-care expenditures, 1960, 1980, 1996. (*From:* National Center for Health Statistics. *Health, United States, 1998, with Socioeconomic Status and Health Chartbook.* (Hyattsville, Md., 1998), p. 346)

❧ Trends in Development of the Health-Care System

During the days of the early colonists, our health-care system was a system of superstition and faith. It has evolved into a system predicated on a strong belief in science; the epidemiological model of disease; highly developed technology; and strong values of individuality, competition, and free enterprise. Two major forces—free enterprise and science—have largely shaped the problems we now face. Health problems have evolved from the epidemics of 1850 to the chronic diseases of today, notwithstanding the resurgence of tuberculosis and the AIDS epidemic. In 1850, health-care technology was virtually nonexistent; today it dominates the delivery of health care. We now take for granted such dramatic procedures as kidney, heart, and liver transplants. New technologies and biomedical milestones are materializing daily (Torrens 1988, 3–31). However, the consequences of these events are also rising daily in terms of extraordinary costs and countless errors.

Social organizations to control the use of technology did not exist in 1850; today they proliferate, and the federal government is expected to play a dominant role. The belief that health care is a right for all Americans is still a predominant philosophy, yet the fulfillment of that right is still in question. The trends in the 1980s and early 1990s, such as the cutbacks in federal funding for health services and the attempt to turn the clock back on social programs, have led to a diminished and denigrated role for the government in people's health.

There is growing and grave concern about the realization of this basic human right. Mounting social problems, such as toxic waste, homelessness, and millions of people without health insurance, confound the situation. These factors all affect the delivery of health care. The problems of acquiring and using the health-care system are ongoing.

TIME LINE: 1900–1999

The events that have occurred in the health-care system, whether within the public or medical sector, have happened within the context of the longer societal framework. The public sector events include those related to the collective responsibility for the health of large populations in many dimensions—prevention, surveillance, disease control, and so forth—and those events, positive and negative, that affect large population cohorts. The medical events are those that include the development of diagnostic and/or therapeutic methods that are problem specific and affect limited numbers of people. In some instances it is difficult to determine in which category an event lies, but if is part of the public health sector, it is included in that category. The public health events include government laws and policies that were designed initially to increase the scope of the health-care system and later to control medical events. Thus, the time line highlights sociocultural events from the twentieth century and juxtaposes the public and medical events.

The Twentieth Century: Selected Sociocultural, Public Health, and Medical Events

Period[a]	1901–1914 Seeds of Change	1914–1919 Shell Shock
Socio-cultural Events[a]	1903—"Kitty Hawk" flown by Wright Brothers 1906—San Francisco earthquake 1908—Model T Ford introduced 1909—NAACP organized 1914—Panama Canal opened	1914–1918—World War I 1917—Russian Revolution 1918—Germany surrenders, Armistice signed 1919—Prohibition
Public Health Events[b]	1900—Walter Reed: Mosquitoes transmit yellow fever 1900—Quinine used to cure malaria 1906—Pure Food and Drug Act 1907—Tuberculin testing begun 1910—Flexner Report on Medical Education; Bureau of Mines established 1912—Diphtheria antitoxin immunization developed 1913—Schick test for diphtheria	1915—Smallpox immunization mandatory 1916—Margaret Sanger promotes birth control 1918–1919—Influenza pandemic
Medical Events[b,c]	1900—Freud interprets dreams 1900—Insulin shock therapy begun 1903—Electrocardiography introduced 1903—Radium used to treat cancer 1908—National Institutes of Health founded 1911—Rockefeller Institute founded 1912—X-rays developed 1914—Niacin used to fight pellagra	1914—Mayo Clinic opened 1914—Ether developed 1914—Blood transfusions 1917—Oxygen therapy introduced

Notes: Public health events are events related to the collective responsibility for the health of large populations in many dimensions—prevention, surveillance, disease control, and so forth; and events, positive and negative, that affect large populations.

The Twentieth Century: Selected Sociocultural, Public Health, and Medical Events

Period[a]	1920–1929 Boom to Bust	1929–1936 Stormy Weather
Socio-cultural Events[a]	1920—Women's suffrage 1920—First radio broadcast 1921—First Miss America 1924—4 million Ku Klux Clan members 1925—Scopes Trial 1927—Lindbergh—New York to Paris flight	1929—Stock market crash 1930—Great Southern drought 1932—F. D. Roosevelt elected President 1931—Rise of Nazi Party in Germany 1933—Prohibition ends 1935—New Deal and Social Security Act passed 1936—Olympic Games in Berlin
Public Health Events[b]	1924—Scratch test to determine susceptibility to diphtheria 1924—BCG introduced 1923—Dick test to determine susceptibility to scarlet fever	1929—Blue Cross and Blue Shield created 1931–39—Pertusis immunization introduced 1932—Artificial respiration introduced 1932—Tuskegee syphilis experiment begins 1933—Diphtheria immunization introduced 1933—Tetanus toxoid immunization introduced 1934—Mumps virus isolated 1935—Wagner Act, National Labor Act
Medical Events[b,c]	1923—Mitral valve surgery introduced 1923—Ethylene introduced as an anesthetic 1923—Sodium amytal introduced as an anesthetic 1923—Peritoneal dialysis introduced 1925—Exchange transfusions introduced	1929—First heart catheterization 1929—Theory of Gestalt psychology advanced 1933—Tomography introduced 1933—Grantly Dick-Reed advocates natural childbirth 1933—Divinylether put to clinical use 1935—Sulfa drugs developed with the introduction of sulfonamide 1935—Insulin developed to treat diabetes

Notes: Medical events are development of diagnostic and/or therapeutic methods that are problem specific and affect limited numbers of people.

(continued)

The Twentieth Century: Selected Sociocultural, Public Health, and Medical Events—Continued

Period[a]	1936–1941 Over the Edge	1941–1945 Global Nightmare

Socio-
cultural
Events[a]
	1936—H. G. Wells's *The War of the Worlds*
	1936—Italy seizes Ethiopia
	1936—*Life* magazine born
	1938—Kristallnacht in Germany
	1939—The SS *Saint Louis* turned away from
	    Cuba and the United States
	1939—World's Fair (New York)
	1939—Germany invades Poland
	1940—London burned
		1941—Pearl Harbor bombed; WWII; United States
		    at war with Japan and then Germany
		1944—Normandy Invasion
		May 1945—War ends in Europe
		8/6/1945—Hiroshima—first use of
		    atomic bomb

Public Health Events[b]	1936—Poliomyelitis virus isolated 1936—Cortisone developed 1936—Rabies virus grown in tissue culture 1937—First blood banks and blood transfusions 1937—TB patch test developed 1938—Typhoid antiserum prepared 1938—Measles virus cultivated 1940—Typhus vaccine introduced	1942—Imhoff system of sewage purification 1943—Penicillin used to treat syphilis 1944—DDT insecticide introduced 1944—Hearing tests introduced Mid-40s—Tetanus antitoxin developed 1947—Taft-Hartley Act

Medical
Events[b,c]
	1936—Method of collateral circulation
	    discovered to treat angina and cardiac
	    ischemia
	1938—Angiocardiography introduced
	1938—Stilbestrol introduced
	1939—Heart–lung machine first used on
	    animals
	1938—Electric convulsive therapy introduced
	1941—Penicillin and sulphadiazine developed
	1941—Rh incompatibility between mother and
	    child reported
		1942—Radioisotope bone scanning introduced
		1942—Curare introduced in anesthesia
		1942—Continuous caudal anesthesia used in labor
		    and delivery
		1944—Blalock procedure developed
		1944—Artificial kidney introduced
		1945—Streptomycin used to treat TB

The Twentieth Century: Selected Sociocultural, Public Health, and Medical Events

Period[a]	1946–1952 An Uneasy Peace	1953–1961 Mass Markets
Socio- cultural Events[a]	1946—Transistor discovered 1946—World's first electronic computer assembled 1947—Marshall Plan 1947—Jack R. Robinson plays professional baseball 1948—"Levittown" opened 1950—Korean War/McCarthy hysteria begins 1951—Rosenberg trial	1953—Stalin dies 1954—"One nation under God" added to the pledge of allegiance 1953—Television descends on the nation: *I Love Lucy* 1954—TV dinners 1955—Disneyland opens; Frisbees, wiggleballs, hula hoops, Mickey Mouse ears; Elvis Presley, Marilyn Monroe; Rosa Parks refuses to give up her seat on a Montgomery, Alabama, bus and bus boycott ensues 1956—*Brown v. Board of Education;* desegregation of public schools 1957—Russians first in space with *Sputnik* 1959—Cuban Revolution 1960—JFK elected president
Public Health Events[b]	1946—Hill-Burton Act for hospital construction passed 1948—World Health Organization started	1953—Department of Health, Education, and Welfare established 1954—Salk vaccine for polio 1957—Health Interview Survey (HIS) 1960—Measles vaccine developed 1961—Sabin oral polio vaccine
Medical Events[b,c]	1947—Kolff-Brigham artificial kidney 1948—First shunt for mitral stenosis performed 1948—Exchange blood transfusions for Rh incompatibility 1949—Cortisone discovered	1952/3—Heart-lung machine perfected 1954—Antipsychotics and neuroleptics introduced 1954—First successful organ (kidney) transplant 1957—Valium introduced

(continued)

The Twentieth Century: Selected Sociocultural, Public Health, and Medical Events—Continued

Period[a]	1961–1969 Into the Streets	1969–1981 Years of Doubt
Socio- cultural Events[a]	1961—Peace Corps begun; Bay of Pigs, Cuba 1962—Berlin Wall; ballistic missiles in Cuba—standoff Kennedy/Kruschev; the Beatles lead the youthful rebellion; Civil Rights Movement 1963—JFK assassinated; Viet Nam War builds up; Woodstock; march on Washington with Martin Luther King Jr. 1965—Malcom X assassinated 1968—Chicago riots; Martin Luther King Jr. assassinated; Robert Kennedy assassinated 1965–1968—More than 100 race riots in American cities 1969—Neil Armstrong walks on the moon	1970—SDS Weathermen blow up a townhouse in New York; Kent State protest; My Lai Massacre 1972—Watergate break in; Nixon to China 1973–74—Oil embargo; Nixon resigns; busing in Boston, MA 1975—Vietnam truce 1976—Antitax revolt
Public Health Events[b]	1961—Thalidomide disaster 1962—Rachel Carson's *Silent Spring* published 1963—Mumps live virus vaccine developed 1964—Surgeon General's Report on Smoking; Civil Rights Act passed 1965—War on Poverty; Medicare/Medicaid passed; Health Professionals' Education Assistance Act passed 1965—Regional Medical Program; Indian Health Service established 1966—Rubella vaccine developed 1967—Community health planning; Age Discrimination Act passed	1970—Earth Day; National Environmental Policy Act; EPA founded; Occupational Health and Safety Act passed 1972—PSROs established; Clean Water Act; Tuskegee experiment ends 1973—*Roe v. Wade* decision legalizes abortion; final report written on the Tuskegee Syphilis Study by U.S. Public Health Service 1973—Emerging infections identified 1973—HMO Act 1974—Comprehensive Health Planning; "Certificate of Need" 1976—Toxic Substance Control Act (TSCA) and Resource Conservation and Recovery Act (RCRA) passed 1977—WHO; *Health for All by Y2K* published 1978—Love Canal; hepatitis B (HBV) vaccine developed 1979—Three Mile Island 1980—Comprehensive Environmental Response, Compensation, and Liability Act (CERCLA) passed; "Superfund"; *Promoting Health, Preventing Disease: Objectives for the Nation* published
Medical Events[b,c]	1961—External cardiac pacing 1962—Immunosuppresent drug azathioprine developed 1963—Liver transplant method developed 1967—First human heart transplant	**Biotechnical Explosion** 1971—CT scans developed 1970s—Clotbusters—streptokinase/ urokinase introduced; monoclonals introduced; interferon 1978—First test-tube baby 1979—Cyclosporine developed 1980—Nuclear magnetic resonance introduced

Sources:
[a]From *The Century* by Peter Jennings. Copyright © 1998 by ABC Television Network Group, a division of Capital Cities, Inc. Used by permission of Doubleday, a division of Random House, Inc.
[b]Lasker, R. D. 1997. *Medicine and Public Health.* New York: New York Academy of Medicine; Last, J. M. 1998. *Public Health and Human Ecology,* 2d ed. Stamford, Conn.: Appleton & Lang; Wallace, R. B., ed. 1998. *Public Health and Preventive Medicine* 14th ed. Stamford, Conn.: Appleton & Lang; Yoder-Wise, P. S. 1995. *Leading and Managing in Nursing.* St. Louis: Mosby.

The Twentieth Century: Selected Sociocultural, Public Health, and Medical Events

Period[a]	1981–1989 New Morning	1989–1999 Machine Dreams
Socio-cultural Events[a]	1981—Air traffic controllers strike 1981—Tax cut—Reaganomics 1982—Vietnam Veterans Memorial dedicated 1983—HIV/AIDS epidemic recognized 1986—*Challenger* explosion 1987—10/19—Black Monday—stock market crash; glasnost 1989—Tiananmen Square; Berlin Wall torn down	1991—Desert Storm; beating of Rodney King 1992—L.A. riots 1993—Assault on the Branch Davidians in Waco, Texas 1995—Million Man March; Oklahoma City bombing 1998—President Clinton impeached in the House of Representatives; Desert Fox
Public Health Events[b]	1981—Block grants 1984—Bhopal, India—chemical leak 1985—Emergence of crack cocaine 1986—Superfund Amendments and Reauthorization Act (SARA)—Right to Know and Local Emergency Planning (LEP); Chernobyl, Ukraine—Nuclear reactor meltdown 1988—"The Future of Public Health" published; Hispanic Health & Nutrition Examination Survey	1990—Americans with Disabilities Act passed 1993–1994—Failure of health reform 1993—Family and Medical Leave Act 1996—Assisted suicide; Dr. J. Kevorkian
Medical Events[b,c]	1981—HIV virus isolated at the Institut Pasteur, Paris 1984—Monoclonal antibodies 1985—Retroviral oncogenes	1992—Human Genome Project 1993—Hantavirus pulmonary syndrome 1997—Septuplets born and survive 1998—Octuplets born; seven survive 1998—Stem cell cloning

[b&c]Annas, G. J. and Elias, S. 1998. Thalidomide and the *Titanic*. *American Journal of Public Health* 89(1):98; Friedman, M., and Friedland, G. W. 1998. *Medicine's Ten Greatest Discoveries*. New Haven: Yale University Press; Matarazzo, W. 1998. Through These Eyes. BWH (Brigham and Women's Hospital, Boston, Mass. 3(4)(Fall):2–11; Morton, L. T., and Moore, R. J. 1998. *A Chronology of Medicine and Related Sciences*. Cambridge: University Press; Shorter, E. 1987. *The Health Century*. New York: Doubleday; and Williams, S. J., and Torrens, P. R. 1988. *Introduction to Health Services*, 3d ed. New York: Wiley.

This information is further embedded in the key health system issues of the century and the key health problems, and selected key health strategies of the time. The key issues are professionalization, infrastructure building, improving access, cost control, market forces, and the reinvention of government. The key health problems are infectious disease, chronic diseases, and the modern changes. Key health strategies include maternal and infant health, antibiotics, screen and treat, and managed care.

At the turn of the century, 1900–1930, efforts were underway to identify medicine as a profession and to eradicate all philosophies of care that were not under the umbrella of the Flexner definition of a profession. Agents such as quinine for malaria and the diphtheria antitoxin for immunization were discovered, and the use of radium to treat cancer was begun.

Infectious diseases, including pneumonia and influenza were pandemic. The main health strategy was maternal and child health, given the large numbers of new immigrants. In 1929 third-party payment for health care was begun with the creation of Blue Cross and Blue Shield.

Between 1930 and 1960 the health-care system issue was infrastructure building. The passage of the Hill-Burton Act in 1946 provided funding for the building of hospitals and other health-care resources. The system was on a roll—the development of today's extraordinarily costly tests and treatments was begun, and the settings for their use were built. The development of vaccines and antibiotics paved the way to a decrease in the occurrence of communicable disease, and a false sense of freedom from illness began to develop. At the same time it began to become obvious that for many, access to health care was becoming more and more difficult.

In 1965 Lyndon Johnson's War on Poverty became the focal point of social and health policy and among other laws, Medicare and Medicare came into being. The Health Professionals Education Assistance Act was passed, which led to the proliferation of medical nursing and other allied health programs. In 1967 the first heart transplant was performed by Dr. Christian Barnard in South Africa, and a whole new focus on science and technology was born. Today, transplants have become nearly ordinary events, and an entitlement philosophy is applied to receiving them.

The 1960s were an explosive time—there were too many assassinations, too many riots—yet strides were made in the struggle for civil rights. The war in Vietnam was a nightly television event until the truce in 1975. The 1970s, '80s, and '90s all had their share of strife and progress. Progress in health care was accompanied by escalation of costs and limiting of comprehensive care.

❋ *Health-Care Reform*

In 1993 and 1994 both President and Mrs. Clinton made an extraordinary effort to study our complex health-care system and to reform it. That effort came to little, and the present political energy has shifted from health-care reform to welfare reform and the saving of Social Security and Medicare. The nation's 76 million baby boomers will soon be able to retire, which will necessitate large payouts from Social Security and Medicare, but it is unknown how many workers there will be to contribute to the system. The size of the shortfall depends on the changes in longevity, the birth rate, and immigration rates (Zitner 1999). Efforts such as managed care (Saltus 1999) and the discounting of payments for medications for the elderly are short-term and controversial approaches to managing funds.

Meanwhile, the costs of health care continue to soar, causing some hospitals to downsize their nursing staff in an effort to reduce costs. Throughout President Clinton's campaign to control health-care costs, discussion focused on how to pay for care but not on what to do to address the underlying high costs. The president sought health-care reform in the middle ground between competition and regulation and designed a plan to

- Rely on market forces to hold down costs.
- Ensure a multitiered health-care system by encouraging all but the most wealthy to seek care in health maintenance organizations. (HMOs)
- Install new regulatory measures (Eckholm 1994).

Ultimately, it was believed that the Clinton plan would create a few giant insurers, and HMOs would dominate the market; most people would be forced into low-cost plans, doctors would be employed by the insurers or HMOs, hospitals would be controlled by insurers and HMOs, care would be multitiered, the bureaucracy would increase, costs would not be contained, and financing would be regressive. The overall goal of health-care reform was to make health care accessible, comprehensive, and affordable—a right and not a privilege of all residents of the United States. At this writing, the plans for health-care reform are dead, and the costs of health care continue to climb. Technology is advancing and our use of it is increasing, and we continue to spend vast sums on the care of patients in the last year of life while delivering less and less preventive care. In addition, the costs of for-profit care continue to explode, and the dominant force in managed care is the for-profit health maintenance organization.

The for-profit HMOs compete to provide care for a preset fee, are run by larger insurance companies, and underprice established HMOs. Insurance companies and HMOs are presently dominating the system, and the private sector is creating large linkages. For example, one private hospital chain, Columbia/HCA Healthcare, has grown from a small regional facility to the owner of 311 hospitals—half of all the for-profit hospitals in the country. This chain includes not only private for-profit hospitals but nonprofit hospitals as well.

The quality of care may or may not be better. Fees are paid on fixed amounts, and the doctor is paid whether or not a given patient's symptoms are treated (Eckholm 1994).

❧ *Common Problems in Health-Care Delivery*

Many problems exist within today's health-care delivery system. Some of these problems affect all of us, and others are specific to the poor and to emerging majority populations. It has been suggested that the health-care delivery system fosters and maintains a childlike dependence and depersonalized condition for the consumer. The following sections describe problems experienced by most consumers of health care, as categorized by Ehrenreich and Ehrenreich (1971, 4–12).

"FINDING WHERE THE APPROPRIATE CARE IS OFFERED AT A REASONABLE PRICE"

It may be difficult for even a knowledgeable consumer to receive adequate care. One summer, I was on vacation with my 11-year-old daughter. She complained of a sore throat for 2 days, and when she did not improve on the third day, I decided to take her to a pediatrician and have a throat culture taken. She was running a low-grade fever, and I suspected a strep infection. I phoned the emergency room of a local teaching hospital for the name of a pediatrician, but I was instructed to "bring her in." I questioned the practicality of using an emergency room, but the friendly voice on the other end of the line assured me: "If you have health insurance and the child has a sore throat, this is the best place to come." After a rather long wait, we were seen by an intern who was beginning his first day in pediatrics. To my dismay and chagrin, the young man appeared to have no idea of how to proceed. The resident entered and patiently demonstrated to the fledgling intern—using my daughter—how to go about doing a physical examination on a child. Since I had brought the child to the emergency room merely for a throat culture, I felt that what they were doing was unnecessary and said so. After much delay, the throat culture was taken; we were told we could leave and should call back in 48 hours for the report. As we left the cubicle, we had to pass another cubicle with an open curtain—where a woman was vomiting all over herself, the bed, and the equipment while another intern was attempting to insert a gastric tube. Needless to say, my daughter was distressed by the sight, which she could not help but witness. The reward for this trial was an inflated bill.

Two days later, I called back for the report. It could not be located. When it was finally "found," the result was negative. I took issue with this because it took 30 minutes for them to find the report. Perhaps this sounds a bit overstated; however, I had the feeling that they told me it was negative just to get me off the phone.

I related this personal experience to bring out two major points. First, it is not easy to obtain what I, as a health-care provider, consider to be a rather minor procedure. Second—and perhaps more important—it was expensive!

The average health-care consumer in such a circumstance may very well have no idea of what is really going on. When health care is sought, one should have access to professionally performed examinations and treatment. When one is seeking the results of a laboratory test, the results should be available immediately at the agreed-on time and place instead of being lost in a jungle of bureaucracy.

"FINDING ONE'S WAY AMIDST THE MANY AVAILABLE TYPES OF MEDICAL CARE"

A friend's experience illustrates how hard it may be to find appropriate medical care. She had minor gastric problems from time to time and initially sought help from a family physician. He was unable to treat the problem adequately; therefore, she decided to go elsewhere. However, for many reasons—including anger, embarrassment, and fear of reprisal—she chose not to tell the family physician that she was dissatisfied with his care, nor did she request a referral. She was essentially on her own in terms of securing an appointment with either a gastroenterologist or a surgeon. She very quickly discovered that no physician who was a specialist in gastroenterology would see her on a self-referral. In order to get an appointment, she had to ask her own general practitioner for a referral or else seek initial help from another general practitioner or internist. Since she had little money to spend on a variety of physicians, she decided to wait to see what would happen. In this instance, happily, she was fortunate and has had few further problems.

As a teaching and learning experience, I ask students to describe how they go about selecting a physician and where they go for health care. The younger students in the class generally seek the services of their families' physicians. The older or married students often have doctors other than those with whom they "grew up." These latter students generally are quite willing to share the trials and tribulations that they have experienced. When given the freedom to express their actions and reactions, most admit to having a great deal of difficulty in getting what they perceive to be *good* health care. A number of the older students state that they select a physician on the staff of the institution where they are employed. They have had an opportunity to see him at work and can judge, first hand, whether he is "good" or "bad." One mother stated that she worked in pediatrics during her pregnancy solely to discover who was the best pediatrician. A newly married student stated that she planned to work in the delivery room to see which obstetrician delivered a baby with the greatest amount of concern for both the mother and the child.

That is an ideal situation for members of the nursing profession, but what about the average lay person who does not have access to this resource? This question alerts the students to the specialness of their personal situations and exposes them to the immensity of the problem that the average person experiences. After individual experiences are shared, the class can move on to work through a case study such as the following.

Ms B. is a new resident in this city. She discovers a lump in her breast and does not know where to turn. How does she go about finding a doctor? Where does she go?

One initial course of action is to call the American Cancer Society for advice. From there, she is instructed to call the County Medical Society, since the

American Cancer Society is not allowed to give out physicians' names. During a phone call to the County Medical Society, she is given the names of three physicians in her part of the city. From there she is on her own in attempting to get an appointment with one of them. It is not uncommon for a stranger to call a physician's office and be told (1) "The doctor is no longer seeing any additional new patients," (2) "There is a 6-month wait," or (3) "He sees no one without a proper referral."

The woman, of course, has another choice: she can go to an emergency room or a clinic, but then she discovers that the wait in the emergency room is intolerable for her. She may rationalize that because a "lump" is not really an "emergency," she should choose another route. She may then try to secure a clinic appointment, and once again she may experience a great deal of difficulty in getting an appointment at a convenient time. She may finally get one and then discover that the wait in the clinic is unduly long—which may cause her to miss a day of work.

"FIGURING OUT WHAT THE PHYSICIAN IS DOING"

It is not always easy for members of the health professions to understand what is happening to them when they are ill. Alas, what must it be like for the average person who has little or no knowledge of health-care routines and practices?

Pretend that you are a lay person who has just been relieved of all your clothes and given a paper dress to put on. You are lying on a table with strange eyes peering down at you. A sheet is thrown over you, and you are given terse directions—"breathe," "cough," "don't breathe," "turn," "lift your legs." You may feel without warning a cold disk on your chest or a cold hand on your back. As the physical examination process continues, you may feel a few taps on the ribs, see a bright light shining in your eye, feel a cold tube in your ear, and gag on a stick probing the inside of your mouth. What is going on? The jargon you hear is unfamiliar. You are being poked, pushed, prodded, peered at and into, jabbed, and you do not know why. If you are female and going for your first pelvic examination, you may have no idea what to expect. Perhaps you have heard only hushed whisperings, and your level of fear and discomfort is high. Insult is added to injury when you experience the penetration of a cold, unyielding speculum: "What is the doctor doing now and why?"

These hypothetical situations are typical of the usual physical examinations that you may encounter routinely in a clinic or private physician's office. Suppose you have a more complex problem, such as a neurological condition, for which the diagnostic procedures may indeed be painful and complicated. Have you ever had a CT scan? A magnetic resonance image (MRI)? An angioplasty? Quite often, those who deliver care have not experienced the vast number of procedures that are performed in diagnostic workups and in treatment. They have little awareness of what the patient is thinking, feeling, and experiencing. Similarly, because the names and the purposes of the procedures are familiar to health-care workers—don't forget, this is *their* culture—they may take their own understanding of the procedures for granted and have difficulty appreciating why the patient cannot understand what is happening.

"Finding Out What Went Wrong"

What did you do the last time a patient asked to read the chart? Traditionally, you uttered an authoritative "tsk," turned abruptly on white-heeled shoes, and walked briskly away. Who ever heard of such nerve? A patient asking to read a chart! In recent years, a "patient's bill of rights" has evolved. One of its mandates is that the patient has the right to read his or her own medical record. Experience, however, demonstrates that this right is still not always granted. Suppose one enters the hospital for what is deemed to be a simple medical or surgical problem. All is well if everything goes according to routine. However, what happens when complications develop? The more determined the patient is to discover what the problem is or why there are complications, the more the patient believes that the health-care providers are trying to hide something. The cycle perpetuates itself, and a tremendous schism develops between provider and consumer. Quite often, "the conspiracy of silence" tends to grow as more questions are asked. This unpleasant situation may continue until the patient is locked inside his or her subjective world. It is rare for a person truly to understand unforeseen complications. Nurses all too often enter into this collusion and play the role of a silent partner with the physician and the institution.

"Overcoming the Built-in Racism and Male Chauvinism of Doctors and Hospitals"

Students tend to have little difficulty in describing many incidents of racism and male chauvinism: that they are mostly women suffices, and that they are nurses adds meaning to the problem. Classroom discussion helps to identify subtle incidents of racism and to identify them as such. For example, students may realize that black patients may be the last to receive morning or evening care, meal trays, and so forth. If this is a normal occurrence on a floor, it is an indictment in itself. Racism may take another tack. Is it an accident that the black person is the last patient to receive routine care or has he consciously been made to wait? Does the fact that the black person may have to wait longest for water or a pill demonstrate racism on a conscious level, or is it subliminal?

Nurses recognize the subtle patronization of both themselves and of female patients. Once the situation is probed and spelled out, the students adopt a much more realistic attitude toward the insensitivity of those who choose a racist or chauvinistic style of giving care. Students have noted that when they are aware of what is happening, they are better able to take steps to block future occurrences. Some have written letters to me after they have begun or returned to the practice of nursing, stating that knowing the phenomenon is common helps them to project a stronger image in their determination to work for change.

❀ *Pathways to Health Services*

When a health problem occurs, there is an established system whereby health-care services are obtained. Suchman (1965) contends that the family is usually the first resource. It is in the domain of the family that the person seeks validation that what he or she is experiencing is indeed an illness. Once the belief is validated, health care outside of the home is sought. When one is dealing with the medical system in general, help is sought from a physician in the private office of a general practitioner, internist, or pediatrician or in a hospital emergency room or clinic.* This is known as the level of first contact, or the *entrance* into the health-care system.

The second level of care, if needed, is found at the specialist's level: in clinics, private practice, or hospitals. Obstetricians, gynecologists, surgeons, neurologists, and other specialists make up a large percentage of those who practice in medicine.

The third level of care is delivered within hospitals that provide inpatient care and services. Care is determined by need, whether long-term (as in a psychiatric setting or rehabilitation institute) or short-term (as in the acute care setting and community hospitals).

An in-depth discussion of the different kinds of hospitals—voluntary or profit-making and nonprofit institutions—is more appropriate to a book dealing solely with the delivery of health care (see the annotated bibliography at the end of this book). In our present context, the issue is: What does the patient know about such settings, and what kind of care can he or she expect to receive?

To many students, the problems of the ward are far removed from the scope of practice they know from nursing school and from what they ordinarily see in a work setting (unless they choose to work in a city or county hospital). Many students assume that the care they observe and deliver in a suburban or community hospital is the universal norm. This is a fundamental error in experience and understanding, which can be corrected if students are assigned to visit first the emergency room of a city hospital and then the emergency room of a suburban hospital in order to compare the two milieus. Unless students visit each setting, they fail to gain an appreciation of the major differences—how vastly such facilities differ in the scope of patients' treatment. Students typically report that in the suburban emergency room, the patients are called by name, their families wait with them, and every effort is made to hasten their visit. The contrast is astounding with people in urban emergency rooms who have waited for extended periods of time, are sometimes not addressed by name, and are not allowed to have family members come with them while they are examined. The noise and confusion are also factors that confront and dismay students when they are exposed to big-city emergency rooms.

❋ *Medicine As an Institution of Social Control*

The people of today's death-denying, youth-oriented society have unusually high expectations of the healers of our time. We expect a cure (or if not a cure, then the prolongation of life) as the normal outcome of illness. The technol-

---

*It is not unusual for a family to be receiving care from many different physicians, with limited or no communication among the attending physicians. Problems and complications erupt when a physician is not aware that other physicians are caring for a patient. Let us not forget that in rural and remote areas, comprehensive health care is difficult to obtain. For patients who are forced to use the clinics of a hospital, there is certainly no continuity of care because intern and resident physicians come and go each year.

ogy of modern health care dominates our expectations of treatment, and our primary focus is on the *curative* aspects of medicine, not on prevention.

As control over the behavior of a person has shifted from the family and church to a physician, "be good" has shifted to "take your medicine." The role that physicians play within society in terms of social control is ever-growing, so that conflict frequently arises between medicine and the law over definitions of accepted codes of behavior and the relative status of the two professions in governing American life. Zola (1966, 1972) uses the following examples to illustrate the "medicalization" of society.

"THROUGH THE EXPANSION OF WHAT IN LIFE IS DEEMED RELEVANT TO THE GOOD PRACTICE OF MEDICINE"

This factor is exemplified by the change from a specific etiological model of disease to a multicausal one. The "partners" in this new model include greater acceptance of comprehensive medicine, the use of the computer, and the practice of preventive medicine. In preventive medicine, however, the medical person must get to the lay person before the disease occurs: clients must be sought out. Thus, forms of social control emerge in an attempt to *prevent* disease: low-cholesterol diets, avoidance of stress, stopping smoking, getting proper and adequate exercise.

"THROUGH THE RETENTION OF ABSOLUTE CONTROL OVER CERTAIN TECHNICAL PROCEDURES"

This step is, in essence, the right to perform surgery and the right to prescribe drugs. In the life span of human beings, modern medicine can often determine life or death from the time of conception to old age through genetic counseling; abortion; surgery; and technological devices such as computers, respirators, and life-support systems. Medicine has at its command drugs that can cure or kill—from antibiotics to the chemotherapeutic agents used to combat cancer. There are drugs to cause sleep or wakefulness, to increase or decrease the appetite, to increase or decrease levels of energy. There are drugs to relieve depression and stimulate interest. (In the United States, those mood-altering drugs are consumed at a rate higher than those medications prescribed and used to treat specific diseases.) In addition, medicine can control what medications are available for legal consumption.

"THROUGH THE EXPANSION OF WHAT IN MEDICINE IS DEEMED RELEVANT TO THE GOOD PRACTICE OF LIFE"

This expansion is illustrated by the use of medical jargon to describe a state of being—such as the "health" of the nation or the "health" of the economy. Any political or economic proposal or objective that enhances the "health" of those concerned wins approval.

There are numerous areas in which medicine, religion, and law overlap. For example, public health practice, law, and medicine overlap in the creation of laws that establish quarantine and the need for immunization. As another example, a child is unable to enter school without proof of having received certain inoculations. Medicine and law also merge in areas of sanitation and rodent control, and insect control. A legal–medical dispute can arise over the guilt or innocence of a criminal as determined by his "mental state" at the time of a crime.

Some diseases carry a social stigma: one must be screened for tuberculosis before employment, a history of typhoid fever permanently prevents a person from commercially handling food, venereal disease must be reported and treated, and even the ancient disease of leprosy continues to carry a stigma.

Abortion represents an area replete with conflict that involves politics, law, religion, and medicine. Those in favor of abortion rights believe that it is a woman's right to have an abortion and that the matter is confidential between the patient and her physician. Opponents argue on religious and moral grounds that abortion is murder. At present, the law sanctions abortion. In many states, however, Medicaid will no longer pay for an abortion unless the mother's life is in danger, a policy that makes it increasingly difficult for the poor to obtain these services.

Another highly charged area of conflict involves the practice of euthanasia. With the burgeoning of technological improvements, the definition of *death* has changed in recent years. It sometimes takes a major court battle to "pull the plug," such as in the Nancy Cruzan case. The recent battles with Dr. Jack Kevorkian have stretched these issues even further.

Finally, one might ponder that although many daily practical activities are undertaken in the name of health—taking vitamins, practicing hygiene, using birth control, engaging in dietary or exercise programs—the "diseases of the rich" (cancer, heart disease, and stroke) tend to capture more public attention and funding than the diseases of the poor (malnutrition, high maternal and infant death rates, sickle-cell anemia, and lead poisoning).

ALTERNATIVE THERAPIES

Alternative, unconventional, or unorthodox therapies cover a broad spectrum of health beliefs and practices. Such therapies, which are medical practices that do not conform to the standards of the medical community, are not taught widely in the medical and nursing communities and are not generally available in the allopathic health-care system, including the hospital settings. These include such therapies as acupuncture, massage therapy, and chiropractic medicine. *Alternative* therapies, in this text, refers to therapies that one may elect to use that are *not* a part of their cultural heritage; *traditional* therapies are those therapies that are a part of one's traditional cultural heritage. In other words, a European American electing to use acupuncture as a method of treatment is seeking alternative treatment; a Chinese American using this treatment modality is using traditional medicine.

The use of alternative therapies is growing rapidly. They are now frequently used by patients with cancer, arthritis, chronic back or other pain, stress-related problems, AIDS, gastrointestinal problems, and anxiety. The most frequent users are educated, upper-income white Americans in the 25–49 age group. They are most likely to live on the West Coast. The total projected out-of-pocket expenditure for unconventional therapy was $10.3 billion in 1990, and ranged from $27.0 to $34.4 billion in 1997. There has been a 380% increase in the use of herbal remedies since 1990 (Eisenberg et al. 1998, 1574).

The Institute of Noetic Sciences, founded in 1973, is a research foundation, an educational institution, and an organization that has over 40,000 members worldwide. It promotes philosophies of self-healing and research into this area.

The remainder of this book portrays these methods as they occur in both the dominant assimilated American culture and in the many traditional or immigrant cultures that now blend with the American whole.

❧ *Goals of Health-Care Delivery*

In this chapter we have explored, in a very limited way, many of the issues surrounding the American health-care delivery system by examining the trends that led to its character today, by looking at the experiences a person may have in attempting to obtain care, and by listing many of the issues related to care and the costs of the system. The struggles continue, and a balance between the high technology of the 1990s and the need for primary preventive care follows us into the new century.

❧ *References*

Ad Hoc Committee to Defend Health Care. 1997. For Our Patients, Not for Profits—A Call to Action. *JAMA* 278(21):1733.

Bernstein, N. 1998. Prosecutor Drops Charges in Case of Infant's Death. *New York Times,* 16 July.

Eckholm, E. 1994. While Congress Remains Silent, Health Care Transforms Itself. *New York Times,* 18 December.

Ehrenreich, B., and Ehrenreich, J. 1971. *The American Health Empire: Power, Profits, and Politics.* New York: Random House, Vintage Books. (The headings that follow this reference in the text are quoted from this book.)

Eisenberg, D. M., Davis, R. B., Ettner, S. L., et al. 1998. Trends in Alternative Medicine Use in the United States, 1990–1997. *JAMA* 280(18):1569–1575.

Knowles, J. 1970. It's Time to Operate. *Fortune* (January): 79.

National Center for Health Statistics. 1998. *Health, United States, 1998, with Socioeconomic Status and Health Chartbook.* Hyattsville, Md.

Rodwin, V. G. 1999. Comparative Analysis of Health Systems: An International Perspective. In *Health Care Delivery in the United States,* New York: Springer. edited by S. Jonas and A. R. Kovner

Saltus, R. 1999. Managed, Yes, but Couple Wonders, Is Care?" *Boston Globe,* 18 February.

Suchman, E. A. 1964. Sociomedical Variations among Ethnic Groups. *American Journal of Sociology* 70:319–331.

———. 1965. "Social Patterns of Illness and Medical Care." *Journal of Health and Human Behavior* 6:2–16.

Torrens, P. R. 1988. Historical Evolution and Overview of Health Services in the United States. In *Introduction to Health Services,* 3d ed., edited by S. J. Williams and P. R. Torrens. New York: Wiley.

Tye, L. 1999. Patients at Risk—Mistakes Plaguing System. *Boston Globe,* 15 March.

Zitner, A. 1999. Demographers Caught Looking on US Trends. *Boston Sunday Globe,* 14 March.

Zola I. K. 1966. Culture and Symptoms: An Analysis of Patients Presenting Complaints. *American Sociological Review* 31 (October): 615–630.

———. 1972. Medicine as an Institution of Social Control. *Sociological Review 20* (4) (November): 487–504. (The headings that follow this reference in the text are quoted from this article.)

*Figure 3-1 from page 45

The chapter-opening quilt panel of allopathic health-care system images depicts objects used to protect, maintain, or restore overall health. The **syringe and vials** symbolize immunization, the one nearly absolute method for protecting health. Since 1915, when smallpox immunization became mandatory, the incidence of many once-fatal communicable diseases has been drastically reduced or even eliminated because of highly regulated immunization practices. **Health education brochures** represent the trend to "screen and treat" and to increase the awareness of methods of prevention or screening for early detection spawned an enormous movement for health education. **X-rays** have been used in the diagnosis of health problems since 1912. The highly sophisticated equipment of today is able to detect countless health problems at an early stage. **CT (computerized tomography) scanning techniques** have developed since 1971. **Laboratory equipment** is used in every diagnostic laboratory procedure—general laboratory studies, hematology, bacteriology, and pathology. These procedures have grown increasingly sophisticated over this century. **Blood transfusions** have been administered since 1914, and the technology surrounding the procedure has been enhanced by the development of blood banks in 1937 and the knowledge of grouping and Rh incompatibility. The blood supply has been extremely carefully scrutinized since the discovery of HIV and the reported use of tainted blood in the 1970s. **Emergency room equipment** and **electrocardiogram machines** are widely used in hospitals. The practice of electrocardiography was introduced in 1903. **Paddles** are used in external cardiac pacing, which began to be used in 1961. These paddles may conjure up the image that the modern health-care system has the ability to restore life to the dead. **Clocks** remind us that once the heart stops beating there is a finite amount of time in which a heartbeat can be restored. Life is finite—it is a fatal disease.

Unit

II

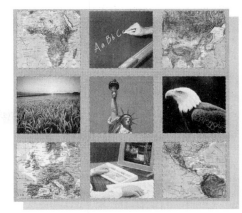

Cultural Awareness

Unit II develops the "plot" of this book by providing background material for the central themes discussed in this text. Chapter 4 explores the concept of "heritage" and discusses culture, ethnicity, religion, and socialization with broad examples relevant to health. Chapters 4 and 5 explore the notion of HEALTH traditions and weave in an exploration of holistic HEALTH and the role it plays in overall health and healing practices. Chapter 7 discusses why this content is so vital in the new millennium.

Unit II will enable you to:

1. Identify and discuss the factors that contribute to heritage consistency—culture, ethnicity, religion and socialization.

2. Describe homeopathic health-care systems.

3. Describe traditional aspects of health care.

4. Understand the demographic changes in the United States.

5. Describe barriers to health care such as poverty and language.

As you proceed through this unit there are several activities that link Unit 1 to this unit and will help the content come alive. These are activities in which several people may participate and share their experiences.

1. Who is the first person you turn to when you are ill? To whom do you go first, and where do you go next?

2. You have just moved to a new location. You do not know a single person in this community. How do you find health-care resources?

3. Visit an emergency room in a large city hospital. Visit an emergency room in a small community hospital. Spend several hours quietly observing what occurs in each setting.

    a. How long do patients wait to be seen?

    b. Are patients called by name?

c. Are relatives or friends allowed into the treatment room with the patient?

4. Determine the cost of a day of hospitalization.

a. How much does a room cost? How much is a day in the intensive care unit or coronary care unit? How much is time in the emergency room? How is a surgical procedure charged?

b. How much is charged for diagnostic procedures, such as a computed tomography (CT) scan or ultrasound? How much is charged for such equipment as a simple intravenous (IV) setup?

c. What are the pharmacy charges?

d. How many days, or hours, are women kept in the hospital after delivery of a child? Is the newborn baby sent home at the same time? If not, why not? What is the cost of a normal vaginal delivery and normal newborn care?

5. Visit a homeopathic pharmacy or a natural food store and examine the shelves that contain herbal remedies and information about alternative health care.

a. What is the cost of a variety of herbal remedies used to maintain health or to prevent common ailments?

b. What is the cost of a variety of herbal remedies used to treat common ailments?

c. What is the range of costs for literature?

Compare and contrast the experience in questions 4 and 5.

6. Attend a worship service in a house of worship with which you are not familiar. Inquire of the clergyperson what is done within this faith tradition to maintain, protect, and restore HEALTH.

7. Visit a community healer other than a physician.

8. Attend a healing service.

9. Explore other methods of healing such as massage or herbal therapy.

10. Explore birth and birthing practices in traditions other than your own.

11. Explore end-of-life practices and mourning in traditions other than your own.

Chapter 4

Culture and Heritage

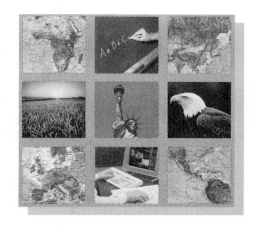

When there is a very dense cultural barrier, you do the best you can, and if something happens despite that, you have to be satisfied with little success instead of total successes. You have to give up total control. . . .

—Anne Fadiman, 1997

In May 1988 Anne Fadiman, the editor of the *American Scholar,* met the Lee family of Merced, California. Her subsequent book, *The Spirit Catches You and You Fall Down,* published in 1997, tells the compelling story of the Lees and their daughter Lia, and their tragic encounter with the American health-care delivery system.

When Lia was 3 months old she was brought to the emergency room of the county hospital with epileptic seizures. The family was unable to communicate in English; the hospital staff did not include competent Hmong interpreters. From the parents' point of view, Lia was experiencing "the fleeing of her soul from her body and the soul had become lost." They knew these symptoms to be *quag dab peg*—"the spirit catches you and you fall down." The Hmong regard this experience with ambivalence yet know that it is serious and potentially dangerous, as it is epilepsy. It is also an illness that evokes a sense of both concern and pride.

The parents and the health-care providers both wanted the best for Lia, yet a complex and dense trajectory of misunderstanding and misinterpreting was set in motion. The tragic cultural conflict lasted for several years and caused considerable pain to each party (Fadiman 1997).

This moving incident exemplifies the extreme events that can occur when two antithetical cultural belief systems collide within the overall environment of the health-care delivery system. Each party comes to a health-care event

Figure 4–1 (From top to bottom—left to right) The four corners: the four corners of the earth—Africa, Asia, Europe, and North and South America; center square: the Statue of Liberty; vertical inner panels: chalkboard and computer; horizontal middle panels: spacious sky, waves of grain, eagle. *(For more information on each picture see explanation at the end of chapter.*)*

with a set notion of what ought to happen—and unless each is able to understand the view of the other, complex difficulties can arise.

How, then, do we prepare ourselves to negotiate these complex sociocultural situations? What is the scope of the conflict? How do we broker compatible methods of providing health care when there are opposing health-related beliefs? This chapter addresses these questions by exploring the issues of immigration, culture, and heritage from a broad perspective.

Since the mid-1960s there has been a social explosion in the United States that has resulted in a surge of group consciousness. Blacks first, then Hispanics, Asian Americans, American Indians, and European American (white) ethnic groups began to assert their cultural group identity. The rejuvenation of ethnic identity eroded both the melting pot myth and the belief that an American culture would decrease group awareness (Giordano and Giordano 1977, 1). A second social explosion is being caused by the profound forces of demographic change. The rates of immigration have risen to well over 16 million people since 1980 and the number of residents who were foreign born people in 1997 was 25,779,000 (Bureau of the Census 1998).

Immigrants and their descendants constitute most of the population of the United States. Most Americans who are not themselves immigrants have ancestors who came from elsewhere (Castillo 1979). The only people considered native are the American Indians, the Aleuts, and the Inuit (or Eskimos), for they migrated here thousands of years before the Europeans (Thernstrom 1980, vii).

Immigrants come to the United States seeking religious and political freedom and economic opportunities. The life of the immigrant is fraught with difficulties—going from an "old" to a "new" way of life, learning a new language, and adapting to a new climate, new foods, and a new culture. Socialization of immigrants occurs in American public schools, and Americanization, according to Greeley, (1975) is for some a process of "vast psychic repression," wherein one's language and other familiar trappings are shed. In part, the concept of the melting pot has been created in schools, where children learn English, reject family traditions, and attempt to take on the values of the dominant culture and "pass" as "Americans" (Novak 1973).

Between 1981 and 1996 over 14 million immigrants were admitted to the United States. In 1966 alone, 915,900 people were granted legal permanent resident status. Mexico was the country of birth of 18% of immigrants, and nearly 34% of all immigrants were born in Asia. Tables 4–1 and 4–2 list the numbers of people admitted to this country from 1981 to 1996 and in 1996 alone. Nearly two-thirds of all immigrants reside in California, New York, Florida, Texas, New Jersey, and Illinois; one in five immigrants reside in New York or Los Angeles. The number of new Americans naturalized in 1996—1.045 million people—was double that of 1995, and 1.6 million aliens were deported (Bureau of the Census 1997).

In 1998 President Clinton authorized the entry of 78,000 refugees for fiscal year 1999, including 48,000 from Europe, 9000 from East Asia, 12,000 from Africa, and 3000 from Latin America and the Caribbean (Associated Press 1998). Earlier immigration events are noted in Box 4–1.

Table 4–1	Country of Origin of Immigrants, 1981–1996
All countries	13,484,275
Mexico	3,304,682
Philippines	843,741
Vietnam	719,239
China	539,267
Dominican Republic	509,902
India	498,309
Korea	453,018
El Salvador	362,225
Jamaica	323,625
Cuba	254,193

Source: U.S. Immigration and Naturalization Service. *Statistical Yearbook of the Immigration and Naturalization Service, 1996.* (Washington, DC: U.S. Government Printing Office, 1997.)

Table 4–2	Country of Origin of Immigrants, 1996
All countries	915,900
Mexico	163,572
Philippines	55,876
India	44,859
Vietnam	42,067
China	41,728
Dominican Republic	39,604
Cuba	26,466
Ukraine	21,079
Russia	19,668
Jamaica	19,089

Source: U.S. Immigration and Naturalization Service. *Statistical Yearbook of the Immigration and Naturalization Service, 1996.* (Washington, DC: U.S. Government Printing Office, 1997.)

Box 4–1

Highlights of Immigration History 1798–1996

Year	Event
1798	Alien and Sedition Acts passed
1808	African slave trade prohibited
1819	First immigrant data collected
1824	Naturalization set at 2 years
1844	Nativist riots in Philadelphia
1846	Potato famine in Ireland results in massive Irish influx
1849	California gold rush; imported Chinese labor
1862	Homestead Act opens land to immigrants
1870	Naturalization extended to Africans
1882–1943	Chinese Exclusion Act
1886	Statue of Liberty opens
1892	Ellis Island Immigration Station opens
1898	Immigrants classified by "race"
1903	Political radicals banned from entering the United States
1907	1,004,756 people—a record—pass through Ellis Island
1908	"Gentleman's Agreement" restricts Japanese immigration
1910	Entrance barred to criminals, paupers, and diseased
1917	Literacy required for immigrants over 16
1924	Annual racial quotas established; Border Patrol established

1942–1964	Bracero Program allows temporary workers
1975	Vietnam War ends; Indochinese refugee program
1980	Mariel boatlift from Cuba—125,000 people
1986	Amnesty for illegal aliens
1990	Ellis Island immigration museum opens
1996	Illegal Immigration Reform and Immigrant Responsibility Act of 1996
1996	Personal Responsibility and Work Opportunity Reconciliation Act of 1996
1996	Antiterrorism and Effective Death Penalty Act of 1996

From: Lefcowitz, E. *The United States Immigration History Timeline.* (New York: Terra Firma Press. 1990). Reprinted with permission; U.S. Immigration and Naturalization Services Statistics on the World Wide Web (http://www.ins.usdoj.gov/stats/index.html)

Table 4–3 **Countries of Origin of the Undocumented Population, 1996**

All countries	5,000,000 (approximate)
Mexico	2,700,000
El Salvador	335,000
Guatemala	165,000
Canada	120,000
Haiti	105,000
Philippines	95,000
Honduras	90,000
Poland	70,000
Nicaragua	70,000
Bahamas	70,000
Colombia	65,000
Ecuador	55,000
Dominican Republic	50,000
Trinidad and Tobago	50,000
Jamaica	50,000
Pakistan	41,000
India	33,000
Dominica	32,000
Peru	30,000
Korea	30,000
Other	744,000

From: U.S. Immigration and Naturalization Services Statistics. (http://www.ins.usdoj.gov/stats/index.html)

In addition to the number of people entering the United States legally, there were 4.6 to 5.4 million undocumented immigrants residing here in 1996. It is extremely difficult to count the number of people who are hiding because they are not documented. However, it is widely recognized that the population is growing by about 275,000 people each year. California is the leading state of residence for undocumented people. Other states include Texas, New York, and Florida. Table 4–3 lists the countries of origin of undocumented people.

Given that every immigrant group brings cultural attitudes toward health, health care, and illness, and that widely varying health and illness beliefs and practices exist within each of these groups, the field of cultural conflict takes on a life of its own. We are living in a pluralistic and universal society, and it is becoming more and more evident that cultural differences are increasingly serving to isolate and alienate us one from another. J. D. Hunter (1994, 236) has pointed out that merely educating people about the differences that underlie culturally determined beliefs is not enough; one must first confront competing ideals of truth. "The Differences must be confronted."

❧ Cultural Conflict

Hunter describes cultural conflicts as events that occur when there is polarization between two groups and the differences are intensified by the way they are perceived. The struggles are centered on the control of the symbols of culture. In the case of the conflict between the Lee family and the health-care system, the scope of the conflict is readily apparent and lends itself to further analysis. Hunter describes the fields of conflict as found in family, education, media and the arts, law, and electoral politics. Health care is a sixth field, and the conflict is between those who actively participate in traditional health-care practices—that is, the practices of their given ethnocultural heritage—and those who are progressive and see the answers of contemporary health problems in the science and technology of the present. Chapters 5–6 and 7–12 describe this conflict in greater detail and explore traditional health, illness and healing beliefs and practices.

❧ Acculturation and Heritage Consistency

Health and illness can be interpreted and explained in terms of personal experience and expectations. We can define our own health or illness and determine what these states mean to us in our daily lives. We learn from our own cultural and ethnic backgrounds how to be healthy, how to recognize illness, and how to be ill. Furthermore, the meanings we attach to the notions of health and illness are related to the basic, culture-bound values by which we define a given experience and perception.

To understand and appreciate differences in health and illness beliefs and practices that may be culturally determined, it is necessary to analyze theories relating to the Americanization of beliefs. This chapter presents two sets of theories, the first of which relates to socialization and acculturation and the quasi creation of a melting pot or some other common threads that are part of an American whole. The second, and opposite, set of theories analyzes the degree to which people have maintained their traditional heritage. It then becomes possible to analyze health beliefs by determining a person's ties to the traditional heritage and culture, rather than to signs of acculturation. The assumption is that there is a relationship between people with strong identities—either with their heritage or the level at which they are acculturated into the American culture—and their health beliefs and practices. Support group needs and networks also may relate to the degree that people identify with the traditional heritage. The concept of heritage consistency is a new one in mainstream health-care provider circles. The following discussion focuses on both acculturation and heritage consistency.

SOCIALIZATION

Socialization is the process of being raised within a culture and acquiring the characteristics of that group. Education—be it elementary school, high school, college, or nursing—is a form of socialization. For many people who have been socialized within the boundaries of a "traditional culture" or a non-Western culture, modern "American" culture becomes a second cultural identity. Those who immigrate here, legally or illegally, from non-Western or nonmodern countries may find socialization into the American culture, whether in schools or in society, to be an extremely difficult and painful process. They may experience biculturalism, which is a dual pattern of identification and often of divided loyalty (LaFrombose et al. 1993).

Fundamental to understanding culturally determined health and illness beliefs and practices from different heritages requires moving away from linear models of process to more complex patterns of cultural beliefs and interrelationships. Several models exist to explain the phenomena of second-culture acquisition.

ACCULTURATION

While becoming a competent participant in the dominant culture, a member of a minority culture is always identified as a member of that minority culture. The process of acculturation is involuntary in nature, and the member of the minority group is forced to learn the new culture to survive. Individuals experience second-culture acquisition when they must live within or between cultures (LaFrombose et al. 1993). *Acculturation* also refers to cultural or behavioral assimilation and may be defined as the changes of one's cultural patterns to those of the host society. In the United States, people assume that the usual course of acculturation takes three generations; hence, the adult grandchild of an immigrant is considered fully Americanized.

ASSIMILATION

Acculturation also may be referred to as *assimilation,* the process by which an individual develops a new cultural identity. Assimilation means becoming in all ways like the members of the dominant culture. The process of assimilation encompasses various aspects, such as cultural or behavioral, marital, identification, and civic. The underlying assumption is that the person from a given cultural group loses this cultural identity to acquire the new one. In fact, this is not always possible, and the process may cause stress and anxiety (LaFrombose et al. 1993). Assimilation can be described as a collection of subprocesses: a process of inclusion through which a person gradually ceases to conform to any standard of life that differs from the dominant group standards and, at the same time, a process through which the person learns to conform to all the dominant group standards. The process of assimilation is considered complete when the foreigner is fully merged into the dominant cultural group (McLemore 1980, 4).

There are four forms of assimilation: cultural, marital, primary structural, and secondary structural. One example of cultural assimilation is the ability to speak excellent American English. It is interesting to note that, according to the 1990 census, in the United States 32 million people speak a language other than English as their primary language (Bureau of the Census 1993). Marital assimilation occurs when members of one group intermarry with members of another group. The third and fourth forms of assimilation, those of structural assimilation, determine the extent to which social mingling and friendships occur between groups. In primary structural assimilation, the relationships between people are warm, personal interactions between group members in the home, the church, and social groups. In secondary structural assimilation there is nondiscriminatory sharing, often of a cold impersonal nature, between different groups in settings such as schools and workplaces (McLemore 1980, 39).

The concepts of socialization, assimilation, and acculturation are complex and sensitive. The dominant society expects that all immigrants are in the process of acculturation and assimilation and that the world view that we share as health-care practitioners is commonly shared by our clients. Because we live in a pluralistic society, however, many variations of health beliefs and practices exist.

When cultures clash, many misanthropic feelings, or "isms" can enter into a person's consciousness (Table 4–4). Just as Hunter proclaimed that the "differences" must be confronted, so too must stereotypes, prejudice, and discrimination be confronted. It is impossible to describe traditional beliefs without a temptation to stereotype. But each person is an individual; therefore, levels of heritage consistency differ within and between ethnic groups, as do health beliefs.

Another issue that manifests itself in this arena is that of prejudice. Prejudice occurs either because the person making the judgments does not understand the given person or his or her heritage, or the person making the judgment generalizes an experience of one individual from a culture to all members of that group. Discrimination occurs when a person acts on prejudice and denies another person one or more of their fundamental rights.

The debate still rages between those who believe that America is a melting pot and that all groups of immigrants must be acculturated to an Ameri-

| Table 4–4 | Common "Isms" Plus One Non-"ism" |

Belief	Definition
Racism	The belief that members of one race are superior to those of other races
Sexism	The belief that members of one gender are superior to the other gender
Heterosexism	The belief that everyone is or should be heterosexual and that heterosexuality is best, normal, and superior
Ageism	The belief that members of one age group are superior to those of other ages
Ethnocentrism	The belief that one's own cultural, ethnic, or professional group is superior to that of others. One judges others by his or her "yardstick," and is unable or unwilling to see what the other group is really about. "My group is best!"
Xenophobia	The morbid fear of strangers

From: Proceedings of the Invitational Meeting, Multicultural Issues in the Nursing Workforce and Workplace (Washington, DC: American Nurses' Association, 1993).

can norm, and those who dispute theories of acculturation and believe that the various groups maintain their own identities within the American whole. The concept of "heritage consistency" is one way of exploring whether people are maintaining their traditional heritage and of determining the depth of a person's traditional cultural heritage.

HERITAGE CONSISTENCY

Heritage consistency is a concept developed by Estes and Zitzow (1980) to describe "the degree to which one's lifestyle reflects his or her respective tribal culture." The theory has been expanded in an attempt to study the degree to which a person's lifestyle reflects his or her traditional culture, whether European, Asian, African, or Hispanic. The values indicating heritage consistency exist on a continuum, and a person can possess value characteristics of both a consistent heritage (traditional) and an inconsistent heritage (acculturated). The concept of heritage consistency includes a determination of one's cultural, ethnic, and religious background (see Fig. 4–2).

Culture.   There is not a single definition of culture, and all too often definitions tend to omit salient aspects of culture or to be too general to have any real meaning. Of the countless ideas of the meaning of this term, some are of particular note. Fejos (1959, 43) describes culture as "the sum total of socially inherited characteristics of a human group that comprises everything which one generation can tell, convey, or hand down to the next; in other words, the nonphysically inherited traits we possess." Another way of understanding the concept of culture is to picture it as the luggage that each of us carries around for our lifetime. It is the sum of beliefs, practices, habits, likes, dislikes, norms, customs, rituals, and so forth that we learned from our families during the years of socialization. In turn, we transmit cultural luggage to our children. A

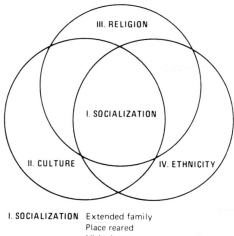

I. SOCIALIZATION Extended family
                  Place reared
                  Visits home
                  Raised with extended family
                  Name

II. CULTURE   Extended family
                  Participation in folkways
                  Language

III. RELIGION   Extended family
                  Church membership and participation
                  Historic beliefs

IV. ETHNICITY   Extended family
                  Resides in ethnic community
                  Participates in folkways
                  Socializes with members of same
                      ethnic group
                  Identifies as ethnic-American

Figure 4–2 Model of heritage consistency.

third way of defining culture, and one that is most relevant in areas of traditional health, is that culture is a "metacommunication system," wherein not only the spoken words have meaning, but everything else as well (Matsumoto 1989, 14).

All facets of human behavior can be interpreted through the lens of culture, and everything can be related to and from this context. Culture includes all the following characteristics:

1. Culture is the medium of personhood and social relationships.
2. Only part of culture is conscious.
3. Culture can be likened to a prosthetic device because it is an extension of biological capabilities.
4. Culture is an interlinked web of symbols.
5. Culture is a device for creating and limiting human choices.
6. Culture can be in two places at once—it is found in a person's mind and also exists in the environment in such form as the spoken word or an artifact (Bohannan 1989, 12).

Culture is a complex whole in which each part is related to every other part. It is learned, and the capacity to learn culture is genetic, but the subject matter is not genetic and must be learned by each person in his or her family and social community. Culture also depends on an underlying social matrix, and included in this social matrix are knowledge, belief, art, law, morals, and custom (Bohannan 1989, 13).

Culture is learned in that people learn the ways to see their environment—that is, they learn from the environment how to see and interpret what they see. People learn to speak, and they learn to learn. Culture, as the medium of our individuality, is the way in which we express our self. It is the medium of human social relationships in that it must be shared and creates social relationships. The symbols of culture—sound and acts—form the basis of all languages. Symbols are everywhere—in religion, politics, and gender— these are cultural symbols, the meaning of which varies between and within cultural groups (Bohannan 1989, 11–14). The society in which we live, and political, economic, and social forces, tend to alter the way in which some aspects of a particular culture are transmitted and maintained. Many of the essential components of a given culture, however, pass from one generation to the next unaltered. Consequently, much of what we believe, think, and do, both consciously and unconsciously, is determined by our cultural background. In this way culture and ethnicity are handed down from one generation to another.

Ethnicity. Cultural background is a fundamental component of one's ethnic background. Before we proceed with this discussion, though, we need to define some terms so that we can proceed from the same point of reference.

> **ethnic:** *adj* **1** of or pertaining to a social group within a cultural and social system that claims or is accorded special status on the basis of complex, often variable traits including religious, linguistic, ancestral, or physical characteristics **2** broadly, characteristic of a religious, racial, national, or cultural group **3** pertaining to a people not Christian or Jewish; heathen; pagan: "These Are Ancient Ethnic Revels of a Faith Long Since Forsaken." (Longfellow) (*American Heritage Dictionary* 1976, paperback ed.).

The term *ethnic* has for some time aroused strongly negative feelings and often is rejected by the general population. One can speculate that the upsurge in the use of the term stems from the recent interest of people in discovering their personal backgrounds, a fact used by some politicians who overtly court "the ethnics." Paradoxically, in a nation as large as the United States and comprising as many different peoples as it does—with the American Indians being the only true native population—we find ourselves still reluctant to speak of ethnicity and ethnic differences. This stance stems from the fact that most foreign groups that came to this land often shed the ways of the "old country" and quickly attempt to assimilate themselves into the mainstream, or the so-called melting pot (Novak, 1973).

matching game + Religion   at La Mayte - African
Bar/ culture + Religion   province
Ethnicity

- **ethnicity:** *n* **1** the condition of belonging to a particular ethnic group **2** ethnic pride
- **ethnocentrism:** *n* **1** belief in the superiority of one's own ethnic group **2** overriding concern with race
- **xenophobe:** *n* a person unduly fearful or contemptuous of strangers or foreigners, especially as reflected in his political or cultural views
- **xenophobia:** a morbid fear of strangers

The behavioral manifestations of these phenomena occur in response to people's needs, especially when they are foreign-born and must find a way to function (1) before they are assimilated into the mainstream and (2) in order to accept themselves. The people cluster together against the majority, who in turn may be discriminating against them.

Indeed, the phenomenon of ethnicity is "complex, ambivalent, paradoxical, and elusive" (Senior 1965, 21). Ethnicity is indicative of the following characteristics a group may share in some combination:

1. Common geographic origin
2. Migratory status
3. Race
4. Language and dialect
5. Religious faith or faiths
6. Ties that transcend kinship, neighborhood, and community boundaries
7. Shared traditions, values, and symbols
8. Literature, folklore, and music
9. Food preferences
10. Settlement and employment patterns
11. Special interest with regard to politics in the homeland and in the United States
12. Institutions that specifically serve and maintain the group
13. An internal sense of distinctiveness
14. An external perception of distinctiveness

There are at least 106 ethnic groups and more than 200 American Indian groups in the United States that meet many of these criteria. People from every country in the world have immigrated to this country and now reside here. Some nations, such as Germany, England, Wales, and Ireland, are heavily represented; others, such as Japan, the Philippines, and Greece have smaller numbers of people living here. People continue to immigrate to the United States, with the present influx coming from Vietnam, Laos, Cambodia, Cuba, Haiti, Mexico, and South and Central American countries (Thernstrom, 1980, vii).

Religion.   The third major component of heritage consistency is religion. Religion, "the belief in a divine or superhuman power or powers to be obeyed and worshipped as the creator(s) and ruler(s) of the universe; and a system of beliefs, practices, and ethical values," is a major reason for the development of

Table 4–5	Membership in Religious Bodies in North America, 1996 (in thousands)

Religious Group	Membership (in thousands)
Protestant	72,773
Baptist	33,892
Methodist	11,995
Lutheran	2,601
Presbyterian	3,637
Episcopal	2,537
Other	18,111
Catholic	61,208
Jewish	5,836
None	23,165
Other—not Christian	6,089

From: Compiled from http://www.infoplease.com/ipa/A000148.html. as attributed to *Britannica Book of the Year, 1997,* and *Yearbook of American and Canadian Churches, 1998.*

ethnicity (Abramson 1980, 869–875). The practice of religion is revealed in numerous cults, sects, denominations, and churches. Ethnicity and religion are clearly related, and one's religion quite often is the determinant of one's ethnic group. Religion gives a person a frame of reference and a perspective with which to organize information. Religious teachings vis-à-vis health help to present a meaningful philosophy and system of practices within a system of social controls having specific values, norms, and ethics. These are related to health in that adherence to a religious code is conducive to spiritual harmony and health. Illness is sometimes seen as the punishment for the violation of religious codes and morals.

The U.S. census has resisted asking questions about religion. However, data of religious affiliations are available on the Internet, and Table 4–5 lists religious affiliations in North America, including the United States and Canada, in 1996.

EXAMPLES OF HERITAGE CONSISTENCY

The factors that constitute heritage consistency are listed in Table 4–6. The following are examples of each factor:

1. The person's childhood development occurred in the person's country of origin or in an immigrant neighborhood in the United States of like ethnic group. For example, the person was raised in a specific ethnic neighborhood, such as an Italian, Black, Hispanic, or Jewish one, in a given part of a city and was exposed only to the culture, language, foods, and customs of that particular group.

| *Table 4–6* | **Factors Indicating Heritage Consistency** |

 1. Childhood development occurred in the person's country of origin or in an immigrant neighborhood in the United States of like ethnic group.
 2. Extended family members encouraged participation in traditional religious or cultural activities.
 3. Individual engages in frequent visits to country of origin or to the "old neighborhood" in the United States.
 4. Family homes are within the ethnic community.
 5. Individual participates in ethnic cultural events, such as religious festivals or national holidays, sometimes with singing, dancing, and costumes.
 6. Individual was raised in an extended family setting.
 7. Individual maintains regular contact with the extended family.
 8. Individual's name has not been Americanized.
 9. Individual was educated in a parochial (nonpublic) school with a religious or ethnic philosophy similar to the family's background.
10. Individual engages in social activities primarily with others of the same ethnic background.
11. Individual has knowledge of the culture and language of origin.
12. Individual possesses elements of personal pride about heritage.

2. Extended family members encouraged participation in traditional religious and cultural activities. For example, the parents sent the person to religious school, and most social activities were church-related.

3. The individual engages in frequent visits to the country of origin or returns to the "old neighborhood" in the United States. The desire to return to the old country or to the old neighborhood is prevalent in many people; however, many people, for various reasons, cannot return. The people who came here to escape religious persecution or whose families were killed during either world war or during the Holocaust may not want to return to European homelands. Other reasons why people may not return to their native country include political conditions in the homeland or lack of relatives or friends in that land.

4. The individual's family home is within the ethnic community of which he or she is a member. For example, as an adult the person has elected to live with family in an ethnic neighborhood.

5. The individual participates in ethnic cultural events, such as religious festivals or national holidays, sometimes with singing, dancing, and costumes.

6. The individual was raised in an extended family setting. For example, when the person was growing up, there may have been grandparents living in the same household, or aunts and uncles living in the same house or close by. The person's social frame of reference was the family.

7. The individual maintains regular contact with the extended family. For example, the person maintains close ties with members of the same generation, the surviving members of the older generation, and members of the younger generation.

8. The individual's name has not been Americanized. For example, the person has restored the family name to its European original if it had been changed by immigration authorities at the time the family immigrated or if the family changed the name at a later time in an attempt to assimilate more fully.

9. The individual was educated in a parochial (nonpublic) school with a religious or ethnic philosophy similar to the family's background. The person's education plays an enormous role in socialization, and the major purpose of education is to socialize a given person into the dominant culture. Children learn English and the customs and norms of American life in the schools. In the parochial schools, they not only learn English but also are socialized in the culture and norms of the particular religious or ethnic group that is sponsoring the school.

10. The individual engages in social activities primarily with others of the same religious or ethnic background. For example, the major portion of the person's personal time is spent with primary structural groups.

11. The individual has knowledge of the culture and language of origin. The person has been socialized in the traditional ways of the family and expresses this as a central theme of life.

12. The individual expresses pride in his or her heritage. For example, the person may identify him- or herself as ethnic American and be supportive of ethnic activities to a great extent.

It is not possible to isolate the aspects of culture, religion, and ethnicity that shape a person's world view. Each is part of the other, and all three are united within the person. When one writes of religion, one cannot eliminate culture or ethnicity, but descriptions and comparisons can be made. Referring to Figure 4–3 (pages 86–87) to assess heritage consistency can help determine ethnic group differences in health beliefs and practices. Understanding such differences can help enhance the health-care provider's understanding of the needs of patients and their families and the support systems that people may have or need.

❋ *Cultural Phenomena Affecting Health*

Giger and Davidhizar (1995) have identified six cultural phenomena that vary among cultural groups and affect health care. These are environmental control, biological variations, social organization, communication, space, and time orientation.

ENVIRONMENTAL CONTROL

Environmental control is the ability of members of a particular cultural group to plan activities that control nature or direct environmental factors. Included in this concept are the complex systems of traditional health and illness beliefs, the practice of folk medicine, and the use of traditional healers. This particular cultural phenomenon plays an extremely important role in the way patients respond to health-related experiences, including the ways in which they define health and illness and seek and use health-care resources and social supports.

BIOLOGICAL VARIATIONS

The several ways in which people from one cultural group differ biologically (i.e., physically and genetically) from members of other cultural groups constitute their biological variations. The following are significant examples:

- Body build and structure, including specific bone and structural differences between groups, such as the smaller stature of Asians
- Skin color, including variations in tone, texture, healing abilities, and hair follicles
- Enzymatic and genetic variations, including differences in response to drug and dietary therapies
- Susceptibility to disease, which can manifest itself as a higher morbidity rate of certain diseases within certain groups
- Nutritional variations, countless examples of which include the "hot and cold" preferences found among Hispanic Americans, the yin and yang preferences found among Asian Americans, and the rules of the kosher diet found among Jewish and Islamic Americans. A relatively common nutritional disorder, lactose intolerance, is found among Mexican, African, Asian, and Eastern European Jewish Americans

SOCIAL ORGANIZATION

The social environment in which people grow up and live plays an essential role in their cultural development and identification. Children learn their culture's responses to life events from the family and its ethnoreligious group. This socialization process is an inherent part of heritage—cultural, religious, and ethnic background. Social organization refers to the family unit (nuclear, single-parent, or extended family), and the social group organizations (religious or ethnic) with which clients and families may identify. Countless social barriers, such as unemployment, underemployment, homelessness, lack of health insurance, and poverty, can also prevent people from entering the health-care system.

COMMUNICATION

Communication differences present themselves in many ways, including language differences, verbal and nonverbal behaviors, and silence. Language differences are possibly the most important obstacle to providing multicultural health care because they affect all stages of the client–caregiver relationship. Clear and effective communication is important when dealing with any client, especially if language differences create a cultural barrier. When deprived of the most common medium of interaction with clients—the spoken word—health-care providers often become frustrated and ineffective. Accurate diagnosis and treatment is impossible if the health-care professional cannot understand the patient. When the provider is not understood, he or she often avoids verbal communication and does not realize the effect of nonverbal communication,

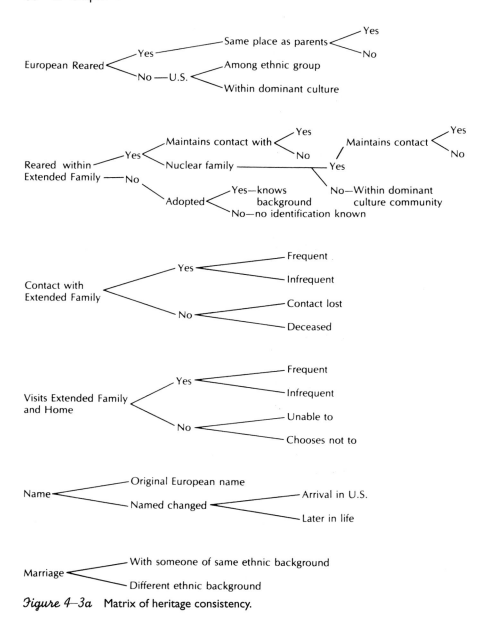

Figure 4–3a Matrix of heritage consistency.

which is all too often the painful isolation of patients who do not speak the dominant language and who are in an unfamiliar environment. Consequently, patients experience cultural shock and may react by withdrawing, becoming hostile or belligerent, or being uncooperative.

Language differences can be bridged, however, with the use of competent interpreters. If the patient does not speak the dominant language, a skilled interpreter is mandatory.

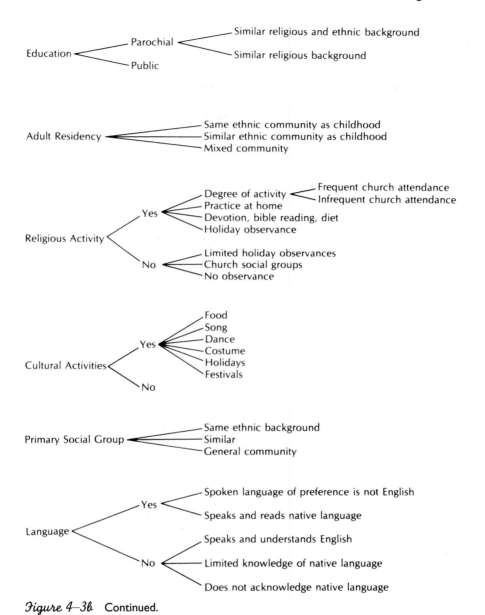

Figure 4–3b Continued.

SPACE

Personal space refers to people's behaviors and attitudes toward the space around themselves. *Territoriality* is the term for the behavior and attitude people exhibit about an area they have claimed and defend or react emotionally about when others encroach on it. Both personal space and territoriality are influenced by culture, and thus different ethnocultural groups have varying norms related to the use of space. Space and related behaviors have different meanings in the following zones:

- *Intimate zone*—extends up to 1½ feet. Because this distance allows adults to have the most bodily contact for perception of breath and odor, incursion into this zone is acceptable only in private places. Visual distortions also occur at this distance.
- *Personal distance*—extends from 1½ to 4 feet. This is an extension of the self that is like having a "bubble" of space surrounding the body. At this distance the voice may be moderate, body odor may not be apparent, and visual distortion may have disappeared.
- *Social distance*—extends from 4 to 12 feet. This is reserved for impersonal business transactions. Perceptual information is much less detailed.
- *Public distance*—extends 12 feet or more. Individuals interact only impersonally. Communicators' voices must be projected, and subtle facial expressions may be lost.

It must be noted that these generalizations about the use of personal space are based on studies of the behavior of European North Americans. Use of personal space varies among individuals and ethnic groups. The extreme modesty practiced by members of some cultural groups may prevent members from seeking preventive health care.

TIME ORIENTATION

The viewing of time in the present, past, or future varies among different cultural groups. Certain cultures in the United States and Canada tend to be future-oriented. People who are future-oriented are concerned with long-range goals and with health-care measures in the present to prevent the occurrence of illness in the future. They prefer to plan in making schedules, setting appointments, and organizing activities. Others are oriented more to the present than the future and may be late for appointments because they are less concerned about planning to be on time. This difference in time orientation may become important in health-care measures such as long-term planning and explanations of medications schedules.

Figure 4–4 illustrates how a given person, with his or her unique ethnic, religious, and cultural background is affected by cultural phenomena. The discussions in Chapters 8 to 12 highlight these phenomena, and examples are presented within the text and in tabular form. The examples used in the text to illustrate health traditions in different cultures are not intended to be stereotypical. With careful listening, observing, and questioning, the provider should be able to sort out the traditions of a given person. Table 4–7 suggests selected examples of etiquette relevant to each of the cultural phenomena.

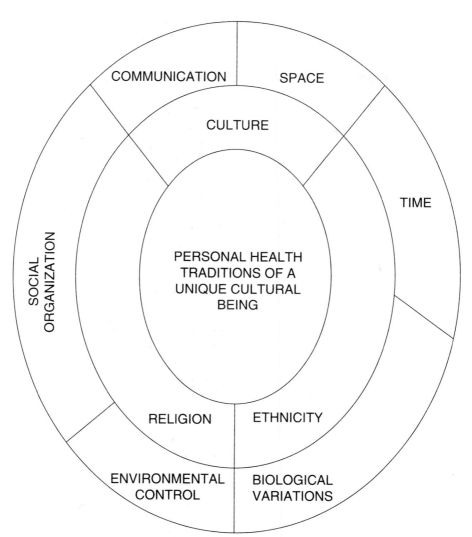

Figure 4–4 Personal health traditions of a unique cultural being.

❋ *Culture and Health-Care Providers*

The United States was once considered a melting pot of diverse ethnic and cultural groups. One aspect of the American dream was that all these diverse groups would blend into one common whole. This blending did not really occur, and today many groups cling to and identify more closely with their ethnic heritage. In fact, among third-, fourth-, or even subsequent-generation Americans, some desire to know where they come from (who they are). The phenomenon of seeking one's heritage is widespread in today's society. A fine example of this is Alex Haley's classic book and the movie based on it, *Roots,* which documents his search for his family's roots.

Table 4–7	**Selected Examples of Etiquette as Related to Selected Cultural Phenomena**	

Time	Visiting	Inform person when you are coming.
	Being on time	Avoid surprises.
		Explain your expectations about time.
	Taboo times	Ask people from other regions and cultures what they expect.
		Be familiar with the times and meanings of person's ethnic and religious holidays.
Space	Body language and distances	Know cultural and/or religious customs regarding contact, such as eye and touch, from many perspectives.
Communication	Greetings	Know the proper forms of address for people from a given culture and the ways by which people welcome one another.
		Know when touch, such as an embrace or handshake, is expected and when physical contact is prohibited.
	Gestures	Gestures do not have universal meaning; what is acceptable to one cultural group is taboo with another.
	Smiling	Smiles may be indicative of friendliness to some, taboo to others.
	Eye contact	Avoiding eye contact may be a sign of respect.
Social organization	Holidays	Know what dates are important and why, whether or not to give gifts, what to wear to special events, what the customs and beliefs are.
	Special events Births Weddings Funerals	Know how the event is celebrated, meaning of colors used for gifts, expected rituals at home or religious services.
Biological variations	Food customs	Know what can be eaten for certain events, what foods may be eaten together or are forbidden, what and how utensils are used.
Environmental control	HEALTH practices and remedies	Know what the general HEALTH traditions are for a given person and question observations for validity.

Adapted from: Dresser, N. *Multicultural Manners.* (New York: Wiley, 1996). Copyright © 1996 John Wiley & Sons, Inc. Reprinted by permission of John Wiley & Sons, Inc.

Because the melting pot—which carried with it the dream of assimilation into a common culture—has proved to be a myth, it is now time to identify and both accept and appreciate the differences among people. It is suggested that this be done not to change people so that they are all alike but to better understand both one's own ethnic culture and the ethnic culture of other people living in this society. Within the health professions, this is mandatory. Since health-care providers learn from their own culture the why and the how of being healthy or ill, it behooves them to treat each patient with deference to his or her own cultural background.

Health-care professionals who have been socialized into a given culture and subsequently resocialized into what I define as the provider culture come into intimate contact with people who may choose to maintain their traditional perceptions and beliefs regarding health and illness. Here lies the paradox: One culture may believe, for example, that people should starve a cold and feed a fever; another may believe the opposite. Such differences in belief can result in elopements from clinics, broken appointments, and failures to follow prescribed regimens.

THE HEALTH-CARE PROVIDER'S CULTURE

The providers of health care-physicians, nurses, social workers, dietitians, laboratory and departmental professionals—are socialized into the culture of their profession. Professional socialization teaches the student a set of beliefs, practices, habits, likes, dislikes, norms, and rituals (components already described as factors that make up a given culture). This newly learned information regarding health and illness differs in varying degrees from that of the individual's background. As students become more and more knowledgeable they usually move farther and farther from their past belief systems and, indeed, farther from the population at large in terms of its understanding and beliefs regarding health and illness. It is not uncommon to hear patients say things like, "I have no idea what the nurses and doctor are saying!" "They speak a foreign language!" "What they are doing is so strange to me."

As a result, health-care providers can be viewed as a foreign culture or ethnic group. They have a social and cultural system; they experience "ethnicity" in the way they perceive themselves in relation to the health-care consumer. Even if they deny the reality of the situation, health-care providers must understand that they are ethnocentric. Not only are they ethnocentric but many of them are also xenophobic. To appreciate this critical issue, consider the following. A principal reason for the difficulty experienced between the health-care provider and the consumer is that health-care providers, in general, adhere rigidly to the Western system of health-care delivery. With few exceptions, they do not publicly sanction any methods of protection or healing other than scientifically proved ones. They ordinarily fail to recognize or use any sources of medication other than those that have been proved effective by scientific means. The only types of healers that are sanctioned are those that have been educated and certified according to the requirements of this culture.

What happens, then, when people of one belief system encounter people who have other beliefs regarding health and illness (either in protection or in treatment)? Is the provider able to meet the needs as perceived and defined by the patient? More often than not, a wall of misunderstanding arises between the two. At this point a breakdown in communications occurs, and the consumer ends up at a disadvantage.

Providers think that they comprehend all facets of health and illness. Granted that in training and education health-care providers have a significant advantage over the consumer-patient; I nevertheless suggest and insist that it is entirely appropriate for them to explore alternative ideas regarding health and illness and to adjust their approach to coincide with the needs of the specific patient. In the past, health-care providers have tried to force Western medicine on one and all, regardless of result. It is time that health care coincided with the needs of the patient instead of inducing additional conflict.

The following list outlines the more obvious aspects of the health-care provider's culture. In connection with later chapters it can be referred to as a framework for comparing various other ethnic and cultural beliefs and practices.

1. Beliefs
   a. Standardized definitions of health and illness
   b. The omnipotence of technology
2. Practices
   a. The maintenance of health and the protection of health or prevention of disease through such mechanisms as the avoidance of stress and the use of immunizations
   b. Annual physical examinations and diagnostic procedures such as Pap smears
3. Habits
   a. Charting
   b. The constant use of jargon
   c. Use of a systematic approach and problem-solving methodology
4. Likes
   a. Promptness
   b. Neatness and organization
   c. Compliance
5. Dislikes
   a. Tardiness
   b. Disorderliness and disorganization
6. Customs
   a. Professional deference and adherence to the pecking order found in autocratic and bureaucratic systems
   b. Handwashing
   c. Employment of certain procedures attending birth and death
7. Rituals
   a. The physical examination
   b. The surgical procedure
   c. Limiting visitors and visiting hours

CULTURE AND EPIDEMIOLOGY

Another area in which culture plays a broad role is in the interpretation of the causation of illness, or epidemiology. Science is inherent in the health-care educational process. In the study of epidemiology, the relationships among the host, agent, and environment are explored. The modern approach attributes the cause of disease (the agent) to bacteria, viruses, chemical carcinogens, pollutants, and so forth. The disorders have names such as pneumonia, meningitis, influenza, polycystic kidney disease. Unless students delve further into study of the field, they may well never become familiar with more traditional theories of epidemiology. For example, the concepts of "soul loss," "spirit possession," and "spells" are rarely, if ever, described and discussed during the educational process of health-care providers, yet these ideas, too, contribute to people's perceptions of the cause of a given disease.

I have found many students who were not only familiar with such concepts as the "evil eye" but in some instances also took precautions to protect themselves against its effect. As discussed in Chapter 2, they often felt forced to take these precautions because of the beliefs of their mothers or grandmothers. After much thought, the acquisition of new facts, and further learning, many of the students chose to shed such beliefs and do not consciously practice what they were taught by their families. Others, however, admitted to still holding such beliefs but were constantly experiencing conflict. These groups of students can be viewed as a microcosm of the larger society. It is known that many people cling to familiar belief systems, a fact that lends comfort to them. (In what other way can some of the hardships of life be explained in a more satisfactory or acceptable manner?)

Another facet of epidemiology that one does not ordinarily encounter in academia is that the causative agent can be another person and not a microbe. The idea that another person can make someone ill by the use of witchcraft or voodoo (or some other form of magic) is an unusual subject within the constraints of a traditional medical curriculum. If the student is to study the cultural perceptions of health and illness, however, some knowledge of a belief in magic is important. The environment that fosters the use of these agents is one in which hate, envy, or jealousy may exist. The way of preventing illness involves not provoking the wrath of one's friends, neighbors, and enemies. A victim of disease may believe that his or her success provoked the envy of friends, that it attracted a witch's attention, or that someone was jealous of a new possession and put a hex on him or her. In the minds of people who still believe and practice traditional health beliefs, these contributing factors are as real as the bacteria and viruses of modern epidemiology are to health-care providers. Regardless of the provider's belief system, the provider needs to keep an open mind in order to provide useful care to consumers who retain traditional beliefs.

CULTURE AND RESPONSE TO PAIN

- "Mr. Smith in room 222 is the ideal patient. He never has a single complaint of pain."
- "Mrs. Cohen in room 223 is a real complainer. She is constantly asking for pain medication and putting on her light."
- "Mrs. O'Mally in room 224 is an ideal patient. She never complains about pain. For that matter, she never complains."
- "Mr. Chen in room 225 says nothing. I often wonder what he is feeling."
- "Mrs. Petrini in room 226 dramatically cries every time I look at her and complains of pain at every opportunity."

These statements (however stereotypical) are descriptions of behaviors observed concerning patients' responses to the subjective feeling of pain. Social scientists, health-care researchers, and other professionals maintain that pain is a culture-bound phenomenon. How pain and discomfort—or, for that matter, most emotions—are presented varies among cultures. A person raised in one cultural background may be allowed the free and open expression of feelings, whereas a person from another culture may have been taught that (for a multitude of reasons) true feelings must never be revealed. Let us say that the preceding statements were all made by the same nurse. Let us go one step further and say that each patient had the same operation on the same day. It would not be unusual, within the limits of general expectations, to see the different patients from differing cultures and ethnic groups exhibit the behaviors described.

The fact that culture plays a role in behavior during illness was aptly demonstrated and strongly documented by Mark Zborowski (1952) in his study on pain. Briefly, his findings were that Jewish and Italian patients generally responded to pain in an emotional fashion, and they tended to exaggerate the response, "old American Yankees" tended to be more stoic, and the Irish tended to ignore pain. Presentation of this type of data often can lead to a major problem—stereotyping. I want to emphasize strongly that such descriptions are general; the results of one study are not necessarily applicable to a specific patient. Even within my own clinical experiences, however, I have observed events such as those described by the quotations. It is preferable to include and discuss such material rather than to ignore it, particularly inasmuch as numerous classical studies in anthropology, sociology, psychology, and social psychology support these data [see, for instance, findings reported by David Mechanic (1963), the late Edward Suchman (1964, 1965), and the late Irving Zola (1966)].

This chapter has served to delineate the cultural conflict that occurs between health-care providers and many of those who have difficulty with the health-care system. It has presented basic and classical definitions and explanations of the foundation of this conflict.

❧ *References*

Abramson, H. J. 1980. Religion. In *Harvard Encyclopedia of American Ethnic Groups*, edited by S. Thernstrom. Cambridge: Harvard University Press.

Associated Press. 1998. President says U.S. will accept fewer refugees. *Boston Globe*, 1 October.

Bohannan, P. 1992. *We, the Alien—An Introduction to Cultural Anthropology*. Prospect Heights, Ill.: Waveland Press.

Castillo, L. J. 1979. Communicating with Mexican Americans—por su buena salud. Keynote address, Houston: Baylor College of Medicine.

Dresser, N. 1996. *Multicultural Manners*. New York: Wiley.

Estes, G., and Zitzow, D. 1980. Heritage Consistency as a Consideration in Counseling Native Americans. Paper read at the National Indian Education Association Convention, Dallas, Texas, November.

Fadiman A. 1997. *The Spirit Catches You and You Fall Down*. New York: Farrar, Straus, Giroux.

Fejos, P. 1959. Man, Magic, and Medicine. In *Medicine and Anthropology*, edited by L. Goldston. New York: International University Press.

Giger, J. N., and Davidhizar, R. E. 1995. *Transcultural Nursing Assessment and Intervention*, 2d ed. St. Louis: Mosby Year Book.

Giordano, J., and Giordano, G. P. 1997. *The Ethno-Cultural Factor in Mental Health*. New York: Institute of Pluralism and Group Identity.

Greeley, A. 1978. *Why Can't They Be Like Us? America's White Ethnic Groups*. New York: E. P. Dutton.

Hunter, J. D. 1994. *Before the Shooting Begins—Searching for Democracy in America's Culture Wars*. New York: Free Press.

LaFrombose T., Coleman L. K., and Gerton, J. 1993. Psychological Impact of Biculturalism: Evidence and Theory. *Psychological Bulletin* 114(3):395.

Matsumoto, M. 1989. *The Unspoken Way*. Tokyo: Kodahsha International.

McLemore, S. D. 1980. *Racial and Ethnic Relations in America*. Boston: Allyn and Bacon.

Mechanic, D. 1963. Religion, Religiosity, and Illness Behavior: The Special Case of the Jews. *Human Organization* 22:202–208.

Novak, M. 1973. How American Are You If Your Grandparents Came from Serbia in 1888? In *The Rediscovery of Ethnicity: Its Implications for Culture and Politics in America*, edited by S. Te Selle. New York: Harper and Row.

Senior, C. 1965. *The Puerto Ricans: Strangers Then Neighbors*. Chicago: Quadrangle Books.

Suchman, E. A. 1964. Sociomedical Variations Among Ethnic Groups. *American Journal of Sociology* 70:319–331.

———. 1965. Social Patterns of Illness and Medical Care. *Journal of Health and Human Behavior* 6:2–16.

Thernstrom, S. ed. 1980. *Harvard Encyclopedia of American Ethnic Groups* (Cambridge: Harvard University Press.

U.S. Commerce, Bureau of the Census. 1993. *1990 Census of Population—Social and Economic Characteristics*. Washington, DC: Government Printing Office.

Zborowski, M. 1952. Cultural Components in Responses to Pain. *Journal of Social Issues* 8:16–30.

———. 1969. *People in Pain*. San Francisco: Jossey-Bass.

Zola I. K. 1966. Culture and Symptoms: An Analysis of Patients Presenting Complaints. *American Sociological Review* 31 (October): 615–630.

———. 1972. The Concept of Trouble and Sources of Medical Assistance: To Whom One Can Turn, with What and Why. *Social Science and Medicine* 6:673–679.

INTERNET SOURCES

http://www.infoplease.com/ipa/A000148.html

U.S. Bureau of the Census—The Official Statistics. 1997. Country of Origin and Year of Entry into the U.S. of the Foreign Born, by Citizenship Status. http://www.bis.census.gov/cps/pub/1997/for_born.htm.

*Figure 4–1 from page 71

The images in the chapter-opening quilt panel represent the processes of acculturation and assimilation: the changes that immigrants experience, the effects of biculturalism, and the pain and promise of a new home. The **four corners** represent the four corners of the earth—Africa, Asia, Europe, and North and South America. People have immigrated to the United States from each of these places for thousands of years. The center square, the **Statue of Liberty**—the most familiar icon of immigration, represents the lure of America. The words of Emma Lazarus echo in this image. "Give me your huddled masses. . . ." The vertical inner panels—a **chalkboard** and **computer**—represent education, learning English, the media, and the total process of acculturation to the dominant culture. The horizontal middle panels—the **spacious sky and waves of grain** and the **eagle**—represent the majesty and power of this land. They speak to our shared dreams and cultural diversity.

Chapter 5

Health Traditions

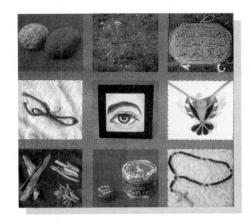

You can do nothing to bring the dead to life; but you can do much to save the living from death.

—*B. Frank School, 1924*

Health-care providers have the opportunity to observe the most incredible phenomenon of life: HEALTH and the recovery from illness. In today's society, the healer is primarily thought by many to be the physician, and the other members of the health team all play a significant role in the prevention, detection, and treatment of disease. Yet human beings have existed, some sources suggest, for 2 million years. How, then, did the species *Homo sapiens* survive before the advent of modern technology? What did the people of other times do to maintain, protect, and restore their HEALTH? It is quite evident that numerous forms of HEALTH care and healing existed long before the methodologies that we apply today.

In the natural course of any life, a person can expect to experience the following set of events: He or she becomes ill; the illness may be acute, with concomitant symptoms or signs such as pain, fever, nausea, bleeding. On the other hand, the illness may be insidious, with a gradual progression and worsening of symptoms, which might encompass slow deterioration of movement or a profound intensification of pain.

If the illness is mild, the person relies on self-treatment or, as is often the case, does nothing, and gradually the symptoms disappear. If the illness is more severe or is of longer duration, the person may consult expert help from a healer of one type or another, usually a physician.

The person recovers or expects to recover. As far back as historians and interested social scientists can trace in the history of humankind, this phenomenon of recovery has occurred. In fact, it made very little difference what mode of treatment was used; recovery was usual. It is this occurrence of nat-

Figure 5–1 (From left to right, top to bottom) Thousand-year eggs, nature, Islamic prayer, red string, eye, thunderbird, herbal remedy, tiger balm, rosary beads. *(For more information on each picture see explanation at the end of chapter.*)*

ural recovery that has given rise to all forms of *healing* that attempt to explain a phenomenon that is natural. That is, one may choose to rationalize the success of a healing method by pointing to the patient's recovery. Over the generations, natural healing has been attributed to all sort of rituals, including trepanning (puncturing the skull), cupping, magic, leeching, and bleeding. From medicine man to sorcerer, the art of healing has passed through succeeding generations. People knew the ailments of their time and devised treatments for them. In spite of ravaging plagues, natural disasters, and pandemic and epidemic diseases, human beings as a species have survived!

In Chapter 3, the dominant health-care system in the United States was discussed: this system is called "allopathic." The word *allopathy* has two roots. One comes from Greek roots meaning "other than disease" because drugs are prescribed on a basis that has no consistent or logical relationship to the symptoms. The second definition for allopathy is derived from German roots and means "all therapies." Allopathy is a "system of medicine that embraces all methods of proven value in the treatment of diseases" (Weil 1983, 17). After 1855, the American Medical Association (AMA) adopted the second definition of allopathy and has since that time exclusively determined who can practice medicine in the United States. For example, in the 1860s the AMA refused to admit women doctors to medical societies, practiced segregation, and demanded the purging of homeopaths. Today, allopaths show little tolerance or respect for such other providers of health care such as homeopaths, osteopaths, and chiropractors and for such traditional healers as lay midwives, herbalists, and medicine men (Weil, 22–25).

This chapter explores the concept of HEALTH, the HEALTH traditions model, the choices people have in terms of complementary and natural methods of HEALTH restoration, other schools of health care in contemporary American society, and examples of herbal (natural) remedies. The understanding of HEALTH, in the traditional context, is fundamental to the development of CulturalCare.

❧ HEALTH *Traditions*

The HEALTH traditions model uses the concept of holistic health—including body, mind, and spirit—and explores what people do from a traditional perspective to maintain HEALTH, protect HEALTH or prevent illness,* and restore HEALTH.

Imagine HEALTH as a complex, interrelated, twofold phenomenon—the balance of all facets of the person—the body, mind, and spirit. The body includes all *physical* aspects, such as genetic inheritance, body chemistry, gender, age, nutrition, physical condition; the *mind* includes cognitive process, such as thoughts, memories, and knowledge of such emotional processes as feelings, defenses, and self-esteem. The *spiritual* facet includes both positive and negative learned spiritual practices and teachings, dreams, symbols, stories; gifts and intuition; grace and protecting forces; as well as positive and negative metaphysical or innate forces. These facets are in constant flux and change over

---

*The phrase "protect health" is synonymous with "prevent illness."

time, yet each is completely related to the others and also related to the context of the person. The context includes the person's family, culture, work, community, history, and environment.

The person must be in a state of balance with the family, community, and the forces of the natural world around him or her. This is what is perceived as HEALTH in a traditional sense and the way in which it is determined within most traditional cultures. *Illness*, in contrast, is the imbalance of one or all parts of the person (body, mind, and spirit); this person may be in a state of imbalance with the family, community, or the forces of the natural world. The ways in which this balance, or harmony, is achieved, maintained, protected or restored often differ from the prevailing scientific health philosophy of our modern societies. Yet, many of the traditional health-related beliefs and practices exist today among people who know and live by the traditions of their own ethnoreligious cultural heritage.

HEALTH, in this traditional context, has nine interrelated facets, represented by the

1. Traditional methods of maintaining HEALTH—physical, mental, and spiritual
2. Traditional methods of protecting HEALTH
3. Traditional methods of restoring HEALTH

The traditional methods of HEALTH maintenance, HEALTH protection, and HEALTH restoration require the knowledge and understanding of HEALTH-related resources from within a given person's ethnoreligious cultural heritage. These methods may be used instead of or along with modern methods of health care. They are not alternative methods of health care because they are methods that are an integral part of a person's given heritage. Alternative medicine is a system of health care that persons may elect to use that is generic and not a part of their particular heritage. The burgeoning system of alternative medicine must not be confused with traditional health and illness beliefs and practices. In subsequent chapters of this book *traditional* health and illness beliefs and practices are discussed, following, in part, these models (Figs. 5–2 and 5–3).

TRADITIONAL HEALTH MAINTENANCE

The traditional ways of maintaining HEALTH are the active, everyday ways people go about living and attempting to stay well, that is, ordinary functioning within society. These include such actions as wearing proper clothing—boots when it snows and sweaters when it is cold, long sleeves in the sun, and scarves to protect from drafts and dust. Many traditional ethnic groups or religions may also prescribe special clothing or head coverings.

The food that is eaten and the methods for preparing it contribute to people's health. Here, too, one's ethnoreligious heritage plays a strong role in the determination of how foods are cooked, what combinations they may be eaten in, and what foods may or may not be eaten. Foods are prepared in the homes and follow the recipes from the family's tradition. Traditional cooking methods do not use preservatives, and traditional cooks don't worry about vi-

	PHYSICAL	MENTAL	SPIRITUAL

MAINTAIN HEALTH	Proper clothing
	Proper diet
	Exercise/Rest
		Concentration
		Social and Family
		  support systems
		Hobbies
			Religious
			  worship
			Prayer
			Meditation

PROTECT HEALTH	Special foods and
	  food combination
	Symbolic clothing
		Avoid certain
		  people who can
		  cause illness
		Family activities
			Religious
			  customs
			Superstitions
			Wearing amulets
			  and other
			  symbolic
			  objects to pre-
			  vent the "Evil
			  Eye" or defray
			  other sources
			  of harm

RESTORE HEALTH	Homeopathic
	  remedies
	  lineaments
	Herbal teas
	Special foods
	Massage
	Acupuncture/
	  moxibustion
		Relaxation
		Exorcism
		Curanderos and
		  other traditional
		  healers
		Nerve teas
			Religious
			  Rituals—spe-
			  cial prayers
			Meditation
			Traditional
			  healings
			Exorcism

Figure 5–2 The nine interrelated facets of health (physical, mental, and spiritual) and *personal* methods of maintaining health, protecting health, and restoring health.

tamins. Most foods are fresh and well prepared. Traditional diets are followed, and food taboos and restrictions obeyed. Cleanliness of the self and the environment is vital.

Mental HEALTH in the traditional sense is maintained by concentrating and using the mind—reading and crafts are examples. There are countless games, books, music, art, and other expressions of identity that help in the maintenance of mental well-being. Hobbies also contribute to mental well-being.

The key to maintaining health is, however, the family and social support systems. Spiritual HEALTH is maintained in the home with family closeness—prayer and celebrations. Rights of passage and kindred occasions are also family and community events. The strong identity with and connections to the "home" community are a great part of traditional life and the life cycle, and factors that contribute to health and well-being.

Many "special objects," such as hats to protect the eyes and face, long skirts to keep the body clean, down comforters to keep warm, special shoes for work and comfort, glasses to improve vision, and canes to facilitate walking, are used to maintain health, and they can be found in many traditional homes.

	PHYSICAL	MENTAL	SPIRITUAL
MAINTAIN HEALTH	Availability of Proper shelter, clothing, and food Safe air, water, soil	Availability of traditional sources of entertainment, concentration, and "rules" of the culture.	Availability and promulgation of rules of ritual and religious worship Meditation
PROTECT HEALTH	Provision of the knowledge of necessary special foods and food combinations, the wearing of symbolic clothing, and avoidance of excessive heat or cold	Provision of the knowledge of what people and situations to avoid, family activities; Family activities	The teaching of: Religious customs Superstitions Wearing amulets and other symbolic objects to prevent the "Evil Eye" or how to defray other sources of harm
RESTORE HEALTH	Resources that provide Homeopathic remedies, lineaments, Herbal teas, Special foods, Massage, and other ways to restore the body's balance of hot and cold	Traditional healers with the knowledge to use such modalities as: relaxation exorcism, storytelling, and/or Nerve teas	The availability of healers who use magical and supernatural ways to restore health: including religious rituals, special prayers, meditation, traditional healings, and/or Exorcism

Figure 5–3 The nine interrelated facets of health (physical, mental, and spiritual) and *communal* methods of maintaining health, protecting health, and restoring health.

❀ *Traditional Etiology*

The protection of HEALTH rests in the ability to understand the cause of a given illness or set of symptoms. Some of the traditional HEALTH and illness beliefs regarding the causation of illness differ from the modern model of etiology. Here illness is most often attributed to the "evil eye." The evil eye is primarily a belief that someone can project harm by gazing or staring at another's property or person (Maloney 1976, 14).

The belief in the evil eye is probably the oldest and most widespread of all superstitions, and it is found to exist in many parts of the world, such as Southern Europe, the Middle East, and North Africa (Maloney, vi).

It is thought by some to be merely a superstition, but what is seen by one person as superstition may well be seen by another as religion. Various evil-eye beliefs were carried to this country by immigrant populations. These beliefs have persisted and may be quite strong among newer immigrants and heritage-consistent peoples (Maloney, vii).

The common beliefs in the evil eye assert that

1. The power emanates from the eye (or mouth) and strikes the victim.
2. The injury, be it illness or other misfortune, is sudden.
3. The person that casts the evil eye may not be aware of having this power.
4. The afflicted person may or may not know the source of the evil eye.
5. The injury caused by the evil eye may be prevented or cured with rituals or symbols.
6. This belief helps to explain sickness and misfortune (Maloney, vii).

The nature of the evil eye is defined differently by different populations. The variables include how it is cast, who can cast it, who receives it, and the degree of power that it has. In the Philippines, the evil is cast through the eye or mouth; in the Mediterranean, it is the avenging power of God; in Italy, it is a malevolent force like a plague and is warded off by wearing amulets.

In various parts of the world, various people cast it: in Mexico—strangers; in Iran—kinfolk; and in Greece—witches. Its power varies, and in some places, such as the Mediterranean, it is seen as the "devil." In the Near East, it is seen as a deity, and among Slovak Americans as a chronic but low-grade phenomenon (Maloney, xv).

Among Germans the evil eye is known as *aberglobin* or *aberglaubisch* and causes preventable problems, such as evil, harm, and illness. Among the Polish, the evil eye is known as *szatan*, literally, "Satan." Some "evil spirits" are equated with the devil and can be warded off by praying to a patron saint or guardian angel. *Szatan* also is averted by prayer and repentance and the wearing of medals and scapulars. These serve as reminders of the "Blessed Mother and the Patrons in Heaven" and protect the wearer from harm. The evil eye is known in Yiddish as *kayn aynhoreh*. The expression *kineahora* is recited by Jews after a compliment or when a statement of luck is made to prevent the casting of an evil spell on another's health. Often the speaker spits three times after uttering the word (Spector 1983, 126–127).

Agents of disease may also be "soul loss," "spirit possession," "spells," and "hexes." Here prevention becomes a ritual of protecting oneself and one's children from these agents. Treatment requires the removal of these agents from the afflicted person (Zola 1972, 673–679).

Illness also can be attributed to people who have the ability to make others ill, for example, witches and practitioners of voodoo. The ailing person attempts to avoid these people to prevent illness and to identify them as part of the treatment. Other "agents" to be avoided are "envy," "hate," and "jealousy." A person may practice prevention by avoiding situations that could provoke the envy, hate, or jealousy of a friend, acquaintance, or neighbor. The evil-eye belief contributes to this avoidance.

Another source of evil can be of human origin and occurs when a person is temporarily controlled by souls not their own. In the Jewish culture, this controlling spirit is known as *dybbuk*. The word comes from the Hebrew word meaning "cleaving" or "holding fast." A dybbuk is portrayed as a "wandering, disembodied soul which enters another person's body and holds fast" (Winkler 1981, 8–9).

❈ HEALTH *Protection*

Among people who believe in traditional ways, illness is often attributed to the evil eye, *envidia,* and "witches" (Zola 1972). In these instances, health may be protected by external controls, such as the avoidance of people who can bring it about by the evil eye, the avoidance of *envidia,* that is, by not provoking the envy of others, and the avoidance of witches or others who can cast spells and other forms of evil.

Traditional practices used in the protection of HEALTH consist of

1. The use of protective objects—worn, carried, or hung in the home
2. The use of substances that are ingested in certain ways and amounts or eliminated, and substances worn or hung in the home
3. The practices of religion, such as the burning of candles, the rituals of redemption, and prayer

OBJECTS THAT PROTECT HEALTH

Amulets are objects, such as charms, worn on a string or chain around the neck, wrist, or waist to protect the wearer from the evil eye or the evil spirits that could be transmitted from one person to another, or could have supernatural origins. For example, the *mano milagroso* (Figure 5–4) is worn by many people of Mexican origin for luck and the prevention of evil. A *mano negro* (Figure 5–5) is placed on babies of Puerto Rican descent to ward off the evil eye. The *mano negro* is placed on the baby's wrist on a chain or pinned to the diaper or shirt and is worn throughout the early years of life.

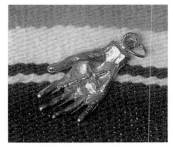

Figure 5–4 *Mano milagroso.* (From the author's personal collection. Photographed by Stephen Vedder.)

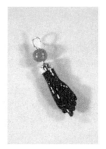

Figure 5–5 *Mano negro.* (From the author's personal collection. Photographed by Stephen Vedder.)

Amulets may also be written documents on parchment scrolls, and these are hung in the home. Figure 5–6 is an example of a written amulet acquired in Jerusalem. It is hung in the home to protect the family from the "evil eye," famine, storms, diseases, and countless other dangers. Table 5–1 describes several practices found among selected ethnic groups to ward off the "evil eye."

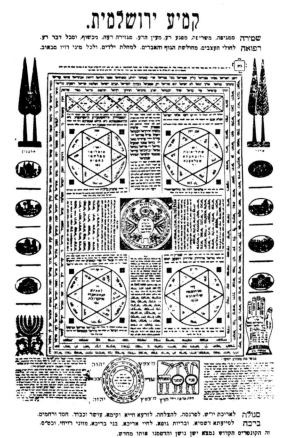

Figure 5–6 The Jerusalem amulet. This amulet serves as protection from pestilence, fire, bad wounds and infection, the evil eye, bad decrees and decisions, curses, witchcraft, and from everything bad; to heal nervous illness, weakness of body organs, children's diseases, and all kinds of suffering from pain; as a talisman for livelihood for success, fertility, honesty, and honor; and for charity, love, mercy, goodness, and grace. It also has the following admonition: "Know before whom you stand—the King of Kings The Holy One, Blessed be He." (Translated by B. Koff, Jerusalem, Israel, 26 December, 1988. From the author's personal collection. Photographed by Stephen Vedder.)

| Table 5–1 | Practices to Ward Off the "Evil Eye" |

Origin	Practices
Scotland	Red thread knotted into clothing
	Fragment of Bible worn on body
South Asia	Knotted hair or fragment of Koran worn on body
Eastern European Jews	Red ribbon woven into clothes or attached to crib
Sephardic Jews	Wearing a blue ribbon or blue bead
Italians	Wearing a red ribbon or the *corno*
Greek	Blue "eye" bead, crucifix, charms
	Phylact—a baptismal charm placed on baby
	Cloves of garlic pinned to shirt
Tunisia	Amulets pinned on clothing consisting of tiny
	figures or writings from the Koran
	Charms of the fish symbol—widely used to ward off evil
Iran	Child covered with amulets—agate, blue beads
	Children often may be left filthy and never washed
	to protect them from the evil eye.
India/Pakistan	Hindus—copper plates with magic drawings rolled in them
	Muslims—slips of paper with verses from the Koran
	Black or red string around the baby's wrist
Guatemala	Small red bag containing herbs placed on baby or crib
Mexico	Amulet with red yarn
Philippines	Wearing of charms, amulets, medals
Puerto Rico	*Mano negro*

Bangles (Figure 5–7) are worn by people originating from the West Indies. The silver bracelets are open to "let out evil" yet closed to prevent evil from entering the body. They are worn from infancy, and as the person grows they are replaced with larger bracelets. These bracelets tend to tarnish and leave a black ring on the skin when a person is becoming ill. When this occurs, the person knows it is important to rest, to improve the diet, and to take other needed precautions. Many people believe they are extremely vulnerable to evil,

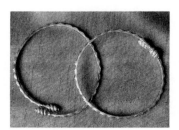

Figure 5–7 Bangles. (From the author's personal collection. Photographed by R. Schadt.)

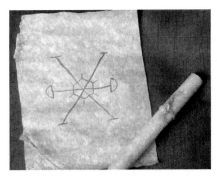

Figure 5–8 Talisman. (From the author's personal collection. Photographed by R. Schadt.)

even to death, when these bracelets are removed. Some people wear numerous bangles. When they move an arm, the bracelets tinkle. It is believed that this sound frightens away the evil spirit. Health-care providers should realize that when these bracelets are removed, the person experiences a great deal of anxiety.

In addition to amulets, there are talismans (Figure 5–8). A talisman is believed to possess extraordinary powers and may be worn on a rope around the waist or carried in a pocket or purse. The talisman illustrated in Figure 5–8 is a marionette, and it protects the wearer from evil. It is recommended that people who wear amulets or carry a talisman *be allowed to do so in health-care institutions.*

SUBSTANCES THAT PROTECT HEALTH

The second practice uses diet to protect HEALTH and consists of many different observances. People from many ethnic backgrounds eat raw garlic or onions (Figure 5–9) in an effort to prevent illness. Garlic or onions also may be worn on the body or may be hung in the Italian, Greek, or Native American home. *Chachayotel* (Figure 5–10), a seed, may be tied around the waist by a Mexican person to prevent arthritic pain. Among traditional Chinese people, thousand-year-old eggs, illustrated in the opening panel, Figure 5–1, are eaten with rice to keep the body healthy and to prevent illness. The ginseng root is

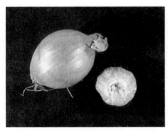

Figure 5–9 Garlic and onion. (From the author's personal collection. Photographed by Stephen Vedder.)

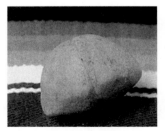

Figure 5–10 Chachayotel. (From the author's personal collection. Photographed by Stephen Vedder.)

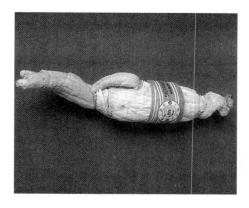

Figure 5–11 Ginseng root. (From the author's personal collection. Photographed by Stephen Vedder.)

the most famous of Chinese medicines. It has universal medicinal applications and is used preventively to "build the blood," especially after childbirth. Tradition states that the more the root looks like a man, the more effective it is. Ginseng is also native to the United States and is used in this country as a restorative tonic (Figure 5–11).

Diet regimens also are used to protect HEALTH. It is believed that the body is kept in balance or harmony by the type of food that one eats.

Traditionalists have strong beliefs about diet and foods and their relationship to the protection of HEALTH. The rules of the kosher diet practiced among Jewish people mandate the elimination of pig products and shellfish. Only fish with scales and fins are allowed, and only certain cuts of meat from animals with a cleft hoof and that chew the cud can be consumed. Examples of this kind of animal are cattle and sheep. Many of these dietary practices, such as the avoidance of pig products, are also adhered to by Muslims. Jews also believe that milk and meat must never be mixed and eaten at the same meal.

In traditional Chinese homes, a balance must be maintained between foods that are *yin* or *yang*. These are eaten in specified proportions. In Hispanic homes, foods must be balanced as to "hot" and "cold." These foods too, must be eaten in the proper amounts, at certain times, and in certain combinations.

SPIRITUAL PRACTICES THAT PROTECT HEALTH

A third traditional approach toward HEALTH protection centers in part on religion. Religion strongly affects the way people choose to protect HEALTH, and it plays a strong role in the rituals associated with HEALTH protection. It dictates social, moral, and dietary practices that are designed to keep a person in balance and healthy. Many people believe that illness and evil are prevented by strict adherence to religious codes, morals, and religious practices. They view illness as a punishment for breaking a religious code. For example, I once interviewed a woman who believed she had cancer because God was punishing her for stealing money when she was a child. An example of a protective

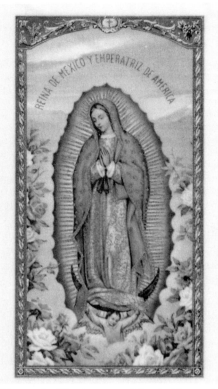

Figure 5–12 Prayer card for the Virgin of
Guadalupe. (From the author's personal
collection. Photographed by Stephen Vedder.)

religious figure is the Virgin of Guadalupe (Figure 5–12), the patron saint of
Mexico, who is pictured on medals that people wear or in pictures hung in the
home. She is believed to protect the person and home from evil and harm, and
she serves as a figure of hope.

Religion can, therefore, help to provide the believer with an ability to understand and interpret the events of the environment and life. This discussion
continues in Chapter 6.

HEALTH RESTORATION

HEALTH restoration in the physical sense can be accomplished by the use of
countless traditional remedies such as herbal teas, liniments, special foods and
food combinations, massage, and other activities.

The restoration of HEALTH in the mental domain may be accomplished
by the use of various techniques such as exorcism, calling on traditional healers, using teas or massage, and seeking family and community support.

The restoration of HEALTH in the spiritual sense can be accomplished by
healing rituals; religious healing rituals; or the use of symbols and prayer, meditation, special prayers, and exorcism.

❧ HEALTH-*Care Choices*

There are countless ways to describe and label health-care beliefs, practices, and systems. "Health care" may be labeled as "modern," "conventional," "traditional," "alternative," "complementary," "allopathic," "homeopathic," "folk," and so forth. The use of the word "traditional" to describe "modern health care" is, by definition, a misnomer. Traditional connotes a tradition—"the delivery of opinions, doctrines, practices, rites, and customs from generation to generation by oral communication" or "a long-established custom or practice that has the effect of an unwritten law handed down through the generations and generally observed that is old and has been passed down for generations" (American Heritage Dictionary, paperback edition). The use of this term to connote modern health care is a misnomer as modern, allopathic, health care is a new science and has been passed down in writing for a relatively short amount of time, rather than orally over many generations!

There are also many reasons why patients may choose to use health-care systems other than modern medical care. These include, but are not limited to, access issues such as poverty, availability, and lack of insurance, and preference for familiar and personal care. "Traditional" here connotes health-care beliefs and practices observed among peoples who have steadfastly maintained their heritage and observe health-care practices derived from within their given ethnocultural heritage.

As stated earlier, in nearly every situation when a person becomes ill there is an expectation for the restoration of health, and the person usually recovers. As far back as historians and interested social scientists can trace in the extended history of humankind, the phenomenon of recovery has occurred. It made little difference what mode of treatment was used; health restoration was usual as well as expected. There are established cultural norms that were and are attributed to the recovery from illness and over time the successful methods for treating various maladies were preserved and passed down to each new generation within a given traditional ethnocultural community. It is the occurrence of natural recovery that has given rise to all forms of therapeutic treatments and the attempts to explain a phenomenon that is natural. Over the generations, natural recovery has been attributed to all sort of rituals, including cupping, magic, leeching, and bleeding. Today, the people who are members of many different native, immigrant, and traditional cultural communities in the United States—African, American Indian, Asian, European, and those of Spanish origin—may continue to utilize the practices found within their tradition.

HEALTH-CARE PHILOSOPHIES

There are two distinctly different health-care philosophies that determine the scope of health beliefs and practices: allopathic and homeopathic. Each of these philosophies espouses effective methods of restoring health, and the "battles" between the philosophies have been hard fought in this country (Starr 1982). One manifestation of these struggles is a preference for "complementary" or "alternative" medicine among people from all walks of life.

Allopathic Philosophy   The dominant health-care system in the United States is "allopathic," and it is predicated on a dualistic philosophy that sees the person as "body and mind" and is discussed earlier in this chapter. Allopathy, as pointed out, is a "system of medicine that embraces all methods of proven value in the treatment of diseases" (Weil 1983, 17). Today, health-care providers that espouse the allopathic philosophy show little tolerance or respect for systems of health care that do not adhere to the scientific and technological norms of the system.

Homeopathic Philosophy   The other health-care philosophy in the United States is homeopathic. Homeopathic medicine was developed between 1790 and 1810 by Samuel C. Hahnemann in Germany and is extremely popular in much of Europe and other parts of the world.

Homeopathy, or homoeopathy, comes from the Greek words homoios (similar) and pathos (suffering). In the practice of homeopathy, the person, not the disease, is treated (Starr 1982). This system, as stated, has not been "tolerated" by the allopaths, yet it continues to thrive and is used by countless peoples. It espouses a holistic philosophy—that is, it sees health as a balance of the physical, mental, and spiritual whole. Homeopathic care encompasses a wide range of health-care practices and is often referred to as "complementary medicine" or "alternative medicine." Complementary, alternative, unconventional, or unorthodox therapies are medical practices that do not conform to the scientific standards set by the allopathic medical community; they are not taught widely in the medical and nursing communities and are not generally available in the allopathic health-care system, including the hospital settings. These include such therapies as acupuncture, massage therapy, and chiropractic medicine.

ALLOPATHIC VERSUS HOMEOPATHIC SYSTEMS

Figure 5–13 demonstrates the health-care pathways a given person may follow. The allopathic system comprises the familiar services—acute care, chronic care, rehabilitation, public/community health, and psychiatric/mental health care.

There are two types of care in the homeopathic system—one that is classified as "complementary" or "alternative," and the other, traditional and culture-bound. Alternative, as stated earlier, refers to therapies that one may elect to use that are not a part of their ethnocultural or religious heritage, or interventions neither taught widely in medical schools nor generally available in U.S. hospitals; traditional therapies are those therapies that are a part of one's traditional cultural heritage. In other words, a European American electing to use acupuncture as a method of treatment is seeking alternative treatment; a Chinese American using this treatment modality is using traditional medicine.

The following are selected examples of alternative care:

1. Aromatherapy—an ancient science, presently popular, that uses essential plant oils to produce strong physical and emotional effects in the body

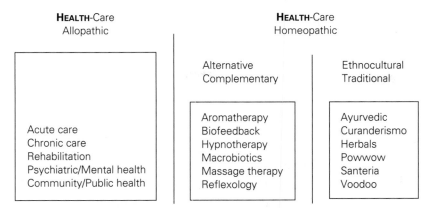

HEALTH-Care Allopathic	HEALTH-Care Homeopathic	
	Alternative Complementary	Ethnocultural Traditional
Acute care Chronic care Rehabilitation Psychiatric/Mental health Community/Public health	Aromatherapy Biofeedback Hypnotherapy Macrobiotics Massage therapy Reflexology	Ayurvedic Curanderismo Herbals Powwow Santeria Voodoo

Figure 5–13 Selected examples of HEALTH-care choices.

2. *Biofeedback*—the use of an electronic machine to measure skin temperatures. The patient controls responses that are usually involuntary.
3. *Hypnotherapy*—the use of hypnosis to stimulate emotions and involuntary responses such as blood pressure
4. *Macrobiotics*—a diet and lifestyle from the Far East and adapted for the United States by Michio Kushif. The principles of this vegetarian diet consists of balancing yin and yang energies of food.
5. *Massage therapy*—use of manipulative techniques to relieve pain and return energy to the body, now popular among many groups both modern and traditional
6. *Reflexology*—the natural science dealing with the reflex points in the hands and feet that correspond to every organ in the body. The goal is to clear the energy pathways and the flow of energy through the body.

TRADITIONAL OR ETHNOCULTURAL CARE

The following list describes selected traditional health care systems:

1. *Ayurvedic*—This 4,000-year-old method of healing originated in India and is the most ancient existing medical system that uses diet, natural therapies, and herbs. Its chief aim is longevity and quality of life. It formed the foundation of Chinese medicine.
2. *Curanderismo*—the traditional Hispanic (Mexican) system of health care that is derived, in part from traditional practices of indigenous Indian and Spanish holistic health practices.
3. *Herbals*—use of the natural environment and substances—herbs, plants, minerals, and animal substances—to prevent and treat illness. For example, the people who are members of North American Indian nations use this system extensively.
4. *Powwow*—A form of traditional health care practiced by German Americans and observed among the Pennsylvania Dutch.

5. *Santeria*—a form of traditional health care observed among the practitioners of Santeria, a syncretic religion that comprises both African and Catholic beliefs. This religion is found practiced among Puerto Ricans and Dominicans.
6. *Voodoo*—a form of traditional health care observed among the practitioners of Voodoo, a religion that is a combination of Christian and African Yoruba religious beliefs.

The use of alternative therapies, defined earlier as interventions neither taught widely in medical schools nor generally available in U.S. hospitals, is growing rapidly. Astin (1998) reported that there are three theories that have been offered to explain why people seek alternative care:

1. *Dissatisfaction*—Patients are not satisfied with allopathic care because it is seen as ineffective, produces adverse effects, or is impersonal, too costly, or too technological.
2. *Need for personal control*—The providers of alternative therapies are less authoritarian and more empowering, as they offer the patient the opportunity to have autonomy and control in their health-care decisions.
3. *Philosophical congruence*—They are compatible with the patients' values, worldview, spiritual philosophy, or beliefs regarding the nature and meaning of health and illness. These therapies are now frequently used by patients with cancer, arthritis, chronic back or other pain, stress-related problems, AIDS, gastrointestinal problems, and anxiety.

Since 1990 Eisenberg and colleagues have studied the trends in the use of alternative medicine in the United States. They reported the results of a national survey of 1539 subjects in 1993 and reported the findings of a 1997 survey in 1998. They found in 1991 that about a third of all American adults use some form of unconventional medical treatment; this number rose to 42.1% in 1997. The most frequent users in both studies were educated upper-income white Americans in the 25–49 age group who were most likely to live on the West Coast. The total projected out-of-pocket expenditure for unconventional therapy was $10.3 billion in 1990 and was conservatively estimated to be $27.0 billion in 1997. The various types of alternative therapies included relaxation techniques, chiropractic, imagery, commercial weight-loss programs, lifestyle diets such as macrobiotics, megavitamin therapy, self-help groups, biofeedback, and hypnosis. Neither study examined the use of traditional healers and therapies by members of the immigrant and traditional communities (Eisenberg et al. 1998, 1574).

HOMEOPATHIC SCHOOLS

The period 1870 through 1930 was when the allopathic health-care model as we know it today was established. During the time that the roots of this system of health care were becoming firmly established, the ideas of the eclectic and other schools of medical thought were also prevalent.

Homeopathic Medicine. As stated earlier in this chapter, homeopathic medicine was developed between 1790 and 1810 by Samuel C. Hahnemann in Germany. Homeopathy, or homoeopathy, comes from the Greek words *homoios* (similar) and *pathos* (suffering). In the practice of homeopathy, the person, not the disease, is treated. The practitioner treats a given person by using minute doses of plant, mineral, or animal substances. The medicines are selected using the principle of the "law of similars." A substance that is used to treat a specific set of symptoms is the same substance that if given to a healthy person would cause the symptoms. The medicines are administered in extremely small doses. These medicines are said to provide a gentle but powerful stimulus to the person's own defense system and, in turn, to help the person heal.

Homeopathy was popular in nineteenth-century America and Europe because it was successful in treating the raging epidemics of those times. In 1900, 20 to 25% of physicians were homeopaths. Due to allopathic efforts to wipe out the homeopaths that began in 1906, the movement has dissipated. A small group of homeopaths still exists in the United States, however, and there are larger practices in India, Great Britain, France, Greece, Germany, Brazil, Argentina, and Mexico (Homeopathic Educational Services).

Osteopathic Medicine. Osteopathy, developed in 1874 by Dr. A. T. Still in Kirksville, Missouri, is the art of curing without the use of surgery or drugs. Osteopathy attempts to discover and correct all mechanical disorders in the human machine and to direct the recuperative power of nature that is within the body to cure the disease. It claims that if there is an unobstructed blood and nerve supply to all parts of the body, the effects of a given disease will disappear.

Osteopaths are fully qualified physicians who can practice in all areas of medicine and surgery. They, like the medical doctor, have completed four years of medical school, one year of internship, and generally a further residency in a specialty area. They take the same course work as do medical doctors, often use the same textbooks, and often take the same licensing examinations. There are 14 osteopathic medical schools in the United States and 214 hospitals. The lines of distinction between the medical doctor and the osteopath arise because the osteopath, in addition to using modern scientific forms of medical diagnosis and treatment, uses manipulation of the bones, muscles, and joints as therapy. Osteopaths also employ structural diagnosis and take into account the relationship between body structure and organic functioning when they determine a diagnosis. The osteopathic doctor has the same legal power to treat patients as a medical doctor (Denenberg).

Chiropractic. Chiropractic is a controversial form of healing that has been in existence for well over a century. It, too, adheres to a disease theory and a method of therapy that differs from allopathy. It was developed as a form of healing in 1895 in Davenport, Iowa, by a storekeeper named Daniel David Palmer, also known as a "magnetic healer." Palmer's theory underlying the practice of chiropractic was that an interference with the normal transmission of "mental impulses" between the brain and body organs produced diseases. The interference is caused by misalignment or subluxation of the vertebrae of the spine, which decreases the flow of "vital energy" from the brain through the nerves and spinal cord to all parts of the body. The treatment consists of manipulation to eradicate the subluxation.

Chiropractic is practiced in two ways. One form is that of the "mixers," who use heat therapy, enemas ("colonic irrigation"), exercise programs, and other therapeutic practices. The other group, the "straight" chiropractors, who use only manipulation, disapprove of the practices of the "mixers." They believe that the other techniques are a form of allopathic medicine (Cobb 1977).

Eclectic Medicine. The word *eclectic* means "choosing," and it refers to choosing the means for treating disease. Methods and remedies are selected from all other systems. This school of medicine believes that nature has curative powers, and practitioners seek to remove the causes of disease through the natural outlets of the body. They treat the cause of disease rather than the symptoms and do not use bleeding, antimony, or poisons to treat diseases (School 1924, 1545–1546).

Hydrotherapy. A German farmer, Priessnitz, developed hydrotherapy in 1840. It includes the application of water, internally and externally, in any form at any temperature, with the belief that the water can have a most profound effect on the body (School 1924, 1527).

There were also many popular theories of healing during this era that focused only on the mind. Some examples follow.

Mesmerism. In the late eighteenth century, mesmerism was a popular form of healing by touch and was named for its founder, Friedrich Anton Mesmer. Mesmer believed that illness was a condition in which the body and mind of a person were influenced by a mysterious force emanating from another person. He further believed that the stars exerted an influence on people and that this force was the same as electricity and magnetism. Initially, he believed that stroking the body with magnets would bring about a cure for illness. He later modified this to the belief that touch alone could heal (School 1924, 1592).

Hypnotism. Hypnotism artificially creates a condition in which the person apparently is asleep and acts in obedience to the will of the operator as regards both motion and sensation. It was developed in 1841 by James Braid, an English surgeon (School 1924, 1595).

Mind Cure. Mind cure is the cure of disease by means of the mind alone, in which *faith* influences the cure of disease. Two prerequisites in faith healing are the desire to get well and faith in the treatment (School 1924, 1598).

Christian Science. The religious philosophy of scientism lies outside allo-pathic and most homeopathic philosophies and delivery systems, yet it is one of the forms of mind cure. It rejects allopathic practices and uses only spiritual means for healing. Christian Science was developed by Mary Baker Eddy in 1879 in Boston to "commemorate the word and works of our Master, which should reinstate primitive Christianity and its lost element of healing" (adver-tisement 1990). Furthermore, the doctrine teaches that those who really fol-low Jesus should follow Him in healing, which can be done through the mind. The definition of illness is that sickness is merely a false impression conveyed by an erring mortal mind. The fundamental propositions of Christian Science are (advertisement 1990):

1. God is all.
2. God is good. Good is mind.
3. God, Spirit, being all, nothing is matter.
4. Life, God, omnipotent good, deny death, evil, sin, disease. Disease, sin, evil, death, deny good, omnipotent God, life.

To the people who believe, Christian Science is a way based on the laws of God. It is devoted to lifting the burdens of sin and suffering from all hu-manity. It is an established church and deeply committed to the belief in the inspired teaching of Jesus and His disciples. Further consideration of this reli-gious philosophy is found in Chapter 6.

❧ HEALTH *Restoration*

NATURAL REMEDIES

The use of natural products such as wild herbs and berries accessible to the healers developed into today's science of pharmacology. Early humankind had a wealth of knowledge about the medicinal properties of the plants, trees, and fungi in their environment. They knew how to prepare concoctions from the bark and roots of trees and from berries and wild flowers. As an example, pur-ple foxglove, which contains the cardiotonic digitalis, was used for centuries to slow the heart rate.

The current popularity of wholistic options includes health foods and has given rise to the popular use of various diets to protect health. In addition, health-food stores make available a number of medicinal teas and herbs. (A listing of commonly used herbs is presented in Table 5–2.) Almost 100 herbal teas are listed in a small paperback entitled *Herbal Tea Book* (Adrian and Den-nis 1976). The herbs are listed alphabetically, and the source and use of each are given. An even larger listing is given in *Herbs: Medicine and Mysticism* by Sybil Leek, who is known as one of the "world's foremost astrologers and witches." This book has a wide audience. Countless other sources are available.

It is difficult to sort out which aspects of folk medicine have merit and which are a hoax. From the viewpoint of the consumer—if he or she has faith

Table 5-2 Commonly Used Herbal Remedies

Herb	Action	Use	Administration
Alfalfa (or Lucerne)	Stimulant, nutritive	Arthritis; weight gain; strength-giving	1 oz herb to 1 pint water; drink 1 cupful as tea
Anise (seed used)	Stimulant; aromatic; relaxant	Flatulence; dry coughs	2 tsp of seed to ½ pint water; dose: 1–3 tsp often
Bayberry (bark used)	Astringent; stimulant; emetic	Sore-throat gargle; cleanses stomach; douche; rinse for bleeding gums	1 oz powdered bark to 1 pint water; drink as tea
Blessed thistle	Diaphoretic; stimulant emetic	Reduces fevers; breaks up colds; digestive problems	1 oz herb to 1 pint water; small doses as desired
Bugleweed	Romatic; sedative; tranquilizer; astringent	Coughs; relieves pulmonary bleeding; increases appetite	1 oz herb to 1 pint water; drink by glassful often
Catnip (leaves)	Diaphoretic; tonic; antispasmodic	Helpful in convulsions; produces perspiration	1 oz leaves to 1 pint water
Cayenne pepper (fruit and seed)	Stimulant	Purest and most positive stimulant in herbal medicine; healing of burns and other wounds; relieves toothaches	Powder in small doses; by mouth or topical (measured by teaspoonful); tsp
Chestnut, horse (bark and fruit)	Astringent; narcotic; tonic	Bark used for fevers; fruit to treat rheumatism	Bark: 1 oz to 1 pint water, tsp 4 times per day; fruit: tincture 10 drops twice per day
Chicory (root)	Diuretic; laxative	Liver enlargement; gout; rheumatic complaints	1 oz root to 1 pint water; take freely
Corn silk	Diuretic; mild stimulant	Irritated bladder; urinary stones; trouble with prostate gland	2 oz in 1 pint water; take freely

Herb	Properties	Uses	Preparation/Dosage
Dandelion (root)	Diuretic; tonic	Used in many patent medicines; general body stimulant; used chiefly with kidney and liver disorders	Roasted roots are ground and used like coffee; small cup once or twice per day
Ergot (fungus)	Uterine stimulant; sedative hemostatic	Menstrual disorders; stops hemorrhage	Liquid extract 10–20 minims by mouth
Eucalyptus	Antiseptic; antispasmodic, stimulant	Inhale for sore throat; apply to ulcers and other wounds	Local application or fluid extract in small doses by mouth
Fennel (seeds)	Aromatic; carminative (expels air from bowels)	Gas; gout; colic in infants; increases milk in nursing mothers	Pour water (½ pint) or 1 tsp of seeds; take freely
Garlic (juice)	Diaphoretic; diuretic; stimulant; expectorant	Treats colds; diuretic; antiseptic	Juice, 10–30 drops
Goldenrod (leaves)	Aromatic; stimulant	Sore throat; general pain; colds; rheumatism	1 oz leaves to 1 pint water; small dose often
Hollyhock (flowers)	Diuretic	Chest complaints	1 oz flowers to 1 pint water; drink as much as needed
Ivy (leaves)	Cathartic; diaphoretic	Poultices on ulcers and abscesses	As a poultice
Ivy, poison (leaves)	Irritant; stimulant; narcotic	Rheumatism; sedative for the nervous system	Liquid extract 5–30 drops
Juniper berries	Diuretic; stimulant	Bladder and kidney problems; gargles; digestive aid	Oil of berries 1–5 drops
Licorice (root)	Demulcent	Coughs; prevents thirst	Powdered root
Lily of the valley (flower)	Cardiac stimulant; diuretic; stimulant	Headaches	½ oz of flowers to 1 pint water; tablespoon doses

(continued)

Table 5-2—Continued

Herb	Action	Use	Administration
Marigold (flowers and leaves)	Diaphoretic; stimulant	Flowers and leaves made into a salve for skin eruptions; relieves sore muscles, amenorrhea	1 oz herbs and petals to 1 pint water; 1 tbsp on mouth or topical application
Mistletoe (leaves)	Nervine; antispasmodic; tonic; narcotic	Epilepsy and hysteria; painful menstruation; induces sleep	2 oz to ½ pint water; 1 tbs often
Mustard (leaves)	Cooling; sedative	Hoarseness (excellent aid in recovering the voice)	Liquid extract; small doses
Nightshade, deadly (poison) (leaves and root)	Narcotic; diuretic; sedative; antispasmodic	Eye diseases; increases urine; stimulates circulation	Powdered leaves and root; small amounts
Papaya leaves	Digestive	Digestive disorders; fresh leaves; dry wounds	Papain; small doses
Rosemary (leaves) (herb)	Astringent; diaphoretic; tonic; stimulant	Prevents baldness; cold; colic; nerves; strengthens eyes	1 oz herb to 1 pint water; small doses
Saffron (flower pistils)	Carminative; diaphoretic	Amenorrhea; dysmenorrhea; hysteria	1 dram flower pistils in 1 pint water; teacup doses
Thyme (dried herb)	Antiseptic; antispasmodic; tonic	Perspiration; colds; coughs; cramps	1 oz herb to 1 pint water; 1 tbs doses often

From: Leek S. *Herbs and Mysticism* (Chicago: Henry Regnery, 1975). pp. 73–235. Reprinted with permission.

in the efficacy of an herb, a diet, a pill, or a healer—it is not a hoax. From the viewpoint of the medical establishment, jealous of its territorial claim, this same herb, diet, pill, or healer is indeed a hoax if it is *ineffective* and *prevents* the person from using the method of treatment the physician-healer believes is effective.

The tensions between allopathic and homeopathic philosophies have been going on since the late nineteenth century. In this chapter we explored traditional ways of maintaining, protecting, and restoring HEALTH, choices available to patients, and HEALTH-care philosophies.

❀ *References*

Adrian, A., and Dennis, J. 1976. *Herbal Tea Book.* San Francisco: Health.

Advertisement. 1990. Why Is Prayer Being Prosecuted in Boston? *Boston Globe,* 11 April.

Astin, J. A. 1998. Why Patients Use Alternative Medicine: Results of a National Study. *JAMA* 279, no. 19 (May 20): 1548–1553.

Cobb, A. K. 1977. Pluralistic Legitimation of an Alternative Therapy System: The Case of Chiropractic. *Medical Anthropology* 6(4) (Fall):1–23.

Denenberg, H. n.d. Pamphlet. *Shopper's Guide to Osteopathic Physicians.*

Eisenberg, D. M., Davis, R. B., Ettner, S. L., et al. 1998. Trends in Alternative Medicine Use in the United States, 1990–1997. *JAMA* 280(18):1569–1575.

Homeopathic Educational Services. 1979. *Educational pamphlet.* Berkeley, Calif. Reprint, Harrisburg, Penn.: Pennsylvania Osteopathic Association.

Leek, S. 1975. *Herbs: Medicine and Mysticism.* Chicago: Henry Regnery.

Leeson, J. 1967. Paths to Medical Care in Lasaka, Zambia. Master's thesis, University of Manchester, England. Preliminary findings, 12 July, p. 14.

Maloney, C., ed. 1976. *The Evil Eye.* New York: Columbia University Press.

School, B. F., ed. 1924. *Library of Health Complete Guide to Prevention and Cure of Disease.* Philadelphia: Historical.

Spector, R. E. 1983. A Description of the Impact of Medicare on Health–Illness Beliefs and Practices of White Ethnic Senior Citizens in Central Texas. Ph.D. diss. University of Texas at Austin School of Nursing. Ann Arbor, Mich.: University Microfilms International, 126–127.

Starr, P. 1982. *The Social Transformation of American Medicine.* New York: Basic Books, 79, 145.

Weil, A. 1983. *Health and Healing.* Boston: Houghton Mifflin.

Winkler, G. 1981. *Dybbuk.* New York: Judaica Press.

Zola, I. K. 1972. The Concept of Trouble and Sources of Medical Assistance to Whom One Can Turn with What. *Social Science and Medicine* 6: 673–679.

*Figure 5–1 from page 97
The chapter-opening panel of HEALTH-related images depicts objects that may used to protect, maintain, and/or restore physical, mental, or spiritual HEALTH by people of many different heritages. This panel is symbolic of the HEALTH traditions model and its themes, which will be discussed later in the chapter. **Thousand-year eggs,** from China, represent traditional foods that may be eaten daily to maintain physical HEALTH. **Nature**—the enjoyment of nature, the natural environment, may be a universal way of maintaining mental HEALTH.

The **Islamic prayer,** from East Jerusalem represents prayer, a way of maintaining spiritual HEALTH. **Red string,** obtained from the Tomb of Rachel in Bethlehem, Israel, may be worn to protect physical HEALTH. The **eye,** from Cuba, represents the plethora of eye-related objects that may be worn or hung in the home to protect the mental HEALTH of people by shielding them from the envy and bad wishes of others. The **thunderbird,** from the Hopi Nation may be worn for spiritual protection and good luck. The *herbal remedy* from Africa represents herbs that may be used by people from all ethnocultural traditional backgrounds as one method of restoring physical HEALTH. **Tiger balm,** from Singapore, represents substances that are used in massage therapy that may be used as a way of restoring mental HEALTH. **Rosary beads,** from Italy, symbolize prayer and meditation methods used in the spiritual restoration of HEALTH.

Chapter 6

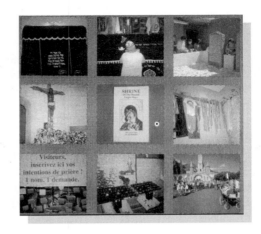

Healing: Magico-religious Traditions

In the early summer of 1990, a Christian Scientist couple was convicted in Suffolk (Boston, Massachusetts) Superior Court of involuntary manslaughter in the death of their 2-year-old son. They had relied solely on prayers to heal their son of a bowel obstruction. The verdict was applauded by the prosecutor, for it set a precedent for children's rights. The Christian Scientists denounced it as an attack on their faith.

What is healing? What is the connotation of this word from a magicoreligious perspective? This chapter explores these questions by introducing a wide range of ideas and magicoreligious practices.

The professional history of nursing was born with Florence Nightingale's knowledge (1860) that "nature heals." In more recent times, Blattner (1981) has written a text designed to help nurses assist patients to upgrade their lives in a holistic sense and to heal the person—body, mind, and spirit. Krieger (1979), in the *Therapeutic Touch,* has developed a method for teaching nurses how to use their hands to heal. Wallace (1979) has described methods of helping nurses to diagnose and to deliver spiritual care. She points out that the word

> spiritual is often used synonymously with religion, but that the terms are not the same. If they are used synonymously as a basis for assessment of nursing needs some of the patient's deepest needs may be glossed over. Spiritual care implies a much broader grasp of the search for meanings that goes on within every human life.

In addition to answers to these questions from nursing, one is able to explore the concept from the classical and historical viewpoints of anthropology, sociology, psychology, and religion.

Figure 6–1 (From left to right, top to bottom) The Tomb of Rachel in Bethlehem, Israel; the Tomb of David in Jerusalem, Israel; the Tomb of Menachem Mendel Scheerson in Queens, New York; the Black Jesus in the San Fernando Cathedral in San Antonio, Texas; the Shrine of the Blessed Virgin Mary in the Orthodox Christ of the Hills Monastery in Blanco, Texas; the Church of Our Lady of San Juan in San Juan, Texas; The Church in Yverdon-Les-Bains in Switzerland; St. Phillippe Du Roule Church in Paris, France; Lourdes, France. *(For more information on each picture see explanation at the end of chapter.*)*

From the fields of anthropology and sociology come texts that describe rituals, customs, beliefs, and practices that surround healing. Shaw (1975, 121) contends that "for as long as man has practiced the art of magic, he has sought to find personal immortality through healing practices." Buxton (1973) describes traditional beliefs and indigenous healing rituals in Mandari and relates the source of these rituals with how man views himself in relation to God and earth. In this culture, the healer experiences a religious calling to become a healer. Healing is linked to beliefs in evil and the removal of evil from the sick person. Naegele (1970, 18) describes healing in our society as a form of "professional practice." He asserts, however, that "healing is not wholly a professional monopoly and that there are several forms of non-professional healing such as the 'specialized alternatives.'" These include Christian Science and the marginally professional activities of varying legitimacy, such as chiropractic, folk medicine, and quackery. He states: "To understand modern society is to understand the tension between traditional patterns and self-conscious rational calculations devoted to the mastery of everyday life."

Literature from the field of psychology abounds with references to healing. Shames and Sterin (1978) describe the use of self-hypnosis to heal, and Progoff (1959), a depth-psychologist, describes *depth* as the "dimension of wholeness in man." He has written extensively on how one's discovery of the inner self can be used for both healing and creation.

Krippner and Villaldo (1976, viii) contend that there is a "basic conflict between healing and technology" and that "the reality of miracles, of healing, of any significant entity that could be called God is not thought to be compatible with the reality of science." They further contend that healings are psychosomatic in origin and useful only in the sense of the placebo effect.

The literature linking religion to healing is bountiful. The primary source is the Bible and prayers. Bishop (1967, 45) discusses miracles and their relationship to healing. He states that the "miracles must be considered in relation to the time and place in which they occur." He further describes faith and its relationship to healing and states that "*something* goes on in the process of faith healing." He also points out that healing "is the exception rather than the rule." Healing through faith generally is not accepted as a matter of plain fact, but it is an event to rejoice over.

Ford (1971, 6) describes healing of the spirit and methods of spiritual healing for spiritual illness. He describes suffering in three dimensions: that of body, mind, and spirit. He fully describes telotherapy—spiritual healing—which is both a means and an invitation. His argument is that full healing takes place only when there is agape love—divine love—and no estrangement from God. Russell (1937, 221) and Cramer (1923, 11) assert that healing is the work of God alone. Russell asserts that "God's will normally expresses itself in health," and Cramer focuses on the unity of man with God and claims that permanent health is truth, that healing is the gift of Jesus, and that it is a spiritual gift.

✿ *Religion and Healing*

Religion plays a vital role in one's perception of health and illness. Just as culture and ethnicity are strong determinants in an individual's interpretation of the environment and the events within the environment, so, too, is religion. In fact, it is often difficult to distinguish between those aspects of a person's belief system arising from a religious background and those that stem from an ethnic and cultural heritage. Some people may share a common ethnicity, yet be of different religions; a group of people can share the same religion, yet have a variety of ethnic and cultural backgrounds. It is never safe to assume that all individuals of a given ethnic group practice or believe in the same religion. The point was embarrassingly driven home when I once asked a Chicano woman if she would like me to call the priest for her while her young son was awaiting a critical operation. The woman became angry with me. I could not understand why until I learned that she was a Methodist and not a Catholic. I had made an assumption, and I was wrong. She later told me that not all Chicanos are Catholic. After many years of hearing people make this assumption, she had learned to react with anger.

Religion strongly affects the way people interpret and respond to the signs and symptoms of illness. Today, just as it did in antiquity, religion also plays a role in the rites surrounding both birth and death. So pervasive is religion that the diets of many people are determined by their religious beliefs. Religion and the piety of a person determine not only the role that faith plays in the process of recovery but also in many instances the response to a given treatment and to the healing process. Each of these threads—religion, ethnicity, and culture—is woven into the fabric of each person's particular response to treatment and healing.

ANCIENT RITUALS

Many of the rituals that we observe at the time of birth and death have their origins in the practices of ancient human beings. Close your eyes for a few moments and picture yourself living thousands and thousands of years ago. There is no electricity, no running water, no bathroom, no plumbing. The nights are dark and cold. The only signs of the passage of time are the changing seasons and the apparent movement of the various planets and stars through the heavens. You are prey to all the elements, as well as to animals and the unknown. How do you survive? What sort of rituals and practices assist you in maintaining your equilibrium within this often hostile environment? It is from this milieu that many of today's practices sprang.

Generally speaking, three critical moments occur in the life of almost every human being: birth, marriage, and death (Morgenstern 1966, 3). One needs to examine the events and rites that were attendant on birth and death in the past and to demonstrate how many of them not only are relevant to our lives today but also are still practiced.

BIRTH RITUALS

In the minds of early human beings, the number of evil spirits far exceeded the number of good spirits, and a great deal of energy and time was devoted to thwarting these spirits. They could be defeated by the use of gifts or rituals, or, when the evil spirits had to be removed from a person's body, with redemptive sacrifices. Once these evil spirits were expelled, they were prevented from returning by various magical ceremonies and rites. When a ceremony and incantation were found to be effective, they were passed on through the generations. It has been suggested and supported by scholars that from this primitive beginning, organized religion came into being. Today, many of the early rites have survived in altered forms, and we continue to practice them.

The power of the evil spirits was believed to endure for a certain length of time. The 3rd, 7th, and 40th days were the crucial days in the early life of the child and new mother. Hence it was on these days, or on the 8th day, that most of the rituals were observed. It was believed that during this period, the newborn and the mother were at the greatest risk from the power of supernatural beings and thus in a taboo state. "The concept underlying taboo is that all things created by or emanating from a supernatural being are his, or are at least in his power" (Morgenstern 1966, 31). The person was freed from this taboo by certain rituals, depending on the practices of a given community. When the various rites were completed and the 40 days were over, both the mother and child were believed to be redeemed from evil. The ceremonies that freed the person had a double character: they were partly magic and partly religious.

I have deliberately chosen to present the early practices of Semitic peoples because their beliefs and practices evolved into the Judaic, Christian, and Islamic religions of today. Because the newborn baby and mother were considered vulnerable to the threats of evil spirits, many rituals were developed to protect them. For example, in some communities, the mother and child were separated from the rest of the community for a certain length of time, usually 40 days. Various people performed precautionary measures, such as rubbing the baby with different oils or garlic, swaddling the baby, and lighting candles. In other communities, the baby and mother were watched closely for a certain length of time, usually 7 days. (During this time span, they were believed to be intensely susceptible to the effects of evil—hence, close guarding was in order.) Orthodox Jews still refer to the 7th night of life as the "watch night" (Morgenstern 1966, 22–30).

The birth of a male child was considered more significant than that of a female, and many rites were practiced in observance of this event. One ritual sacrifice was cutting off a lock of the child's hair and then sprinkling his forehead with sheep's blood. This ritual was performed on the 8th day of life. In other Semitic countries, when a child was named, a sheep was sacrificed and asked to give protection to the infant. Depending on regional or tribal differences, the mother might be given parts of the sheep. It was believed that if this sacrificial ritual was not performed on the 7th or 8th day of life, the child would die (Morgenstern 1966, 87). The sheep's skin was saved, dried, and placed in the child's bed for 3 or 4 years as protection from evil spirits.

Both the practice of cutting a lock of a child's hair and the sacrifice of an animal served as a ceremony of redemption. The child could also be redeemed from the taboo state by giving silver—the weight of which equaled the weight of the hair—to the poor. Although not universally practiced, these rites are still observed in some form in some communities of the Arab world.

Circumcision is closely related to the ceremony of cutting the child's hair and offering it as a sacrifice. Some authorities hold that the practice originated as a rite of puberty: a body mutilation performed to attract the opposite sex. (Circumcision was practiced by many peoples throughout the ancient world. Alex Haley's *Roots* describes it as a part of initiating boys into manhood in Africa.) Other sources attribute circumcision to the concept of the sanctity of the male organ and claim that it was derived from the practice of ancestor worship. The Jews of ancient Israel, as today, practiced circumcision on the 8th day of life. The Moslems of Palestine circumcise their sons on the 7th day in the tradition that Mohammed established. In other Moslem countries, the ritual is performed anywhere from the 10th day to the 7th year of life. Again, this sacrifice redeemed the child from being taboo in his early stages of life. Once the sacrifice was made, the child entered the period of worldly existence. The rite of circumcision was accompanied by festivals of varying durations. Some cultures and kinship groups feasted for as long as a week.

The ceremony of baptism is also rooted in the past. It, too, symbolically expels the evil spirits, removes the taboo, and is redemptive. It is practiced mainly among members of the Christian faith, but the Yezidis and other non-Christian sects also perform the rite. Water was thought to possess magical powers and was used to cleanse the body from both physical and spiritual maladies, which included evil possession and other impurities. Usually, the child was baptized on the 40th day of life. In some communities, however, the child was baptized on the 8th day. The 40th (or 8th) day was chosen because the ancients believed that, given performance of the particular ritual, this day marked the end of the evil spirits' influence (Morganstern, 1966).

Some rituals also involved the new mother. For example, not only was she (along with her infant) removed from her household and community for 40 days, but in many communities she had to practice ritual bathing before she could return to her husband, family, and community. Again, these practices were not universal, and they varied in scope and intensity from people to people. Table 6–1 illustrates examples of birth-related religious rituals.

EXTENSIONS OF BIRTH RITUALS TO TODAY'S PRACTICES

Early human beings, in their quest for survival, strove to appease and prevent the evil spirits from interfering with their lives. Their beliefs seem simple and naive, yet the rituals that began in those years have evolved into those that exist today. Attacks of the evil spirits were warded off with the use of amulets, charms, and the like. People recited prayers and incantations. Because survival

Religion	Practice	Time	Method
Baptist (27 bodies)	Baptism	Older child	Immersion
Church of Christ	Baptism	8 years	Immersion
Church of Jesus Christ of Latter Day Saints (Mormons)	Baptism	8 years or older	Immersion
Eastern Orthodox Churches	Baptism	Infants	Total immersion
Episcopalian	Baptism	Infant	
Friends (Quaker)	No baptism	Named	
Greek Orthodox	Baptism	40 days	Sprinkle or immersion
Islam	Circumcision	7th day	
Jewish	Circumcision	8th day	
Lutheran	Baptism	6–8 weeks	Pouring, sprinkling, immersion
Methodist	Baptism	Childhood	
Pentecostal	Baptism	Age of accountability	
Roman Catholic	Baptism	Infant	Pour water
Russian Orthodox	Baptism	Infant	Immerse three times
Unitarian	Baptism	Infant	

Table 6–1 Birth-Related Religious Rituals

was predicated on people's ability to appease evil spirits, the prescribed rituals were performed with great care and respect. Undoubtedly, this accounts in part for the longevity of many of these practices through the ages. For example, circumcision and baptism still exist, even when the belief that they are being performed to release the child from a state of being taboo may not continue to be held. It is interesting also that adherence to a certain timetable is maintained. For example, as stated, the Jewish religion mandates that the ritual of circumcision be performed on the eighth day of life.

The practice, too, of closely guarding the new mother and baby through the initial hours after birth is certainly not foreign to us. The mother is closely watched for hemorrhage and signs of infection; the infant initially is watched for signs of choking or respiratory distress. This form of observation is very intense. Could factors such as these have been what our ancestors watched for? If early human beings believed that evil spirits caused the frequent complications that surrounded the birth of a baby, it stands to reason that they would seek to control or prevent these complications by adhering to astute observation, isolation, and rituals of redemption.

Table 6–2 lists birth rites from selected nations.

Table 6–2 Cross-Cultural Guide to Birth Rites from Selected Nations

If your client/family is of the following national origin	The rites you may observe before, when, and/or after birth occurs may include
Afghanistan (population 89% Muslim)	Use of traditional birth attendant (dais) Breast feeding nearly universal BCG at birth
Albania (population 70% Muslim, 20% Orthodox, Catholic 10%)	BCG at birth
Algeria (population 99% Muslim)	Father not present at delivery Baby wrapped in swaddling clothes Breast feeding common BCG at birth
Australia (population 76% Christian)	Physician delivers, father usually present Breast feeding BCG at birth
Bahrain (population 100% Muslim)	BCG at birth
Bangladesh (population 83% Muslim, 16% Hindu, 1% other)	Mother prays postpartum, remains indoors up to 40 days Only husband visits Objects placed over door to prevent evil spirits Breast feeding BCG at birth
Belize (population 90% Christian)	50% of children born out of wedlock Christened before visitors allowed, to prevent evil eye Bottle feeding preferred BCG at birth
Brazil 70% Catholic, 30% other	Fathers not present during labor and delivery 40-day rest period for mother Short-term breast feeding BCG at birth
Cambodia Kampuchea (population 95% Buddhist)	Seek prenatal care at 5 to 6 months of pregnancy Do not compliment newborn to prevent evil spirits Breast feeding BCG at birth
Chad (population 44% Muslim)	Female circumcision BCG at birth
China (population 97% Atheist and Eclectic)	Fathers do not come into labor and delivery Newborn considered 1 year at birth Breast feeding

(continued)

Table 6–2 —Continued	
Cuba (population 85% Catholic)	Avoid loud noises and looking at deformed people when pregnant Stay home for 41 days Breast feeding BCG at birth
Egypt (population 94% Muslim)	Sugar water and foods offered after 40 days Newborn swaddled Celebration held on seventh day of life
Ethiopia (population 45% Muslim, 35% Ethiopian Orthodox, and 20% Animist and other)	Pregnancy is a dangerous time because of evil eye Unfulfilled cravings may cause miscarriage Mother confined 14–40 days postpartum Father may not attend labor and delivery
France (population 90% Catholic)	BCG at birth
Germany (population predominantly Christian)	Breast feeding BCG at birth
Greece (population 98% Greek Orthodox)	Amulets may be placed on baby or crib BCG at 5–6 years
Haiti (population 80% Catholic, 10% Protestant, 10% Voodoo)	Avoid exposure to cold air during pregnancy May bury placenta beneath the doorway to the home or burn it Infants named after a 1-month confinement Nutmeg, castor oil, or spider webs may be placed on umbilical stump; bellybands may be used
India (population 83% Hindu, 11% Muslim, 6% other)	Cravings during pregnancy are satisfied—seen as baby's Birth of son may be festively celebrated BCG at birth
Indonesia (population 88% Muslim)	Many children valued Breast feeding BCG at birth
Iran (population 98% Muslim)	May place amulets on baby or in room BCG at birth
Iraq (population 97% Muslim)	Fertility of five children rewarded May place amulets on baby or in room BCG at birth
Ireland (population 94% Catholic)	BCG at birth Baptism at 40 days
Israel (population 83% Jewish)	Orthodox Jews do not allow men into labor and delivery Newborn vulnerable to evil first week of life—amulets used Male circumcision on eighth day of life

Table 6-2 —**Continued**

Italy (population 99% Catholic)	Grandmother may want to give grandson his birth bath Amulets and/or medals may be placed on the baby or in the room
Japan (population 84% Buddhist)	Midwives may be used Mother may stay confined up to 100 days Mother may not shower or wash hair for a week
Jordan (population 95% Muslim)	Mother has a 40-day confinement postpartum Males are circumcised on the seventh day Infant rubbed with salt and oil after birth and swaddled
Korea (South) (population 72% Buddhist and Confucianist, 28% Christian)	Father not present at birth Mother avoids exposure to cold and does not drink cold liquids Breast feeding
Kuwait (population 85% Muslim)	Breast feeding Amulets used to prevent evil eye BCG at 3½ to 4 years
Laos (population 85% Buddhist)	Newborns not complimented to avoid evil spirits Colostrum believed maybe to cause diarrhea BCG at birth
Malaysia (population 58% Muslim, 30% Buddhist, 8% Hindu)	Many birth taboos Amulets used Breast feeding BCG at birth
Mali	BCG at birth
Mexico (population 97% Catholic)	Avoid cold air Be active to have a small, easy-to-deliver baby Coin may be strapped to navel to keep it attractive
Morocco (population 99% Muslim)	BCG at birth
Netherlands	Home births common
Nigeria (population 50% Muslim)	Traditional birth attendants are frequently used BCG at birth
Norway (population 94% Lutheran)	Kangaroo care Father may attend delivery Breast feeding
Pakistan (population 97% Muslim)	Traditional birth attendants BCG at birth

(continued)

Table 6–2	—Continued
Philippines (population 83% Catholic, 9% Protestant, 5% Muslim)	Symbolic unlocking ritual performed during labor Showers and bathing prohibited for 10 days postpartum New mother dresses in warm clothing BCG at birth
Portugal (population 97% Catholic)	Midwives Mother may consume chicken soup or melted butter after delivery to help uterus return to normal
Russia	Breast feeding May use amulets
Sweden (population 94% Lutheran)	Low infant mortality rate Breast feeding
Thailand (population 95% Buddhist)	Mother keeps warm to increase milk supply BCG at birth
Tunisia (population 98% Muslim)	Use of henna to decorate body before going into labor BCG at birth
Vietnam (population 60% Buddhist, 13% Confucianist, 12% Taoist, 3% Catholic, 12% other)	Some type of blossom may be used during labor to symbolically open the cervix Mother drinks only warm liquids during labor Child 1 year old at birth BCG at birth

Adapted from: Geissler, E. M. *Pocket Guide: Cultural Assessment,* 2d ed. (St. Louis: Mosby, 1998). Used with permission.

DEATH RITUALS

It was believed that the work of evil spirits and the duration of their evil—whether it was 7 or 40 days—surrounded the person, family, and community at the time of and after death. Rites evolved to protect both the dying and dead person and the remaining family from these evil spirits. The dying person was cared for in specific ways (ritual washing), and the grave was prepared in set ways (storing food and water for the journey after death). Further rituals were performed to protect the deceased's survivors from the harm believed to be rendered by the deceased's ghost. It was believed that this ghost could return from the grave and, if not carefully appeased, gravely harm surviving relatives (Morgenstern 1966, 117–60).

Countless ethnocultural and religious differences can be found in the ways we observe dying, death, and mourning. Table 6–3 displays a sampling of the ways death is talked about at various locations in the United States. The expressions for death have been collected over several years of randomly reading the local newspapers' death notices. It is interesting to observe the regional differences in expressions and that in some locations deaths are merely listed by the person's name and in other locations the event of death

Table 6-3 Ways of Expressing Death: Death Expressions from Selected Locations: Bangor, Maine; Boston, Massachusetts; Dallas, Houston, and San Antonio, Texas; Des Moines, Iowa; Elk Horn, Iowa; Los Angeles, California; and New York City

Expression	Location	Religion[a]
"Nothing"	New York, Dallas, Boston, Los Angeles	Catholic, Episcopalian
Passed Away	New York, Dallas, Boston, San Antonio, Bangor, Houston, Elk Horn, Los Angeles	Catholic, Jewish, Baptist, Church of Christ
Died	New York, Dallas, Boston, San Antonio, Bangor, Houston, Des Moines	Baptist, Catholic, Congregational, Christian
Died peacefully	Houston, Bangor, Los Angeles	Catholic, Episcopalian, Jewish
Suddenly	New York	
Passed away peacefully	Houston, Los Angeles	
Entered into the arms of his Lord	San Antonio	Catholic
Departed this life	Dallas	
Went to be with her heavenly father	Houston	
Went to be with her (or his or our) Lord	San Antonio	Catholic
Went home to be with God	Houston	
Sunrise. . .sunset. . .	Houston	Methodist
Departed this life	Houston	Baptist
Passed from this life	Houston	
Deceased	Dallas	Baptist
Expired	Houston	
Unexpectedly	Boston, Bangor	
With his Lord	Houston	
Entered into rest	Boston, San Antonio	Jewish, Catholic

[a]Most death notices do not list the religion of the deceased, and it is difficult to tell unless the funeral is held in a church or synagogue.

evokes comments such as "sun rise. . . . sun set" and "departed this life." Table 6–4 is a guide to death rites from selected nations. Table 6–5 lists beliefs that people from different religious backgrounds may have regarding death. Finally, Table 6–6 lists selected cultural traditions in after-death rituals and mourning.

Expressions of death and death rituals are also found in objects. Figure 6–2, designed as a panel for the HEALTH traditions quilt, depicts several objects that may be used.

| Table 6–4 | Cross-Cultural Guide to Death Rites from Selected Nations |

If your client/family is of the following national origin	The rites you may observe when death occurs may include
Afghanistan (population 89% Muslim)	Muslim rites: Body generally remains at home—cared for, washed, wrapped in white cloth Mullah often in attendance Friends and family visit Buried in 24 hours Ceremony held 2 days after burial and is followed by a meal
Albania (population 70% Muslim, 20% Orthodox, and 10% Catholic)	Muslim rites
Algeria (population 99% Muslim)	Muslim rites
Australia (population 76% Christian)	Cremation and burial are both practiced Grieving may be reserved—crying with no wailing
Bahrain (population 100% Muslim)	Muslim rites
Bangladesh (population 83% Muslim, 16% Hindu, 1% other)	Muslim rites
Belize (population 90% Christian)	Demonstrative in grief May have spectacular funerals
Burma (population 85% Buddhist)	May prefer quality rather than quantity of life Dying may be helped to recall past good deeds Cremation may be preferred
Cambodia Kampuchea (population 95% Buddhist)	Buddhist beliefs as above White clothing worn during 3-month mourning period Some mourners may shave their heads
Chad (population 44% Muslim)	Muslim rites
China (population 97% Atheist and Eclectic)	Initial burial in a coffin; after 7 years, body is exhumed, cremated, and the urn is reburied in a tomb
Cuba (population 85% Catholic)	Family and friends stay with body through night Burial in 24 hours May have holy hour each night for 9 consecutive days
Egypt (population 94% Muslim)	Muslim rites

Table 6-4	—Continued	

Ethiopia (population 45% Muslim, 35% Ethiopian Orthodox, 20% Animist and other)	Muslim rites Loud wailing may be a normal grief reaction
France (population 90% Catholic)	Chrysanthemums are used exclusively for funerals
Germany (population predominantly Christian)	Crying in private is expected Cremation may be selected
Greece (population 98% Greek Orthodox)	May isolate dying person and withhold truth Death at home important Person buried; exhumed in 5 years and bones reburied in urn or vault Widow wears dark mourning clothes for rest of life
Haiti (population 80% Catholic, 10% Protestant, 10% Voodoo)	Burial in 24 hours White clothing represents death
India (population 83% Hindu, 11% Muslim, 6% other)	Non-Hindus ought not touch body; wash body themselves Cremation is preferred Reincarnation is a Hindu belief
Indonesia (population 88% Muslim)	Muslim rites
Iran (population 98% Muslim)	Muslim rites Mourning may be loud, obvious, and expressive
Iraq (population 97% Muslim)	Muslim rites
Ireland (population 94% Catholic)	Practice of watching or "waking" the dead originates from keeping vigil to keep evil spirits away from the deceased—now a religious ritual
Israel (population 83% Jewish)	Relatives remain with dying person Eyes must be closed at death Body is never left alone Buried in ground in 24 hours except if Sabbath (Saturday)
Italy (population 99% Catholic)	Before death fatal diagnosis is not discussed with patient and family Chrysanthemums used for funeral
Japan (population 84% Buddhist)	Control public expressions of grief
Jordan (population 95% Muslim)	Muslim rites
Korea (North) (population 95% Atheist)	Confucian funeral—elaborate Chief mourner and relatives weep

(continued)

Table 6–4	—Continued
Korea (South) (population 72% Buddhist and Confucianist, 28% Christian)	Buddhist accept death as birth into another life Family members observe last breath; may respond with loud wailing and display intense emotion
Kuwait (population 85% Muslim)	Muslim rites
Laos (population 85% Buddhist)	Beliefs in reincarnation White flowers or candles may be placed in the deceased's hands Cremation and burial are practiced
Lebanon (population 75% Muslim)	Muslim rites
Libya	Muslim rites
Malaysia (population 58% Muslim, 30% Buddhist, 8% Hindu)	Muslim rites
Mali	Muslim rites
Mexico (population 97% Catholic)	Family members stay with dying person around the clock Grief may be expressive "Day of the Dead" celebrated in November
Morocco (population 99% Muslim)	Muslim rites
Netherlands	Active euthanasia permitted under certain circumstances
Nigeria (population 50% Muslim)	Muslim rites
Norway (population 94% Lutheran)	Close family members stay with person; no one should die alone Cremation and/or burial
Oman	Muslim rites
Pakistan (population 97% Muslim)	Muslim rites
Philippines (population 83% Catholic, 9% Protestant, 5% Muslim)	Muslim rites Protect person from knowing prognosis Emotional grief may occur after death
Portugal (population 97% Catholic)	Widow wears black and never remarries Visit grave frequently
Russia	Family is told of serious illness and decides if patient should know
Sweden (population 94% Lutheran)	Quiet and open grief acceptable Dying person not left alone Body usually not viewed after death

Table 6–4	—Continued
Thailand (population 95% Buddhist)	Beliefs in reincarnation
Tunisia (Population 98% Muslim)	Muslim rites
Vietnam (population 60% Buddhist, 13% Confucianist, 12% Taoist, 3% Catholic, 12% other)	Death at home preferred Body washed and wrapped in white sheets Burial in ground

Adapted from: Geissler, E. M. *Pocket Guide: Cultural Assessment* (St. Louis: Mosby, 1994), and Lipson, J. G., Dibble, S. L., and Minarik, P. A. *Culture and Nursing Care: A Pocket Guide* (San Francisco: UCSF Nursing Press, 1996). Used with permission.

| Table 6–5 | Religious Groups and Death Beliefs |

Religious Group	Is There a Heaven?	What Is It Like?	Belief In Resurrection?	Recognition of Friends and Relatives	Is Cremation Allowed?
Assemblies of God	Heaven is a real place	A pleasant place	Of the body	Yes	Not encouraged
Baha'is	Heaven designates spiritual proximity to God	An eternal spiritual evolution of the soul	Spiritual	Yes	No
Baptists	A place where the redeemed go	Depicted as being filled with mansions and golden streets	Physical	Yes	Allowed but not encouraged
Buddhists	Numerous heavens	It has no independent existence	No future time is foreseen	See living friends and relatives but are not seen	Preferred
Churches of Christ	Dwelling place of God and future residence of the righteous	A realm of peace and love	Consciousness leaves body at death and takes rebirth until enlightened	Yes	Permitted

(continued)

__Table 6–5__ —Continued

Religious Group	Is There a Heaven?	What Is It Like?	Belief In Resurrection?	Recognition of Friends and Relatives	Cremation Allowed?
Hindus	A relative plane of existence to which souls go to after death	Dwellers in heaven enjoy long life and are free from thirst, hunger and old age	Liberation of the soul	Visions	Most common method for disposing of body
Jews	Place where anxiety and travail are ended	Quiet, peaceful intellectual activity takes place here	Yes; some only in soul	Yes	Not practiced
Lutherans	Believe in heaven	Nature unknown	Physical	Yes	Yes
Mormons	There are three "degrees of glory"	Places of continuing growth and progress	Yes	Yes	Yes, but not encouraged
Muslims	Several layers, usually seven	A garden	Describe afterlife as physical pains and pleasures	Some believe families are reunited	Not practiced
Roman Catholics	A condition: eternal fullness of life	Supreme happiness flowing from intimacy with God	Physical	Entire community together	Disposal of body does not affect afterlife
Seventh Day Adventism	A being in the presence of God	Will be located in the renewed earth	Glorified body will be resurrected for life to come	Yes	No objection
United Methodism	Heaven exists	Being in the presence of God	Body and spirit	Yes	Yes

Adapted from: Johnson, C. J., and McGee, M. G., eds. *How Different Religions View Death and Afterlife.* (Philadelphia: The Charles Press, 1991).

Table 6–6	Cultural Traditions in Mourning and After-Death Rituals
If your client/family is of the following religion	**The rituals you may observe when death occurs may include**
American Indian religions	Beliefs and practices vary widely Seeing an owl is omen of death
Buddhism	Believe in impermanence Last-rite chanting at bedside Cremation common Pregnant women should avoid funerals to prevent bad luck for baby
Catholicism	Obligated to take ordinary, not extraordinary, means to prolong life Sacrament of the sick Autopsy, organ donation acceptable Burial usual
Christian Science	Euthanasia contrary to teachings Do not seek medical help to prolong life Do not donate body parts Disposal of body and parts decided by family
Hinduism	Seen as opposite of birth—a passage—expect rebirth Autopsy, organ donation—acceptable Religious prayers chanted before and after death Men and women display outward grief Cremation common; ashes disposed in holy rivers Thread is tied around wrist to signify a blessing; do not remove
Islam	Euthanasia prohibited Organ donation acceptable Autopsy only for medical or legal reasons Body is washed only by Muslim of same gender
Jehovah's Witness	Euthanasia forbidden Autopsy acceptable if legally necessary Donations of body parts forbidden Burial determined by family preference
Judaism	Autopsy, organ donation not acceptable Euthanasia prohibited Life support not mandated Body ritually washed Burial as soon as possible Seven-day mourning period
Mormonism	Euthanasia not practiced Promote peaceful and dignified death Organ donation individual choice Burial in "temple clothes"

(continued)

Table 6–6 —Continued	
If your client/family is of the following religion	**The rituals you may observe when death occurs may include**
Protestantism	Organ donation, autopsy, and burial or cremation usually individual decisions Prolonging life may have restrictions Euthanasia—varies
Seventh Day Adventism	Prefer prolonging life Euthanasia—no Autopsy, organ donation acceptable Disposal of body and burial—individual decisions

Adapted from: Lipson, J. G., Dibble, S. L., and Minarik, P. A. *Culture and Nursing Care: A Pocket Guide.* (San Francisco: UCSF Nursing Press, 1996). Used with permission.

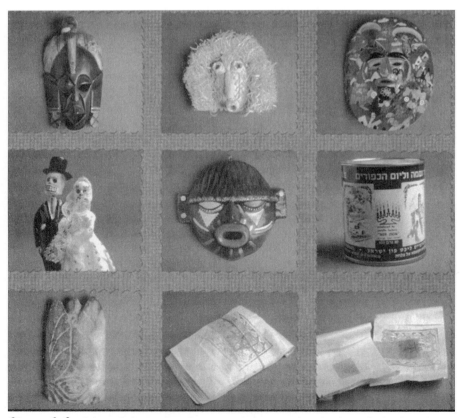

Figure 6–2 Selected objects found in situations surrounding death: masks, bride and groom skeletons, candle, jade stone, ghost money.

- *Masks* represent methods people may use to hide from the "Angel of Death." Masks may also be placed on the face of the deceased. These masks are from Africa, North American Indians, Mexico, and Columbia.
- A *bride and groom skeleton* convey the message that marriage is forever, even unto death. The souls of the bride and groom are united for eternity. Statues such as this one are frequently displayed during the celebration of *Dia de las Muertos*, the Mexican Day of the Dead, on November 2.
- *Candles* are used by many people after death as a way of lighting the way for the soul of the deceased.
- *Jade stone,* from China, is placed in orifices of the body to block the entrance of the evil spirits after death.
- *Ghost money,* from China, is burned to send payments to a deceased person and to ensure their well-being in the afterlife.

❋ *Beliefs That Can Affect Therapy*

ANCIENT FORMS OF HEALING

The crises of birth and death were certainly not the only ones to affect our ancestors. Illness also caused crises. Just as the people of ancient times developed ways of dealing with the events that surrounded birth and death, they evolved elaborate systems of healing. The cause of an illness, once again, was attributed to the forces of evil, which originated either within or outside the body. Early forms of healing dealt with the removal of evil. Once a method of treatment was found effective, it was passed down through the generations in slightly altered forms.

The people who healed often were those who received the gift of healing from a "divine" source. They frequently received this gift in a vision and were unable to explain to others how they knew what to do. Other healers learned their skills from their parents. Most of the healers with acquired skills were women, who subsequently passed their knowledge on to their daughters. People who used herbs and other preparations to remove the evil from the sick person's body were known as herbalists. Other healers included bone setters and midwives, and although early humankind did not separate ills of the body from those of the mind, some healers were more adept at solving problems by using early forms of "psychotherapy."

If the source of sickness-causing evil was within the body, treatment involved drawing the evil out of the body. This may have been accomplished through the use of purgatives that caused either vomiting or diarrhea, or by blood-letting: "bleeding" the patient or "sucking out" blood. (The barbers of medieval Europe did not originate this practice; bleeding was done in ancient times.) Leeching was another method used to remove corrupt humors from the body, and the reader may recall that in Chapter 2 leeching was mentioned by a student whose grandmother had treated illness by that method.

If the source of the evil was outside the body, there were a number of ways to deal with it. One source of "external" evil was witchcraft. In a community, there were often many people (or a single person) who were "different" from the other people. Quite often, when an unexplainable or untreatable illness occurred, it was these people (or person) who were seen as the causative agents. In such a belief system, successful treatment depended on the identification and punishment of the person believed responsible for the disease. (Certainly, the practice of scapegoating is in part derived from this belief.) By removing or punishing the guilty person from the community, the disease would be cured. In some communities, the healers themselves were seen as witches and the possessors of evil skills. How easy it was for ancient humankind to turn things around and blame the person with the skills to treat the disease for causing the disease!

Various rituals were involved in the treatment of ill people. Often, the sick person was isolated from the rest of the family and community. In addition, it was customary to chant special prayers and incantations on the invalid's behalf. Sacrifices and dances often were performed in an effort to cure the ills. Often the rituals of the healer involved reciting incantations in a language foreign to the ears of the general population ("speaking in tongues") and using practices that were strange to the observers. Small wonder, then, as superstition abounded, that at times the healers themselves were ostracized by the population.

Another cause of illness was believed to be the *envy* of people within the community. The best method, consequently, of preventing such an illness was to avoid provoking the envy of one's friends and neighbors. The treatment was to do away with whatever was provoking the envy—even though the act might have prevented a person from accomplishing a "mission in life," and the fear of being "responsible" might have been psychologically damaging.

Today we tend to view the healing methods of ancient people as primitive, yet to fully appreciate their efficacy, we need only make the simple observation that these methods in many forms exist today and have aided the survival of humankind!

RELIGIOUS BELIEFS AND HEALING

There are far too many religious beliefs and practices related to healing to include in this chapter. A discussion of religious healing beliefs from the Judeo-Christian background, however, is possible.

The Old Testament does not focus on healing to the extent the New Testament does. God is seen to have total power over life and death and is the healer of all human woes. God is the giver of all good things and of all misfortune, including sickness. Sickness represented a break between God and humans. In Exodus 15:26 God is proclaimed the supreme healer ("I will put none of the diseases upon you which I put upon the Egyptians; for I am the Lord, your healer.") and in another passage from Deuteronomy 32:39 it is stated "I kill, and I make alive. I have wounded and I heal." The traditionalist Jew believes that the "healing of illness comes from God through the mediation of His 'messenger,' the doctor." The Jew who is ill combines hope for a cure with faith in God and faith in the doctor (Ausubel 1964, 192–195).

The healing practices of the Roman Catholic tradition include a variety of beliefs and numerous practices, both of a preventive and healing nature. For example, Saint Blaise, an Armenian bishop who died in A.D. 316 as a martyr, is revered as the preventer of sore throats. The blessing of the throats on his feast day (February 3) derives from the tradition that he miraculously saved the life of a boy by removing a fishbone that he had swallowed (*Monthly Missalette* 1980, 38).

The saints concerned with other aspects of illness include the following (Foy 1980, 305–313 and Hallam 1994):

Saint	Problem
St. Anthony of Padua	Barrenness
St. Odilia	Blindness
Our Lady of Lourdes	Bodily ills
St. Peregrine	Cancer
St. Francis de Sales	Deafness
St. Joseph	Dying
St. Vitus	Epilepsy
St. Raymond Nonnatus	Pregnancy
St. Lucy	Eye disease
St. Teresa of Avila	Headache
St. John of God	Heart disease
St. Roch	Being bedridden
St. Dymphna	Mental illness
St. Bruno	Possession

Many more saints could be included. I refer you to other sources for information, and I also recommend that you ask patients for information.

In the United States people make pilgrimages to a number of shrines in search of special favors and petitions.

The oldest is the Shrine of Our Lady of La Leche, located in St. Augustine, Florida (Fig. 6–3). This shrine was founded in 1620 by Spanish settlers as a sign of their love for the Mother of Christ. The shrine is visited by thousands of mothers to ask for the blessings of motherhood, a safe and happy delivery, a healthy baby, and holy children. Countless letters can be read at the shrine attesting to the powers of Our Lady of La Leche (Informational brochure).

Another shrine is that of Our Lady of San Juan (Fig. 6–3) located in San Juan, Texas. This shrine houses a statue of the Virgin that was brought to Mexico by the Spanish missionaries in 1623. The statue was responsible for causing a miracle, and devotion to *La Virgin de San Juan* spread. The statue was brought to Texas in the 1940s after a woman claimed to have seen an image of the Virgin in the countryside around San Juan. The statue is presently housed in a beautiful new church, and pilgrims arrive daily to ask for healing and other favors. Again, countless letters are displayed attesting to the healing powers of this statue (Informational brochure).

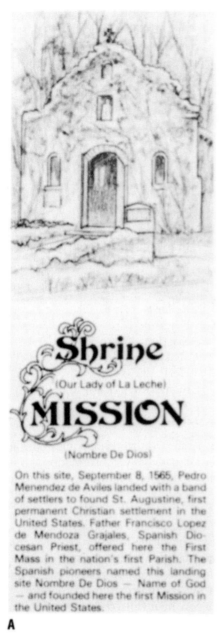

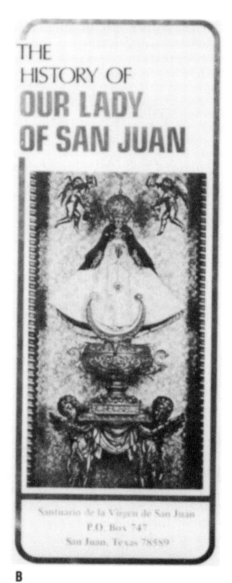

Figure 6–3 A. Our Lady of La Leche Shrine and Mission. B. Our Lady of San Juan Shrine. (From the author's collection.)

A third shrine is that of St. Peregrine for Cancer Sufferers (Fig. 6–4), located in the Old Mission San Juan Capistrano in California. This statue is housed in a small grotto in the shrine. St. Peregrine was born in Italy in 1265

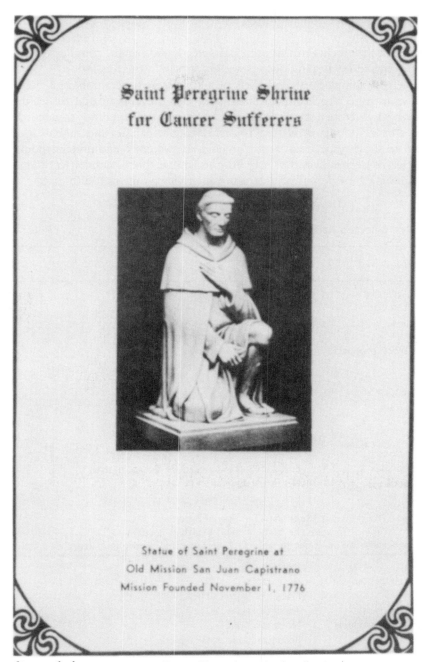

Figure 6–4 Saint Peregrine Shrine. (From the author's collection.)

and died in 1345. He was believed to have miraculous powers against sickness and could cure cancer. This won for him the title "official patron for cancer victims." Once a woman was afflicted with cancer and a lady gave her a prayer to St. Peregrine. The woman prayed for 6 months, and her cancer was arrested. In gratitude for this, the woman had a statue of the saint placed in the mission. Today, the belief in this saint has spread, and, again, countless documents attesting to his healing powers are on display in the mission.

Table 6–7 summarizes the beliefs of people from several religious backgrounds with respect to health, healing, and several events related to health-care delivery. Remember, this is a *summary*, and you are urged not to generalize from this guide when relating to an individual patient and family. It is important to show respect and sensitivity and an awareness and understanding of the different perspectives that may exist and to be able to convey to the patient and family your desire to understand their viewpoint on health care.

Table 6–7 | **Selected Religions' Responses to Health Events**

Baha'i "All healing comes from God."	
Abortion	Forbidden
Artificial insemination	No specific rule
Autopsy	Acceptable with medical or legal need
Birth control	Can choose family planning method
Blood and blood products	No restrictions for use
Diet	Alcohol and drugs forbidden
Euthanasia	No destruction of life
Healing beliefs	Harmony between religion and science
Healing practices	Pray
Medications	Narcotics with prescription
	No restriction for vaccines
Organ donations	Permitted
Right-to-die issues	Life is unique and precious—do not destroy
Surgical procedures	No restrictions
Visitors	Community members assist and support

Buddhist Churches of America "To keep the body in good health is a duty— otherwise we shall not be able to keep our mind strong and clear."	
Abortion	Patient's condition determines
Artificial insemination	Acceptable
Autopsy	Matter of individual practice
Birth control	Acceptable
Blood and blood products	No restrictions
Diet	Restricted food combinations
	Extremes must be avoided
Euthanasia	May permit
Healing beliefs	Do not believe in healing through faith
Healing practices	No restrictions
Medications	No restrictions
Organ donations	Considered act of mercy; if hope for recovery, all means may be taken
Right-to-die issues	With hope, all means encouraged

| *Table 6–7* | —Continued |

Buddhist Churches of America—Continued
"To keep the body in good health is a duty—
otherwise we shall not be able to keep our mind strong and clear."

Surgical procedures	Permitted, with extremes avoided
Visitors	Family, community

Roman Catholics
"The prayer of faith shall heal the sick, and the Lord shall raise him up."

Abortion	Prohibited
Artificial insemination	Illicit, even between husband and wife
Autopsy	Permissible
Birth control	Natural means only
Blood and blood products	Permissible
Diet	Use foods in moderation
Euthanasia	Direct life-ending procedures forbidden
Healing beliefs	Many within religious belief system
Healing practices	Sacrament of sick, candles, laying-on of hands
Medications	May be taken if benefits outweigh risks
Organ donations	Justifiable
Right-to-die issues	Obligated to take ordinary, not extraordinary, means to prolong life
Surgical procedures	Most are permissible except abortion and sterilization
Visitors	Family, friends, priest
	Many outreach programs through Church to reach sick

Christian Science

Abortion	Incompatible with faith
Artificial insemination	Unusual
Autopsy	Not usual; individual or family decide
Birth control	Individual judgment
Blood and blood products	Ordinarily not used by members
Diet	No restrictions
	Abstain from alcohol and tobacco, some from tea and coffee
Euthanasia	Contrary to teachings
Healing beliefs	Accepts physical and moral healing
Healing practices	Full-time healing ministers
	Spiritual healing practiced
Medications	None
	Immunizations/vaccines to comply with law
Organ donations	Individual decides
Right-to-die issues	Unlikely to seek medical help to prolong life
Surgical procedures	No medical ones practiced
Visitors	Family, friends, and members of the Christian Science community and Healers, Christian Science nurses

Church of Jesus Christ of Latter Day Saints

Abortion	Forbidden

(continued)

Table 6-7 —Continued

Church of Jesus Christ of Latter Day Saints—Continued

Artificial insemination	Acceptable between husband and wife
Autopsy	Permitted with consent of next of kin
Birth control	Contrary to Mormon belief
Blood and blood products	No restrictions
Diet	Alcohol, tea (except herbal teas), coffee, and tobacco are forbidden
	Fasting (24 hours without food and drink) is required once a month
Euthanasia	Humans must not interfere in God's plan
Healing beliefs	Power of God can bring healing
Healing practices	Anointing with oil, sealing, prayer, laying-on of hands
Medications	No restrictions; may use herbal folk remedies
Organ donations	Permitted
Right-to-die issues	If death inevitable, promote a peaceful and dignified death
Surgical procedures	Matter of individual choice
Visitors	Church members (Elder and Sister) family and friends
	The Relief Society helps members

Hinduism
"Enricher, Healer of disease, be a good friend to us."

Abortion	No policy exists
Artificial insemination	No restrictions exist but not often practiced
Autopsy	Acceptable
Birth control	All types acceptable
Blood and blood products	Acceptable
Diet	Eating of meat is forbidden
Euthanasia	Not practiced
Healing beliefs	Some believe in faith healing
Healing practices	Traditional faith healing system
Medications	Acceptable
Organ donations	Acceptable
Right-to-die issues	No restrictions
	Death seen as "one more step to nirvana"
Surgical procedures	With an amputation, the loss of limb seen as due to "sins in a previous life"
Visitors	Members of family, community, and priest support

Islam
"The Lord of the world created me—and when I am sick, He healeth me."

Abortion	Accepted
Artificial insemination	Permitted between husband and wife
Autopsy	Permitted for medical and legal purposes
Birth control	Acceptable
Blood and blood products	No restrictions

Table 6-7 —Continued

Islam—Continued
"The Lord of the world created me—and when I am sick, He healeth me."

Diet	Pork and alcohol prohibited
Euthanasia	Not acceptable
Healing beliefs	Faith healing generally not acceptable
Healing practices	Some use of herbal remedies and faith healing
Medications	No restrictions
Organ donations	Acceptable
Right-to-die issues	Attempts to shorten life prohibited
Surgical procedures	Most permitted
Visitors	Family and friends provide support

Jehovah's Witnesses

Abortion	Forbidden
Artificial insemination	Forbidden
Autopsy	Acceptable if required by law
Birth control	Sterilization forbidden
	Other methods individual choice
Blood and blood products	Forbidden
Diet	Abstain from tobacco, moderate use of alcohol
Euthanasia	Forbidden
Healing beliefs	Faith healing forbidden
Healing practices	Reading scriptures can comfort the individual and lead to mental and spiritual healing
Medications	Accepted except if derived from blood products
Organ donations	Forbidden
Right-to-die issues	Use of extraordinary means an individual's choice
Surgical procedures	Not opposed, but administration of blood during surgery is strictly prohibited
Visitors	Members of congregation and elders pray for the sick person

Judaism
"O Lord, my God, I cried to Thee for help and Thou has healed me."

Abortion	Therapeutic permitted; some groups accept abortion on demand
Artificial insemination	Permitted
Autopsy	Permitted under certain circumstances
	All body parts must be buried together
Birth control	Permissible, except with orthodox Jews
Blood and blood products	Acceptable
Diet	Strict dietary laws followed by many Jews—milk and meat not mixed; predatory fowl, shellfish, and pork products forbidden; kosher products only may be requested
Euthanasia	Prohibited
Healing beliefs	Medical care expected
Healing practices	Prayers for the sick
Medications	No restrictions

(continued)

| Table 6-7 | —Continued |

Judaism—Continued
"O Lord, my God, I cried to Thee for help and Thou has healed me."

Organ donations	Complex issue; some practiced
Right-to-die issues	Right to die with dignity
	If death is inevitable, no new procedures need to be undertaken, but those ongoing must continue
Surgical procedures	Most allowed
Visitors	Family, friends, rabbi, many community services

Mennonite

Abortion	Therapeutic acceptable
Artificial insemination	Individual conscience; husband to wife
Autopsy	Acceptable
Birth control	Acceptable
Blood and blood products	Acceptable
Diet	No specific restrictions
Euthanasia	Not condoned
Healing beliefs	Part of God's work
Healing practices	Prayer and anointing with oil
Medications	No restrictions
Organ donations	Acceptable
Right-to-die issues	Do not believe life must be continued at all cost
Surgical procedures	No restrictions
Visitors	Family, community

Seventh-Day Adventists

Abortion	Therapeutic acceptable
Artificial insemination	Acceptable between husband and wife
Autopsy	Acceptable
Birth control	Individual choice
Blood and blood products	No restrictions
Diet	Encourage vegetarian diet
Euthanasia	Not practiced
Healing beliefs	Divine healing
Healing practices	Anointing with oil and prayer
Medications	No restrictions
	Vaccines acceptable
Organ donations	Acceptable
Right-to-die issues	Follow the ethic of prolonging life
Surgical procedures	No restrictions
	Oppose use of hypnotism
Visitors	Pastor and elders pray and anoint sick person
	Worldwide health system includes hospitals and clinics

Unitarian/Universalist Church

Abortion	Acceptable, therapeutic and on demand
Artificial insemination	Acceptable

| Table 6–7 | —Continued |

Unitarian/Universalist Church—Continued	
Autopsy	Recommended
Birth control	All types acceptable
Blood and blood products	No restrictions
Diet	No restrictions
Euthanasia	Favor nonaction
	May withdraw therapies if death imminent
Healing beliefs	Faith healing: seen as "superstitious"
Healing practices	Use of science to facilitate healing
Medications	No restrictions
Organ donations	Acceptable
Right-to-die issues	Favor the right to die with dignity
Surgical procedures	No restrictions
Visitors	Family, friends, church members

Adapted with permission from: Andrews, M. M., and Hanson, P. A. "Religion, Culture, and Nursing" in *Transcultural Concepts in Nursing Care,* 2d ed., ed. J. S. Boyle and M. M. Andrews. (Philadelphia: J. B. Lippincott, 1995), pp. 371–406. Used with permission.

HEALING AND TODAY'S BELIEFS

It is not an accident or coincidence that today, more so than in recent years, we are not only curious but vitally concerned about the ways of healing that our ancestors employed. Some critics of today's health-care system choose to condemn it, with more vociferous critics, such as Illich (1975), citing its failure to create a utopia for humankind. It is obvious to those who embrace a more moderate viewpoint that diseases continue to occur and that they outflank our ability to cure or prevent them. Once again, many people are seeking the services of people who are knowledgeable in the arts of healing and folk medicine. Many patients may elect, at some point in their lives, more specifically during an illness, to use modalities outside the medical establishment. It is important to understand these healers.

There are numerous healers in the general population, some of whom are legitimate and some of whom are not. They range from housewives and priests to gypsies and "witches." Many people seek their services. I have had occasion to meet with several of these folk healers. Without attempting to make a value judgment, I merely report on their skills and methods (Table 6–8).

One healer has an office in a community near where I live. He charges a nominal fee for consultation with either groups or individuals and then gives advice on how to solve a problem. He does not see physically ill people but prefers to help people who have moderate emotional and practical problems. His primary objective is to help people solve these problems. This man tends to be quite popular with young adults in the area, as he lends a "willing ear" and is "not too expensive." He does not keep his clients waiting long, and often the brief wait proves to be interesting because the waiting room is always the scene of an open discussion about his talents.

| *Table 6–8* | Comparisons: Traditional Homeopathic Healer versus Modern Allopathic Physician |

Healer	Physician
1. Maintains informal, friendly, affective relationship with the entire family	1. Businesslike, formal relationship; deals only with the patient
2. Comes to the house day or night	2. Patient must go to the physician's office or clinic, and only during the day; may have to wait for hours to be seen; home visits are rarely, if ever, made
3. For diagnosis, consults with head of house, creates a mood of awe, talks to all family members, is not authoritarian, has social rapport, builds expectation of cure	3. Rest of family usually is ignored; deals solely with the ill person and may deal only with the sick part of the person; authoritarian manner creates fear
4. Generally less expensive than the physician	4. More expensive than the healer
5. Has ties to the "world of the sacred"; has rapport with the symbolic, spiritual, creative, or holy force	5. Secular; pays little attention to the religious beliefs or meaning of a given illness
6. Shares the world view of the patient, i.e., speaks the same language, lives in the same neighborhood, or in some similar socioeconomic conditions, may know the same people, understands the lifestyle of the patient	6. Generally does not share the world view of the patient, i.e., may not speak the same language, live in the same neighborhood, or understand the socioeconomic conditions; may not understand the lifestyle of the patient

Another healer I knew was a young college student. He believed that he possessed certain spirits and skills that enabled him to heal. He had visions that interpreted for him the problems and ills of his clients. This young man maintained a special altar in his room, where he prayed to the "spirits." At that time, he did not charge for his services because he had just received the "message," and the art of healing was new to him. He admitted that he had formerly been a drug addict but was now enrolled in college and hoped to use his education and healing skills to make life better for the people of the streets.

The third healer I am personally acquainted with is a Catholic priest; he is extremely reluctant to call himself a "healer." He does claim, however, to have witnessed and participated in numerous healings. He conducts prayer meetings in his parish. He comes to my classes and lectures to the students on healing and the charismatic movement within the Catholic Church (MacNutt, 1974 and Kelsey, 1973). He defines healing as the "satisfactory response to crises by a group of people, individually or corporately." "Healing," as he explains it, "is applied in a broad, holistic approach; that is, body, mind, and spirit are not separated." His vision of reality is that of a person being full of the spirit of God. According to this priest, the healer has the ability to *heal* but not really to *cure*. He further explains that there are "three types of illness:

spiritual, physical, and mental." In this context, faith is the underlying basis of healing, although he questions whether faith is the only component. Healing becomes a living process whereby that which is wounded or broken becomes whole.

A review of healing and spiritual literature reveals that there are four types of healing.

Spiritual Healing. When a person is experiencing an illness of the spirit, spiritual healing applies. The cause of suffering is personal sin. The treatment method is repentance, which is followed by a natural healing process.

Inner Healing. When a person is suffering from an emotional (mental) illness, inner healing is used. The root of the problem may lie in the person's conscious or unconscious mind. The treatment method is to heal the person's memory. The healing process is delicate and sensitive, and takes considerable time and effort.

Physical Healing. When a person is suffering from a disease or has been involved in an accident that resulted in some form of bodily damage, physical healing is appropriate. Laying on of hands and speaking in tongues usually accompany physical healing. The person is prayed over by both the leader and members of a prayer group (Fig. 6–5).

The priest referred to previously related an incident in which one of the members of the group was experiencing difficulty with ulcers and was not responding to conventional medical treatment. The man, who initially was embarrassed by the idea, allowed the prayer group and the priest to pray over him. In a short time, to his surprise, he recovered from his ulcers.

Deliverance, or Exorcism. When the body and mind are victims of evil from the outside, exorcism is used. In order to effect treatment, the person must be delivered, or exorcised, from the evil. The popularity of films such as *The Exorcist* gives testimony to the return of these beliefs. Incidentally, the priest who has lectured in my classes stated that he does not, as yet, lend credence to exorcisms; however, he was guarded enough not to discount it either.

OTHER FORMS OF HEALING

Auric Healing. Another form of treatment is auric healing. John Richard Turner of Waltham, Massachusetts, considers himself to be an auric healer. He explains that "from the moment of birth until the last breath is taken, a person has a bioenergetic field surrounding his body," known as an "aura" (Turner 1977). If strong enough, it is believed to be transmittable and to have healing powers. By the use of touch, the person with the auric powers is able to effect cure for an ill person (Personal interview). Mr. Turner, who is fairly well known in the Boston area, also claims to be quite popular in California. He states that he visits patients in the hospital along with the physician and that he has been successful in treating people in that setting.

church of saint ignatius of loyola

Liturgy of Anointing

THE CHURCH OF ST. IGNATIUS WILL PRAY FOR THE SICK AND ELDERLY IN THE PARISH ON THE FEAST OF CHRIST THE KING, NOVEMBER 20th AT THE LITURGY FOR ANOINTING AT 9:30 A.M.. AREA RESIDENTS, ESPECIALLY THOSE WHO ARE SICK, DISABLED OR ELDERLY, ARE WELCOME TO TAKE PART. EACH PERSON WHO DESIRES IT WILL BE BLESSED OR ANOINTED WITH HOLY OIL.

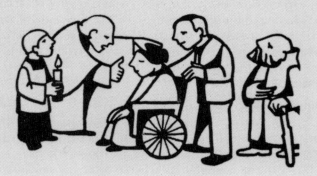

Figure 6–5 Announcement for Liturgy of Anointing of the Sick. (From the author's collection.)

Pilgrimages. The film *We Believe in Niño Fidencio* is a documentary on folk curing and penitent pilgrimages in northern Mexico. Shot in October 1971 in northern Mexico by Dr. and Mrs. John Olson (who were in Mexico doing research), the film is concerned with

> . . . the belief system and ceremonies surrounding a folk curer, Fidencio Constantino, who practiced in Nuevo Leon from the early 1920s until his death in 1938, and who is presently the central figure in a widespread curing cult. Twice each year, upon the anniversaries of his birth and death, Espinazo (a town of about 300 population) is inundated by 10,000 to 15,000 people from Mexico and the United States who make pilgrimages in hopes of a cure and/or help from the Niño. It was during one of these celebrations that the film was made.
>
> Believers combine elements of traditional Catholicism, Indian dances, herbology, and laying on of hands in effecting cures. It is believed that certain individuals receive the Niño's power to heal. They are called "Cajitas" or "Materias" (women), and "Cajones" (men)—"receptacles" of the Niño's power—and they cure in the name of Niño Fidencio and God. During the celebrations they roam Espinazo curing all who wish a cure-blessing. There are several "holy places" in Espinazo where curing is conducted: Fidencio's tomb, "temple," and death bed, two trees, a cemetery hill, the hill of the bell, and the "charco" or mudpond, where Fidencio, conducted baptisms to cure his patients.
>
> The film includes references to other curing alternatives, and attempts to present some of the reasons why the believers continue to select this curing method in the face of modern medical alternatives in nearby towns and cities.
>
> As previously stated, Dr. Olson first learned about this cult in 1968–1969 while doing field research in Mina, a community in the same county as Espinazo. It was during this time that the Olsons met members of the cult (in Mina and Espinazo) including the local "materia," Cayetana, who appear in the film. The narration of the film is based on information and actual recorded interviews given by participants in the cult. Jon Olson is presently an Assistant Professor of Anthropology at California State University at Los Angeles.
>
> Extensive study of the Niño Fidencio complex has been done by Professor June Macklin (Connecticut College) (Informational brochure).

Several healers in the South Texas area are known as *materias* and heal in the name of Niño Fidencio (Fig. 6–6) (Gardner 1992).

This chapter is no more than an overview of the topics introduced. The amount of relevant knowledge could fill many books. The issues raised here are those that, I think, have special meaning to the practice of nursing, medicine, and health-care delivery. We must be aware (1) of what people may be thinking

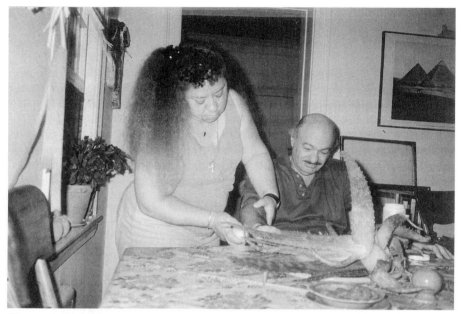

Figure 6–6 Assessment of a client by a *materia*, a healer who heals in the name of Niño Fidencio. (Courtesy of Alma Martinez, Castroville, Texas. Photograph by R. Spector)

that may differ from our own thoughts and (2) that sources of *help* exist outside the traditional medical community. As the beliefs of ethnic communities are explored in later chapters, I shall attempt to delineate who are specifically recognized and used as healers by the members of the community, and I shall describe some of the forms of treatment employed by each community.

❀ *References*

Andrews, M. M., and Hanson, P. A. 1995. Religion, Culture, and Nursing. In *Transcultural Concepts in Nursing Care,* 2d ed., edited by J. S. Boyle and M. M. Andrews. Philadelphia: Lippincott.

Ausubel, N. *The Book of Jewish Knowledge.* 1964. New York: Crown.

Bishop, G. *Faith Healing: God or Fraud?* 1967. Los Angeles: Sherbourne.

Blattner, B. *Holistic Nursing.* 1981. Englewood Cliffs, N.J.: Prentice-Hall.

Boston Indian Council. 1985. Informational pamphlet. Boston, Mass. 1973.

Buxton, J. 1973. *Religion and Healing in Mandari.* Oxford: Clarendon.

Cramer, E. *Divine Science and Healing.* 1923. Denver: The Colorado College of Divine Science.

Ford, P. S. 1971. *The Healing Trinity: Prescriptions for Body, Mind, and Spirit.* New York: Harper and Row.

Foy, F. A., ed. 1980. *Catholic Almanac.* Huntington, Ind.: Our Sunday Visitor.

Gardner, D. 1992. *Niño Fidencio. A Heart Thrown Open.* Santa Fe: Museum of New Mexico Press.

Geissler, E. M. 1994. *Pocket Guide: Cultural Assessment.* St. Louis: Mosby.

———. 1998. *Pocket Guide: Cultural Assessment,* 2d ed. St. Louis: Mosby.

Hallam, E. 1994. *Saints.* New York: Simon and Schuster.

Illich, I. 1975. *Medical Nemesis: The Expropriation of Health.* London: Marion Bogars.

Johnson, C. J., and McGee, M. G., eds. 1991. *How Different Religions View Death and Afterlife.* Philadelphia: The Charles Press.

Kelsey, M. T. 1973. *Healing and Christianity.* New York: Harper and Row.

Krieger, D. 1979. *The Therapeutic Touch.* Englewood Cliffs, N.J.: Prentice-Hall.

Krippner, S., and Villaldo, A. 1976. *The Realms of Healing.* Millbrae, Calif.: Celestial Arts.

Lipson, J. G., Dibble, S. L., and Minarik, P. A. 1996. *Cultural and Nursing Care: A Pocket Guide.* San Francisco: UCSF Nursing Press.

MacNutt, F. 1974. *Healing.* Notre Dame, Ind.: Ave Maria Press.

Maloney, C., ed. 1976. *The Evil Eye.* New York: Columbia University Press, 14.

Monthly Missalette **15,** no. 13 (February 1980): 38.

Morgenstern, J. 1966. *Rites of Birth, Marriage, Death and Kindred Occasions among the Semites.* Chicago: Quadrangle Books.

Naegele, K. 1970. *Health and Healing.* San Francisco: Jossey Bass.

Nightingale, F. [1860] 1946. (A fascimile of the first edition published by D. Appleton and Co.) *Notes on Nursing—What It Is, What It Is Not.* New York: Appleton-Century.

Olson, Jon and Natalie. *We Believe in Niño Fidencio.* Flyer on the film. (P.O. Box 14914, Long Beach, CA 90814).

Progoff, I. 1959. *Depth Psychology and Modern Man.* New York: McGraw-Hill.

Russell, A. J. 1937. *Healing in His Wings.* London: Methuen.

Shames, R., and Sterin, C. 1978. *Healing with Mind Power.* Emmans, Penn.: Rodale Press.

Shaw, W. 1975. *Aspects of Malaysian Magic.* Kuala Lampor, Malaysia: Nazibum Negara.

Steinberg, M. 1947. *Basic Judaism.* New York: Harcourt, Brace and World.

Turner, J. R. 1977. Notes from a lecture delivered at a meeting of the World's Future Society held at Boston College, 16 March.

Wallace, G. 1979. Spiritual Care—A Reality in Nursing Education and Practice. *The Nurses Lamp* 5 (2) (November):1–4.

*Figure 6-1 from page 121

From left to right—top to bottom: The chapter-opening quilt panel contains images of places where people seek healing. The **Tomb of Rachel** in Bethlehem, Israel, is a place where pilgrims go seeking protection, healing, and help, especially for fertility. The **Tomb of David** in Jerusalem, Israel, which is located in the same building as the room of the Last Supper is another frequented place of healing. The **Tomb of Menachem Mendel Schneerson** in Queens, New York, is a holy shrine where Jewish people from around the world gather to seek healing and restore HEALTH. People visit the **Black Jesus** in the San Fernando Cathedral in San Antonio, Texas, to petition for and attest to miraculous healings. It has been reported that the Virgin at the **Shrine of the Blessed Virgin Mary** in Blanco, Texas, cries tears of myrrh. Pilgrims report that they have had mystical and healing experiences in this place. Crutches are left at the **Church Our Lady of San Juan,** in San Juan, Texas, to attest to the miracles that happened in this place. Petitions are placed at the **Church in Yverdon-Les-Bains,** Switzerland, many of which request healing. Petitions expressing gratitude for healing are prominently placed at **St. Phillippe Du Roule Church** in Paris, France. **Lourdes, France** is one of the most famous shrines in the world where documented healings have occurred.

Chapter 7

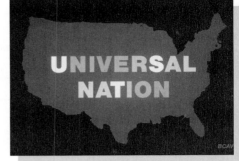

The Influence of Demographics on Health Care

As we enter the 21st century, health-care workers are perched on the cutting edge of enormous demographic, social, and cultural change. Many of these changes will play a dramatic role in both the delivery of health care to patients, their families, and communities, and in the workforce and environment in which the provider practices. The emerging majority constituted 19.7% of the population in 1990 (Bureau of the Census 1992) and is rapidly growing. The charts and comments in this chapter are designed to provide you with a brief overview of the demographic and economic backgrounds of the American population and with a rationale for the importance of knowing about many cultures' HEALTH traditions is.

"Demography is destiny" (Hodgkinson 1986). In order to understand the changes that are taking place in the health-care system, both in the delivery of services and in the profile of the people who are delivering services, we must look at the changes in the American population. The white majority is aging and shrinking; the black, Hispanic, Asian, and American Indian populations are young and growing. In California the demographic theme is that of a "minority majority" by 2005 (Hodgkinson 1986). It is imperative for those of us who deliver health care to be understanding of and sensitive to cultural differences and to the effect of these differences on a given person's health and illness beliefs and practices.

If we look beyond 2000 we observe many interesting demographic shifts. The population of the United States will continue to grow, but more slowly. The young population, ages 0 to 17, grew from 64.4 million in 1990 to 67.4 million in 2000, and then will decline to 64.9 million in 2012. This trend is foreseeable because of the decline in the number of women moving into the childbearing years. The decline will be in the number of white youth (Table 7–1). In addition, Hispanic children, who outnumbered black children in

---

Figure 7–1 Universal nation.   **157**

| Table 7–1 | Projections of the U.S. Population Age 0–17:1990–2010 (in millions of people) | | | |

Youth	1990	2010	Change
Total youth	64.4[a]	64.9[a]	+0.5
White, non-Hispanic	45.2	41.4	−3.8
Hispanic (of any race)	7.2	9.8	+2.6
Black[b]	10.2	11.4	+1.2
Other races[b]	2.2	2.8	+0.6
Increase in total nonwhite youth: +44 million			
Decrease in total white youth: −3.8 million			

From: Hodgkinson, H. L. A Demographic Look at Tomorrow. (Washington, D.C.: Institute for Education Leadership, 1992), p. 5. Reprinted with permission.
[a]Rounding
[b]Includes small number of Hispanics: "other races" are Asian and American Indians.

1997, will be the leading edge of a population trend that will make Hispanics the largest minority group in 2005 (www.census.gov).

❧ Total Population Characteristics

The 1998 census estimated percentages are compared with the 1980 and 1990 census percentages in Table 7–2 and in Figure 7–2. The 1980 census figure for the U.S. total population represented an increase of more than 24 million people over the 1970 census, and 16.8% of the population comprised people of color. It may also be noted that 6.4% of the population claimed Hispanic origin but could be of any race (www.census.gov). In 1990, despite an accepted head count shortfall of 4.7 million people—5% of whom were Hispanic all races, 4.4% black, 2.3% Asian/Pacific Islander, and 0.7% non-Hispanic white (www.census.gov) the population count of the United States represented an increase of 22,167,670 people, over the 1980 census and 19.8% of the population comprised people of color. Again, it may also be noted that 9.0% of the population claimed Hispanic or Spanish origin but could be of any race (Bureau of the Census 1992). Note that the European American majority had shrunk by about 3%, and there is an "emerging majority" of people of color.

In early 1999 the population of the United States was counted as 271,833,873 (Bureau of the Census 1999) people, which represented an increase of 23,124,000 from 1990. Estimates released in December 1998 placed the population at 270,933 (in thousands), and 28.9% of the population comprised people of color. It may also be noted that 11.4% of the population claimed Hispanic or Spanish origin but could be of any race (Bureau of the Census 1999).

Another way to view the census data from 1990 is to examine the breakdown of the non-Hispanic population. Subtracting the Hispanic population data reveals that the white non-Hispanic population in 1990 was 75.2%; the

	1980	%	1990	%	1998 (est.)	%
Total	**226,542**	**100**	**248,710**	**100**	**270,933**	**100**
Hispanic Included						
White		83.2		80.2		82.5
Black		11.7		12.2		12.7
American Indian		0.6		0.8		0.9
Asian/Pacific Islander				1.5		3.9
Other		3.0		3.9		
Hispanic		6.4		9.0		11.4
Non-Hispanic						
White				75.6		72.1
Black				11.8		12.1
American Indian				0.7		0.7
Asian/Pacific Islander				2.8		3.7
Non-Hispanic				90.9		88.6

Table 7–2 Percentage Distributions of the U.S. Population by Race and Hispanic Origin: 1980, 1990, 1998

From: U.S. Bureau of the Census, *1980 Census Population.* Press Release CB81-32 (23 February 1981), and Supplementary Report PC80-S1-1. Washington, D.C.: Government Printing Office, May 1981).
U.S. Bureau of the Census. *1990 Census of the Population, General Population Characteristics United States.* (Washington, D.C.: Government Printing Office. November 1992), p. 4.
U.S. Bureau of the Census. *Resident Population of the United States: Estimates by Sex, Race, and Hispanic Origin, with Median Age.* Internet release date: 28 December. (http://www.census.gov/population/estimates/nation/intfile3-1.txt).

black population, including a small number of Hispanics, was 12.1%; the Native American, Eskimo, and Aleut, including a small number of Hispanics, was 0.8%; and the Asian/Pacific Islander population was 2.9%. The Hispanic population of any race represented 9%. In 1998 the white non-Hispanic population was 72.2%, the black non-Hispanic population, 12.1%; the American Indian, 0.7%; and the Asian/Pacific Islander, 3.7%. This analysis reveals that the white population is shrinking.

PREFERENCE FOR RACIAL OR ETHNIC TERMINOLOGY

Because the remainder of this chapter and text focuses on diverse ethnocultural groups, it has been helpful to locate the following information relating to the preferred term by which a given group of people wants to be called.

- **Hispanic** is the term most preferred by people over Spanish origin, Latino, or some other term.
- **White** is the term most preferred by people over Caucasian, European American, Anglo, or some other term.
- **Black** is the term most preferred by people over African American, Afro-American, Negro, Colored, or some other term.

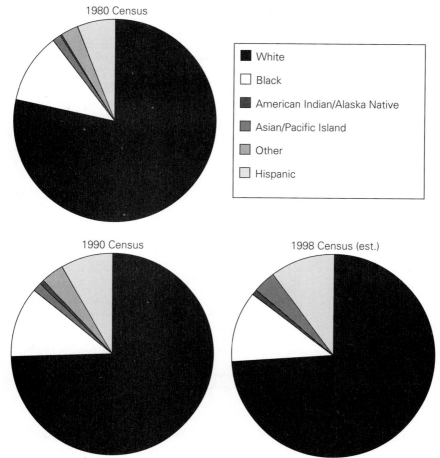

1980 Census

White
Black
American Indian/Alaska Native
Asian/Pacific Island
Other
Hispanic

1990 Census

1998 Census (est.)

Figure 7–2 Percentage Distribution of the Population by Race and Hispanic Origin: 1980, 1990, 1998 (est.).

- **American Indian** is the term most preferred by people over Native American, Alaska Native, or some other term (Infoplease.com 1999).

These terms will be used throughout the text.

AMERICAN INDIAN, ALEUT, AND ESKIMO POPULATIONS

The American Indian, Eskimo, and Aleut populations in the United States constituted 0.9% of the total population in 1998. The greatest percentage (58.6%) of the population were between the ages of 18 and 64, whereas 35.6% were below 18 years of age, and 5.8% were 65 and older in 1990. The median age of the population was estimated to be 27.5 years in 1998.

ASIAN/PACIFIC ISLANDER POPULATION

Members of the Asian/Pacific Island communities in the United States have their origins in China, Hawaii, the Philippines, Korea, Japan, and Southeast Asia (Cambodia, Laos, and Vietnam). The people made up 3.9% of the population in 1998. The greatest percentage of the population (65.1%) were between the ages of 18 and 64, whereas 28.6% were below 18 years of age, and 6.2% were 65 and older in 1990. The median age of the group was estimated to be 31.3 years in 1998.

BLACK POPULATION

The black population in the United States constituted 12.1% of the total population in 1990. Black Americans have their origins in Africa, and their cultural heritage is a mixture of Caribbean cultures (including the West Indian), Native American, and northern European cultures. In 1990 the greatest percentage (59.7%) of this population were between the ages of 18 and 64, 32% were below 18 years of age, and 8.4% were 65 years old and older. The median age of the population in 1998 was estimated to be 30 years.

HISPANIC POPULATION (OF ANY RACE)

Hispanic Americans (of any race) originally came from Spain, Cuba, Central and South America, Mexico, Puerto Rico, and other Spanish-speaking countries. The Hispanic population in the United States made up an estimated 11.4% of the total population in 1998. In 1990 breakdown by country of origin for this population was as follows:

Country of Origin	Percentage of Hispanic Population
Mexico	62.6
Central and South America	13.6
Puerto Rico	11.4
Cuba	4.9
Other	7.6

The estimated median age of the population in 1998 was 26.6 years.

WHITE POPULATION

In 1998 the white population in the United States constituted 82.5% of the total population. This percentage decreased from 83.2% in 1980 but increased a bit from 1990. The greatest percentage (62.2%) of this population were between the ages of 18 and 64, 23.9% of this population were under 18, (the lowest of all groups), and 13.9% (the highest of all groups) were 65 and older. The estimated median age of the population was 35.3 years, the oldest of any group.

Table 7–3 summarizes the estimated median ages of each group.

Table 7–3 | **Estimated Mean Ages of the Population, 1998**

Population Group	Mean Age
American Indian	27.5 years
Asian/Pacific Islander	31.3 years
Black	30.0 years
Hispanic	26.6 years
White	35.3 years

From: National Center for Health Statistics. *Health, United States, 1998, with Socioeconomic Status and Health Chartbook.* (Hyattsville, Md., 1998), 351–352.

❋ *Demographic Barriers to Health Care*

Innumerable demographic barriers restrict access, "the attainment of timely, sufficient, and appropriate health care of adequate quality such that health outcomes are maximized" (Weissman and Epstein 1994) to the health-care system; but, the major such obstacle is poverty. Closely related to, but not necessarily occurring only among the poor, are the problems of access to all types of health-care facilities because of transportation and language barriers.

POVERTY

There are countless ways to answer the question, What is poverty? Poverty may be viewed through many lenses and from anthropological, cultural, demographic, economical, educational, environmental, historical, medical, philosophical, policy, political, racial, sexual, sociological, and theological points of view.

One way of viewing poverty is to list the government programs or subsidies a person receives, such as public housing, government loans to attend college, Medicaid, Aid to Families with Dependent Children (AFDC), or food stamps. Another way of answering this question is with the description used by the United States Bureau of Labor Statistics, which counts the poor and describes the poor by age, education, location, race, family composition, and employment status. A third answer is the federal government definition of the "poverty threshold." This poverty threshold, developed in 1965, is based on pretax income only, excluding capital gains, and does not include the value of noncash benefits, such as employer-provided health insurance, food stamps, or Medicaid. The poverty level figures are used by programs such as Head Start, Low-Income Home Energy, and National School Lunch to determine eligibility. The poverty level for an average family of four was $16,450 in 1998 (*Federal Register* 1998). Table 7–4 lists the poverty guidelines for persons and families for selected years.

The association between socioeconomic status and health status of a given person of family may be explained in part by the reduced access to health

Table 7–4 | **Poverty Guidelines for the Years 1986–1998 for the Contiguous States and the District of Columbia**

Year	First Person	Additional Person	Four-Person Family
1986	$5360	$1880	$11,000
1988	5770	1960	11,650
1990	6280	2140	12,700
1992	6810	2380	13,950
1994	7360	2480	14,800
1996	7740	2620	15,600
1998	8050	2800	16,450

From: Federal Register 63, no. 36 (24, February 1998): 9235–9238.

care among those with lower socioeconomic status. Income may be related to health because it

- increases access to health care
- enables the person and family to live in better neighborhoods;
- enables the person or family to afford better housing;
- enables the person or family to reside in locations not abutting known environmentally degraded locations (heavy industrial pollution or known hazardous waste sites); and,
- increases the opportunity to engage in health promoting behaviors.

Health also may affect income by restricting the type and amount of employment a given person may seek or perhaps by preventing a person from working.

There has been an increase in earning inequality over the last 25 years. Table 7–5 gives the values for median household income for the years 1986–1996, the latest period for which data are available. The income for all races rose, then dipped, in this time period. For blacks and Hispanics it was

Table 7–5 | **Median Household Income for the Years 1986–1996**

Year	All Races	White, Non-Hispanic	Black	Hispanic	Asian or Pacific Islander
1986	$35,642	$38,323	$21,588	$26,272	
1988	36,108	39,224	21,760	27,002	$42,795
1990	35,945	38,349	22,420	26,806	46,158
1992	34,261	37,229	20,974	25,271	42,274
1994	34,158	37,188	22,261	24,796	42,858
1996	35,492	38,787	23,482	24,906	43,276

From: National Center for Health Statistics. Health, United States, 1998, with Socioeconomic Status and Health Chartbook. (Hyattsville, Md., 1998), 144.

much lower than for whites and Asians and people from the Pacific Islands. Much of this change and inequality was due to technological changes that increased income to highly skilled labor. At the same time less skilled workers saw their wages decrease or stagnate. The other factors responsible for this phenomenon include the

- globalization of the economy
- decline in the real minimum wage
- decline in unionization
- increase in immigration
- increase in families headed by women (from 10% in 1970 to 18% in 1996); households headed by women generally have lower incomes.

The following are several other distinct demographic differences in poverty by age, race, ethnicity and household composition:

- In 1996 over one-fifth of all children lived in poverty.
- Between 1970 and 1980 the poverty rate among children increased from 15% to more than 20% and has remained at this figure
- In 1996, 11% of non-Hispanic white children were poor compared with 40% of black and Hispanic children
- Children in households headed by females had the highest rates of poverty, and these rates were higher among black and Hispanic children. (Table 7–6.)

There are also significant geographical variations in the occurrence of poverty. Across the states the average poverty rates from 1994 to 1996 varied from 7 to 24%. Poverty rates were the lowest in New Hampshire (6.5%), Utah (8.0%), Alaska (8.5%), New Jersey (8.7%), and Wisconsin (8.8%). The poverty

Table 7–6 | **Percentages of Persons Poor or Near Poor, 1996**

	All Persons		**Children under 18 in Families**		**Related children under 18 in Female-Headed Families**	
	Poor	*Near Poor*	*Poor*	*Near Poor*	*Poor*	*Near Poor*
All races	13.7	19.8	20.5	22.7	49.3	27.0
White, non-Hispanic	8.6	17.0	11.1	19.7	34.9	29.2
Asian or Pacific Islander	14.5	15.7	19.5	16.4	48.8	17.6
Black[a]	28.4	26.7	39.9	28.1	58.2	26.8
Hispanic	29.4	30.5	40.3	31.7	67.4	21.9

[a]Includes persons of Hispanic origin

From: National Center for Health Statistics. *Health, United States, 1998 with Socioeconomic Status and Health Chartbook.* (Hyattsville, Md., 1998), p. 144.

rates were the highest in New Mexico (24%), District of Columbia (22.5%), Louisiana (22%), Mississippi (21.3%), West Virginia (17.9%), and Texas (17.7%) (National Center for Health Statistics 1998, 145).

CYCLE OF POVERTY

Poverty is more than the absence of money. One way of analyzing the phenomenon is by observing the effects of the "cycle of poverty" as illustrated in Figure 7–3. In this cycle, the poor person lives in a situation that may create poor intellectual and physical development and poor economic production, and in which the birth rate is high; this living situation in turn causes poor production, which creates insufficient salaries and a subsistence economy that forces the person often to reside in densely populated areas or remotely located rural areas where adequate shelter and potable water are scarce, and the person suffers from chronically poor nutrition. These conditions all too often lead to high morbidity and accident rates, precipitating high health-care costs, which, in turn, pre-

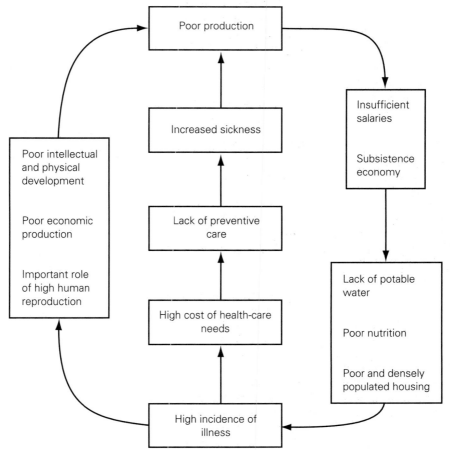

Figure 7–3   The cycle of poverty.

vent the person from seeking health-care services. Thus there is an increase in sickness and poor production, in a cycle that has yet to be broken. Other barriers that are interrelated to this cycle are the lack of access to health-care services, language issues, and transportation issues (Spector 1979, 148–152).

One source of funding available to families in poverty is welfare. This system has, for some time, been under sharp scrutiny by politicians and members of society at large, and efforts have been taken to reform this system of funding the poor. One current plan eliminates able-bodied people from the welfare rolls after 2 years. This will have a profound effect on many mothers with children. The issues of overcrowded housing, poor sanitation, and so forth that are part of the cycle of poverty are not dealt with in any welfare reform plan.

ACCESS

Several factors limit a given family's access to the health-care delivery system, including the availability and location of health-care facilities, transportation to these facilities, and the existence and type of health insurance. The lack of insurance, whether public (Medicaid) or private, is a rapidly increasing problem. A weakness of the current discussion on health-care reform is its lack of concern for coverage and benefits for the poor and minorities.

TRANSPORTATION

The issue of transportation is never ending and never changing. All too frequently, families are not able to get to health-care services because of geographic distance and therefore have to depend on other family members or friends for transportation. In many settings, the hospital responsible for providing free care is not in the same location as the families needing this care. Public transportation may be expensive and, in some locations, nonexistent.

LANGUAGE

Many of the "new Americans" tend to retain their native language, as do many "old Americans" who may have immigrated here a generation ago. More and more immigrants arrive in the United States every year, thereby increasing the need for adequate interpreters, yet all too often these services are not available. It is self-evident that communication is a major necessity in health-care delivery.

Other barriers include depersonalization; hours missed from work, school, and/or home; child care; and excessively long waits for services.

NEW IMMIGRANTS

Since 1972 there has been an explosion in the numbers of people coming to this country, both with and without the necessary documentation. The foreign-born population in 1990 totaled a record 19.8 million (8% of the total population), surpassing the previous highs of 14 million in 1930 and 1980 (Figure 7–4). Foreign-born residents accounted for 8.7% of the population of the United States in 1994. (Table 7–7 lists the top 10 countries of origin for immigrants in 1994.

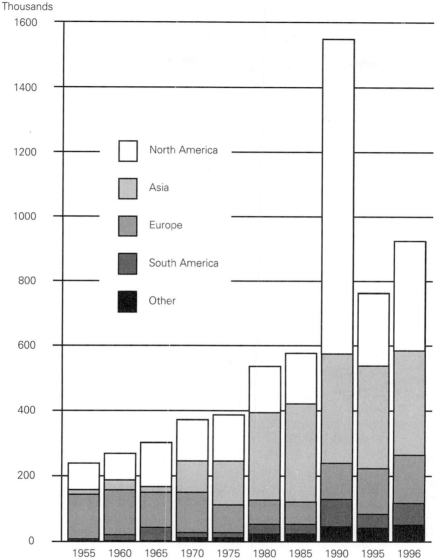

Figure 7–4 Immigrants admitted by Region of Birth: Selected Fiscal Years 1955–1996. (1980–1996, Table 3; 1955–1975, previous *Yearbooks*. See Glossary for fiscal year definitions.)

Other factors relating to immigrants include the following:

- In 1940, 70% of the immigrants came from Europe. In 1992, 15% came from Europe, 37% from Asia, and 44% from Latin America and the Caribbean.
- The foreign born had a higher per capita income than the native born ($15,033 vs. $14,370) in 1989.

| | Table 7–7 | Top 10 Countries of Origin for U.S. Immigrants in Fiscal Year 1994 |

Country	Number of Immigrants (in thousands)
Mexico	6200
Philippines	1000
Cuba	805
El Salvador	718
Canada	679
Germany	625
China	565
Dominican Republic	556
South Korea	533
Vietnam	496

From: Associated Press. U.S. Census Bureau Study, 28 August 1995. Reported in the *Boston Globe,* 29 August 1995.

- The median family income of foreign-born families was almost $4000 less than that of the native born ($31,785 vs. $35,508).
- The unemployment rate for the foreign born was 7.8% in 1990, compared with 6.2% for the native born.
- The percentage of people in large American cities in 1990 under 18 who were foreign born was as follows:

City	Foreign Born (%)
Los Angeles	21
San Francisco	19
Dade County (Miami)	18
New York City	12
Houston	10

- Cities where more than 50% of the residents are foreign born include the following:

City	Foreign Born (%)
Hialeah, Florida	70
Miami, Florida	60
Huntington Park, California	59
Monterey Park, California	52
Miami Beach, Florida	
Santa Ana, California	51

In 1990, there were 230,445,777 people over the age of 5 in the United States. Of this population, more than 198 million (86%) speak only English at home. For the remaining 31,844,979 (14%), the spoken languages are Spanish (54%), French (6%), German (5%), Italian (4%), other Indo-European (13%), Chinese (4%), other Asian (8%), American Indian (1%), and other languages, 5%. Of those who speak other languages, 1,845,243 (or 6%), speak no English at all.

The passage of Proposition 187 in California in November 1994, and earlier laws relating to bilingual education in Texas, demonstrate that many citizens are no longer willing to provide basic human services such as health care and education to the new residents. Thus far, the implementation of these laws has been held up in the courts. Despite such efforts, however, it is evident that immigration to this country will continue. It is predicted that by the year 2020 immigration will be a major source of new people for the United States and will be responsible for whatever growth occurs in the United States after 2030. The United States will continue to attract about two-thirds of the world's immigration, and 85% of the immigrants will be from Central and South America.

❧ Background Information: Ethnic Groups' Traditional Views on HEALTH and Illness

The following information is included in the discussion of the health and illness beliefs and practices of each ethnic group:

- Traditional definitions of HEALTH
- Traditional epidemiological beliefs
- Traditional methods for maintaining, protecting, and restoring HEALTH
- Traditional names and symptoms of a given disease
- Traditional sources of HEALTH care
- Traditional remedies
- Problems the group encounters in dealing with the health-care system
- Current numbers of people enrolled in health professional schools.

It must be kept in mind that this information is general; it is not specific to any one person. Nevertheless, a person's health care and behavior during illness may well have roots in that person's traditional belief system. Problems that arise when caring for a person from one of the ethnic or racial emerging majority groups might be resolved with an understanding of that person's traditional beliefs. Understanding that the beliefs may well differ from those of the dominant culture can help us, as well as the patient, to resolve the problems. In addition, the tendency to disrespect a person whose personal health-care practices differ from those of the dominant culture can be overcome when we understand the underlying reasons for that person's behavior.

All people agree that good health is essential for survival. If we are sick, we cannot work, we cannot provide food for ourselves and families, and we cannot survive and reproduce. Satisfactory health is mandatory for our existence, yet the definition of HEALTH and the means of preserving it vary from people to people. Earlier, we demonstrated that great disagreement exists among health workers about the definition of health, yet we as professionals often expect other people to accept our "nondefinition."

Just as there are differences in the meaning of health, so are there differences in the meaning of illness. What does illness mean to others? Is it simply the symptoms of a disease, or is it more? What causes illness from a traditional viewpoint? Who are the native, traditional healers, and what methods do they use to treat and heal disorders? How do traditional healers differ from physicians and other allopathic providers? What resources are available to a person seeking traditional ethnocultural HEALTH care?

Research has been carried out by nurses, physicians, medical sociologists, anthropologists, and folklorists in the area of HEALTH and illness beliefs to discover and understand the folkways. There is currently much criticism among ethnic groups who have been studied. They question the meaning of these studies and the interpretations of the researchers. Despite these criticisms, however, the work of sociologists and anthropologists is helpful if used as a stepping-stone. In this unit, results of these studies are looked at from a specific standpoint, namely, they are referred to and recommended for further examination in order to help health-care providers understand the behaviors and attitudes of the people for whom they care. In addition, bibliographic resources are included that have been recommended by the members of a given community.

It is important to note that much of the literature regarding the health and illness beliefs of any group of people is contradictory. One research report may indicate that a given group of people view health as a reward for good behavior. Another states that people of the same cultural background believe that health is a matter of chance—something that may be here today, but luck determines how long it remains. Yet another study indicates that some illnesses are believed to be caused by witchcraft, and others by natural elements.

In no way is it implied that any of these findings are universally accurate or that all health care should be based on them. What is important is to note that these studies elucidate, in part, why two (or more) conflicting viewpoints can exist between provider and patient regarding a diagnosis and treatment regimen.

Statements about health practices of chosen ethnic communities are based not only on the existing literature, as noted, but also on the following:

1. Data collected from surveys of students, including ethnic students of color, over a 25-year period
2. Information shared by guest lecturers who are both health-care providers and members of the communities under discussion
3. Data collected from the author's interviews with health-care consumers and providers over a period of 25 years
4. Intense research in both community-based consumer groups and provider groups
5. Extensive travel that includes visits to traditional healers and shrines

In an effort to understand the great complexity of diverse HEALTH and illness beliefs, this book can, of necessity, only touch on the social and culturally related issues of our present population. The text presents the reader with an overview of the traditional HEALTH and illness beliefs and practices of the people who are the patients who use the health-care system and describes only a segment of their lives. The demographic trends described in this chapter indicate that efforts **must** be made now to prepare ourselves for the social changes to come. The problems that arose in the 1990s, particularly those related to health, will continue for many decades, and as Hodgkinson (1992) emphasizes: "More effort should be placed on local prevention of social and medical problems, rather than their expensive and ineffective cures. Tomorrow is an extension of today's trends."

An African proverb says that "to go back to tradition is the first step forward." This first step forward for those of us who will deliver health care in the 21st century is to be culturally aware and to make every effort to recognize and respect the traditional HEALTH beliefs and practices of our patients.

❀ *References*

Federal Register 63, no. 36 (24 February 1998): 9235–9238.

Hodgkinson, H. L. 1986. Reform? Higher Education? Don't Be Absurd! *Higher Education* (December): 273.

———. 1992. *A Demographic Look at Tomorrow.* Washington, DC: Institute for Educational Leadership, 2.

Hollman, F. W. 1990. *United States Population Estimates, by Age, Sex, Race, and Hispanic Origin: 1980–1988.* U.S. Bureau of the Census, January.

National Center for Health Statistics. 1998. *Health, United States, 1998, with Socioeconomic Status and Health Chartbook.* Hyattsville, Md.

Sege, I., and Mashek, J. 1991. Census Total Will Stand Despite Undercounting. *Boston Globe* 16 July.

Spector, M. 1979. Poverty: The Barrier to Health Care. In *Cultural Diversity in Health and Illness,* edited by R. E. Spector. New York: Appleton, Century, and Crofts, 141–162.

U.S. Bureau of the Census. 1981. *1980 Census of Population: Detailed Population Characteristics.* Washington, DC: Government Printing Office, 1–47.

———. 1992a. *1990 Census of the Population, General Population Characteristics United States,* series 1990 CP-1-1 Washington, DC: Government Printing Office, 4.

———. 1992b. *Current Population Reports,* series P-69, no. 181. *Poverty in the United States: 1991,* series 199CP-3-4 Washington, DC: Government Printing Office, 149.

———. 1993a. *1990 Census of the Population, Social and Economic Characteristics American and Alaska Native Areas,* section 2 of 2, 1990 2-1. Washington, DC: Government Printing Office, 1536.

———. 1993b. *1990 Census of the Population, Asians and Pacific Islanders in the United States,* series 1990 CP-3-5. Washington, DC: Government Printing Office, p. 141.

————. 1993c. *1990 Census of the Population, Social and Economic Characteristics, Persons of Hispanic Origin in the United States,* series 1990 CP3-3. Washington, DC: Government Printing Office, 153.

————. 1993d. *1990 Census of the Population, Social and Economic Characteristics United States,* series 1990 CP-2-1 Washington, DC: Government Printing Office, 14.

————. 1994. *1990 Census of the Population. Education in the United States.* series 199CP-3-4. Washington, DC: Government Printing Office, January, 474.

Weissman, J. S., and Epstein, A. M. 1994. *Falling through the Safety Net. Insurance and Access to Health Care.* Baltimore: Johns Hopkins Press.

INTERNET SOURCES

http://www.census.gov/population/estimates/nation/intfile3-1.text
Infoplease.com/ipa/A0762158.html (30 January 99)

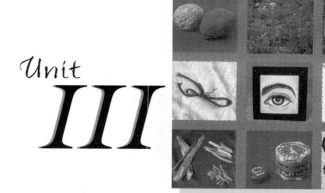

Unit III

Selected Traditional Views of Health and Illness

The chapters in this unit will enable the reader to

1. Develop a level of awareness of the background and health problems of both the emerging majority and white ethnic populations

2. Understand some traditional beliefs of ethnic people with respect to HEALTH and illness

3. Understand the traditional pathways to HEALTH care and the relationship between these pathways and the American health-care system

4. Understand certain manpower problems of each of the communities discussed

5. Be more familiar with the available literature regarding each of the communities

The following exercises are appropriate to all chapters in Unit III.

1. Familiarize yourself with some literature of the given community, that is, read literature, poetry, or a biography of a member of each of the communities.

2. Familiarize yourself with the history and sociopolitical background of each of the communities.

The questions that follow should be thoughtfully considered.

1. What are the traditional definitions of HEALTH and illness in each of the communities?

2. What are the traditional methods of maintaining HEALTH?

3. What are the traditional ways of protecting HEALTH?

4. What are the traditional ways of restoring HEALTH?

5. Who are the traditional healers? What functions do they perform?

Chapter 8

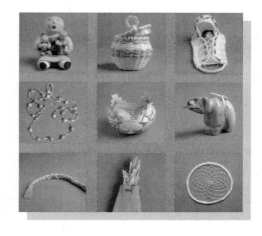

HEALTH and Illness in the American Indian, Aleut, and Eskimo Communities

*The Great Spirit is in all things; he is in the air we breathe.
The Great Spirit is our Father, but the earth is our Mother.
She nourishes us; that which we put into the ground she returns
to us. . . .*

— *Big Thunder, Wabanaki Algonquin*

The descendants of the original inhabitants of the North American continent now are estimated to number 2.0 million people and constitute the smallest of the emerging majority groups. This diverse group comprises numerous tribes and over 400 federally recognized nations, each with its own traditions and cultural heritage. Eskimos, Aleuts, and Indians residing in Alaska are referred to as Alaska Natives; those residing in other states are referred to as American Indians (Bureau of the Census 1998).

To realize the plight of today's American Indian, it is necessary to journey back in time to the years when whites settled in this land. Before the arrival of Europeans, this country had no name but was inhabited by groups of people who called themselves *nations.* The people were strong both in their knowledge of the land and in their might as warriors. The Vikings reached the shores of this country about A.D. 1010. They were unable to settle on the land and left after a decade of frustration. Much later, another group of settlers, since termed the "Lost Colonies," were repulsed. More people came to these shores, however, and the land was taken over by Europeans. As the settlers expanded

Figure 8–1 (From left to right, top to bottom) Storyteller, basket, cradle board, beaded necklace, clay medicine bowl, bear, sweet grass, medicine bag, baby net. *(For more information on each picture see explanation at the end of chapter.*)*

westward, they signed "treaties of peace" or "treaties of land cession" with the Indians. These treaties were similar to those struck between nations, although in this case the agreement was imposed by the "big" nation onto the "small" nation. One reason for treaties was to legitimize the takeover of the land that the Europeans had "discovered." Once the land was "discovered," it was divided among the Europeans, who set out to create a "legal" claim to it. The Indians signed the resultant treaties, ceding small amounts of their land to the settlers and keeping the rest for themselves. As time passed, the number of whites rapidly grew, and the number of Indians diminished because of wars and disease. As these events occurred the treaties began to lose their meaning; the Europeans came to consider them as nothing but a joke. They decided that these "natives" had no real claim to the land and shifted them around like cargo from one reservation to another. Although the Indians tried to seek just settlements through the American court system, they failed to win back the land that had been taken from them through misrepresentation. For example, by 1831, the Cherokees were fighting in the courts to keep their nation in Georgia. They lost their legal battle, however, and, like other Indian nations after the time of the early European settlers, were forced to move westward. During this forced westward movement, many Indians died, and all suffered. Today, many nations are seeking to reclaim their land through the courts (Fortney 1977, Brown 1970; and Deloria 1969, 1974). Several claims, such as those of the Penebscot and Passamaquody tribes in Maine, have been successful.

As the Indians migrated westward they carried with them the fragments of their culture. Their lives were disrupted, their land was lost, and many of their leaders and teachers perished, yet much of their history and culture somehow remain. Today, more and more Indians are seeking to know their history.

Table 8-1	The 10 Largest American Indian Nations

Nation	1990 Population
Cherokee	369,035
Navajo	225,298
Sioux	107,321
Chippewa	105,988
Choctaw	86,231
Pueblo	55,330
Apache	53,330
Iroquois	52,557
Lumbee	50,888
Cree	45,872

From: Zuckoff, M. More and More Claiming American Indian Heritage. *Boston Globe.* 18 April, 1995. Reprinted with permission.

The story of the colonization and settlement of the United States is being re-told with a different emphasis.

American Indians live predominantly in 26 states (including Alaska), with most residing in the western part of the country as a result of the forced westward migration. Although many Indians remain on reservations and in rural areas, just as many people live in cities, especially on the West Coast. Oklahoma, Arizona, California, New Mexico, and Alaska have the largest numbers of Native Americans (Primeaux 1977). Today, more and more people are claiming to have American Indian roots. Since 1970 the Indian population has increased by 140%. By the year 2000, census officials project that there will be roughly 2.3 million Indians, or triple the number in 1970, (Zuckoff 1995). Table 8–1 lists the 10 largest American Indian nations.

❧ *Traditional Definitions of* HEALTH *and Illness*

Although each American Indian nation or tribe had its own history and belief system regarding health and illness and the traditional treatment of illness, some general beliefs and practices underlie the more specific tribal ideas. Certain specifics are noted, either in the text or in footnotes. The data—collected through a review of the literature and from interviews granted by members of the groups—come from the Navajo Nation, the Hopis, the Cherokees, and Shoshones, and New England Indians with whom I have worked closely.

The traditional American Indian belief about HEALTH is that it reflects living in total harmony with nature and having the ability to survive under exceedingly difficult circumstances (Zuckoff 1995). Humankind has an intimate relationship with nature (Boyd 1974, 96).* The earth is considered to be a living organism—the body of a higher individual, with a will and a desire to be well. The earth is periodically healthy and less healthy, just as human beings are. According to the American Indian belief system, a person should treat his or her body with respect, just as the earth should be treated with respect. When the earth is harmed, humankind is itself harmed, and, conversely, when humans harm themselves they harm the earth. The earth gives food, shelter, and medicine to humankind, and for this reason, all things of the earth belong to human beings and nature. "The land belongs to life, life belongs to the land, and the land belongs to itself." In order to maintain HEALTH, Indians must maintain their relationship with Nature. "Mother Earth" is the friend of the Indian, and the land belongs to the Indian (Boyd 1974).

According to Indian belief, as explained by a medicine man, Rolling Thunder, the human body is divided into two halves that are seen as plus and minus (yet another version of the concept that every whole is made of two opposite halves). There are also—in every whole—two energy poles: positive and

---

*This philosophy was reiterated in a lecture at Boston College School of Nursing in April, 1975, by Will Basque, a Micmac Indian and former president of the Boston Indian Council.

negative. The energy of the body can be controlled by spiritual means. It is further believed that every being has a purpose and an identity. Every being has the power to control his or her own self, and from this force and the belief in its potency the spiritual power of a person is kindled (Boyd 1974).

Many American Indians with traditional orientations believe there is a reason for every sickness or pain. They believe that illness is the price to be paid either for something that happened in the past or for something that will happen in the future. In spite of this conviction, a sick person must still be cared for. Everything is seen as being the result of something else, and this cause-and-effect relationship creates an eternal chain. American Indians do not subscribe to the germ theory of modern medicine. Illness is something that must *be*. Even the person who is experiencing the illness may not realize the reason for its occurrence, but it may, in fact, be the best possible price to pay for the past or future event(s) (Boyd 1974).

The Hopi Indians associate illness with evil spirits. The evil spirit responsible for the illness is identified by the medicine man, and the remedy for the malady resides in the treatment of the evil spirit (Leek 1975, 16).

According to legend, the Navaho people originally emerged from the depths of the earth—fully formed as human beings. Before the beginning of time, they existed with holy people, supernatural beings with supernatural powers, in a series of 12 underworlds. The creation of all elements took place in these underworlds, and there all things were made to interact in constant harmony. A number of ceremonies and rituals were created at this time for "maintaining, renewing, and mending this state of harmony" (Bilagody 1969, 21).

When the Navaho people emerged from the underworlds, one female was missing. She was subsequently found by a search party in the same hole from which they had initially emerged. She told the people that she had chosen to remain there and wait for their return. She became known as death, sickness, and witchcraft. Because her hair was unraveled and her body was covered with dry red ochre, the Navahos today continue to unravel the hair of their dead and to cover their bodies with red ochre. Members of the Navaho Nation believe that "witchcraft exists and that certain humans, known as witches, are able to interact with the evil spirits. These people can bring sickness and other unhappiness to the people who annoy them" (Bilagody 1969).

Traditionally, illness, disharmony, and sadness are seen by the Navahos as the result of one or more combinations of the following actions: "(1) displeasing the holy people; (2) annoying the elements; (3) disturbing animal and plant life; (4) neglecting the celestial bodies; (5) misuse of a sacred Indian ceremony; or (6) tampering with witches and witchcraft" (Bilagody 1969). If disharmony exists, disease can occur. The Navahos distinguish between two types of disease: (1) contagious diseases, such as measles, smallpox, diphtheria, syphilis, and gonorrhea, and (2) more generalized illnesses, such as "body fever" and "body ache." The notion that illness is caused by a microbe or other physiological agent is alien to the Navahos. The cause of disease, of injury to people or to their property, or of continued misfortune of any kind must be traced back to an action that should not have been performed. Examples of such infractions are breaking a taboo or contacting a ghost or witch. To the Navahos, the treatment of an illness, therefore, must be concerned with the external causative factor(s) and not with the illness or injury itself (Kluckhohn and Leighton 1962, 192–193).

❦ *Traditional Methods of Healing*

TRADITIONAL HEALERS

The traditional healer of Native America is the medicine man or woman, and Indians, by and large, have maintained their faith in him or her over the ages. The medicine men and women are wise in the ways of the land and of nature. They know well the interrelationships of human beings, the earth, and the universe. They know the ways of the plants and animals, the sun, the moon, and the stars. Medicine men and women take time to determine first the cause of the illness and then the proper treatment. To determine the cause and treatment of an illness, they perform special ceremonies that may take up to several days.

As a specific example, Boyd describes the medicine man, Rolling Thunder, the spiritual leader, philosopher, and acknowledged spokesman of the Cherokee and Shoshone tribes, as being able to determine the cause of illness when the ill person does not himself know it. The "diagnostic" phase of the treatment often may take as long as three days. There are numerous causes of physical illness and a great number of reasons—good or bad—for having become ill. These causes are of a spiritual nature. When modern physicians see a sick person, they recognize and diagnose only the physical illness. Medicine men and women, in contrast, look for the spiritual cause of the problem. To the American Indian, "every physical thing in nature has a spiritual nature because the whole is viewed as being essentially spiritual in nature." The agents of nature, herbs, are seen as spiritual helpers, and the characteristics of plants must be known and understood. Rolling Thunder states that "we are born with a purpose in life and we have to fulfill that purpose" (Boyd 1974, 124, 263). The purpose of the medicine man or woman is to cure, and their power is not dying out.

The medicine man or woman of the Hopis uses meditation in determining the cause of an illness and sometimes even uses a crystal ball as the focal point for meditation. At other times the medicine man or woman chews on the root of jimsonweed, a powerful herb that produces a trance. The Hopis claim that this herb gives the medicine man or woman a vision of the evil that caused a sickness. Once the meditation is concluded, the medicine man or woman is able to prescribe the proper herbal treatment. For example, fever is cured by a plant that smells like lightning; the Hopi phrase for fever is "lightning sickness" (Leek 1975, 16).

The Navajo Indians consider disease as the result of breaking a taboo or the attack of a witch. The exact cause is diagnosed by divination, as is the ritual of treatment. There are three types of divination: motion in the hand (the most common form and often practiced by women), stargazing, and listening. The function of the diagnostician is first to determine the cause of the illness and then to recommend the treatment—that is, the type of chant that will be effective and the medicine man or woman who can best do it. A medicine man or woman may be called on to treat obvious symptoms, whereas the diagnostician is called on to ascertain the cause of the illness. (A person is considered wise if the diagnostician is called first.) Often, the same medicine man or woman can practice both divination (diagnosis) and the singing (treatment). When any form of divination is used in making the diagnosis, the diagnostician meets with the family and discusses the patient's condition and determines the fee.

The practice of motion in the hand includes the following rituals: Pollen or sand is sprinkled around the sick person, during which time the diagnostician sits with closed eyes and face turned from the patient. The hand begins to move during the song. While the hand is moving, the diagnostician thinks of various diseases and various causes. When the arm begins to move in a certain way, the diagnostician knows that the right disease and its cause have been discovered. He or she is then able to prescribe the proper treatment (Wyman 1966, 8–14). The ceremony of motion in the hand also may incorporate the use of sand paintings. (These paintings are a well-known form of art.) Four basic colors are used—white, blue, yellow, and black—and each color has a symbolic meaning. Chanting is performed as the painting is produced, and the shape of the painting determines the cause and treatment of the illness. The chants may continue for an extended time (Kluckhohn and Leighton 1962, 230), depending on the family's ability to pay and the capabilities of the singer. The process of motion in the hand can be neither inherited nor learned. It comes to a person suddenly, as a gift. It is said that people able to diagnose their own illnesses are able to practice motion in the hand (Wyman 1966, 14).

Unlike motion in the hand, stargazing can and must be learned. Sand paintings are often but not always made during stargazing. If they are not made, it is either because the sick person cannot afford to have one done or because there is not enough time to make one. The stargazer prays the star prayer to the star spirit, asking it to show the cause of the illness. During stargazing, singing begins and the star throws a ray of light that determines the cause of the patient's illness. If the ray of light is white or yellow, the patient will recover; if it is red, the illness is serious. If a white light falls on the patient's home, the person will recover; if the home is dark, the patient will die (Wyman 1966, 15).

Listening, the third type of divination, is somewhat similar to stargazing, except that something is heard rather than seen. In this instance, the cause of the illness is determined by the sound that is heard. If someone is heard to be crying, the patient will die (Wyman 1966, 16).

The traditional Navajos continue to use medicine men and women when an illness occurs. They use this service because, in many instances, the treatment they receive from these traditional healers is better than the treatment they receive from the health-care establishment. Treatments used by singers include massage and heat treatment, the sweatbath, and use of the yucca root—

approaches similar to those common in physiotherapy (Kluckhohn and Leighton 1962, 230).

The main effects of the singer are psychological. During the chant, the patient feels cared for in a deeply personal way as the center of the singer's attention, since the patient's problem is the reason for the singer's presence. When the singer tells the patient recovery will occur and the reason for the illness, the patient has faith in what is heard. The singer is regarded as a distinguished authority and as a person of eminence with the gift of learning from the holy people. He is considered to be more than a mere mortal. The ceremony—surrounded by such high levels of prestige, mysticism, and power—takes the sick person into its circle, ultimately becoming one with the holy people by participating in the sing that is held in the patient's behalf. The patient once again comes into harmony with the universe and subsequently becomes free of all ills and evil (Kluckhohn and Leighton 1962, 232).

The religion of the Navajos is one of *good hope* when they are sick or suffer other misfortunes. Their system of beliefs and practices helps them through the crises of life and death. The stories that are told during ceremonies give the people a glimpse of a world that has gone by, which promotes a feeling of security because they see that they are links in the unbroken chain of countless generations (Kluckhohn and Leighton 1962, 233).

Many Navajos believe in witchcraft, and when it is considered to be the cause of an illness, special ceremonies are employed to rid the individual of the evil caused by the witches. Numerous methods are employed to manipulate the supernatural. Although many of these activities may meet with strong social disapproval, Navajos recognize the usefulness of blaming witches for illness and misfortune. Tales abound concerning witchcraft and how the witches work. Not all Navajos believe in witchcraft, but for those who do it provides a mechanism for laying blame for the overwhelming hardships and anxieties of life.

Such events as going into a trance can be ascribed to the work of witches. The way to cure a "witched" person is through the use of complicated prayer ceremonies that are attended by friends and relatives, who lend help and express sympathy. The victim of a witch is in no way responsible for being sick and is, therefore, free of any punitive action by the community if the illness causes the victim to behave in strange ways. However, if an incurably "witched" person is affected so that alterations in the person's established role severely disrupt the community, the victim may be abandoned (Kluckhohn and Leighton 1962, 244).

TRADITIONAL REMEDIES

American Indians practice an act of purification in order to maintain their harmony with nature and to cleanse the body and spirit. This is done by total immersion in water in addition to the use of sweat lodges, herb medicines, and special rituals. Purification is seen as the first step in the control of consciousness, a ritual that awakens the body and the senses and prepares a person for meditation. It is viewed by the participants as a new beginning (Boyd 1974, 97–100).

The basis of therapy lies in nature, hence the use of herbal remedies. Specific rituals are to be followed when herbs are gathered. Each plant is picked to be dried for later use. No plant is picked unless it is the proper one, and only enough plants are picked to meet the needs of the gatherers. Timing is crucial, and the procedures are followed meticulously. So deep is their belief in the harmony of human beings and nature that the herb gatherers exercise great care not to disturb any of the other plants and animals in the environment (Boyd 1974, 101–136).

One plant of interest, the common dandelion, contains a milky juice in its stem and is said to increase the flow of milk from the breasts of nursing mothers. Another plant, the thistle, is said to contain a substance that relieves the prickling sensation in the throats of people who live in the desert. The medicine used to hasten the birth of a baby is called "weasel medicine" because the weasel is clever at digging through and out of difficult territory (Leek 1975, 17).

The following is a list of common ailments and herbal treatments used by the Hopi Indians (Leek 1975, 17–26):

1. Cuts and wounds are treated with globe mallow. The root of this plant is chewed to help mend broken bones.
2. To keep air from cuts, piñon gum is applied to the wound. It is used also in an amulet to protect a person from witchcraft.
3. Cliff rose is used to wash wounds.
4. Boils are brought to a head with the use of sand sagebrush.
5. Spider bites are treated with sunflower. The person bathes in water in which the flowers have been soaked.
6. Snakebites are treated with the bladder pod. The bitter root of this plant is chewed and then placed on the bite.
7. Lichens are used to treat the gums. They are ground to a powder and then rubbed on the affected areas.
8. Fleabane is used to treat headaches. The entire herb is either bound to the head or infused and drunk as a tea.
9. Digestive disorders are treated with blue gillia. The leaves are boiled in water and drunk to relieve indigestion.
10. The stem of the yucca plant is used as a laxative. The purple flower of the thistle is used to expel worms.
11. Blanket flower is the diuretic used to provide relief from painful urination.
12. A tea is made from painted cup and drunk to relieve the pain of menstruation.
13. Winter fat provides a tea from the leaves and roots and is drunk if the uterus fails to contract properly during labor.

The use of Indian cures and herbal remedies continues to be popular. Among the Oneida Indians, the following remedies are used (Knox and Adams 1988):

Illness	Remedy
Colds	Witch hazel, sweet flag
Sore throat	Comfrey
Diarrhea	Elderberry flowers
Headache	Tansy and sage
Ear infection	Skunk oil
Mouth sores	Dried raspberry leaves

Among the Micmac Indians of Canada, the following remedies are used (Boston Indian Council 1984):

Illness	Remedy
Warts	Juice from milkweed plant
Obesity	Spruce bark and water
Rheumatism	Juniper berries
Diabetes	Combination of blueberries and huckleberries
Insomnia	Eat a head of lettuce a day
Diarrhea	Tea from wild strawberry

Table 8–2 summarizes the cultural phenomena affecting American Indians, Aleuts, and Eskimos.

Table 8–2 **Examples of Cultural Phenomena Affecting Health Care Among American Indians, Aleuts, and Eskimos**

Nations of Origin:	200 American Indian nations indigenous to North America; Aleuts and Eskimos in Alaska
Environmental Control:	Traditional health and illness beliefs may continue to be observed by "traditional" people Natural and magicoreligious folk medicine tradition Traditional healer—medicine man or woman
Biological Variations:	Accidents Heart disease Cirrhosis of the liver Diabetes mellitus
Social Organization:	Extremely family oriented to both biological and extended families Children are taught to respect traditions Community social organizations
Communication:	Tribal languages Use of silence and body language
Space:	Space is very important and has no boundaries
Time Orientation:	Present

Adapted from: Spector, R. "Culture, Ethnicity, and Nursing," in *Fundamentals of Nursing,* 3d ed., ed. P. Potter and A. Perry, St. Louis: Mosby-Year Book, 1992), p. 101. Reprinted with permission.

❧ Current Health-Care Problems

Today, American Indians are faced with a number of health-related problems. Many of the old ways of diagnosing and treating illness have not survived the migrations and changing ways of life of the people. Because these skills often have been lost and because modern health-care facilities are not always available, Indian peoples are frequently caught in limbo when it comes to obtaining adequate health care. At least one-third of American Indians exist in a state of abject poverty. With this destitution come poor living conditions and attendant problems, as well as diseases of the poor—including malnutrition, tuberculosis, and high maternal and infant death rates. Poverty and isolated living serve as further barriers that keep American Indians from using limited health-care facilities even when they are available. Many of the illnesses that are familiar among white patients may manifest themselves differently in Indian patients.

❧ Morbidity and Mortality

In fiscal year 1998 the Indian Health Service (IHS) population was estimated to be approximately 1.46 million people, nearly 500,000 fewer than the overall American Indian estimated population. The Indian population residing in the IHS services area is younger than the U.S. population, with 33% of the population younger than 15 years old and 6% of the population older than 65. The median age was estimated to be 28.1, again the youngest median of all population groups. The following is a synopsis of several health statistics (Indian Health Service 1997b, 5–6):

- The birthrate for American Indians and Alaska Natives residing in IHS service areas was 25.6 per 1000 population in 1992–1994, which was 65% greater than the 1993 birthrate for the U.S. population.
- The maternal mortality rate for American Indians and Alaska Natives residing in IHS service areas dropped from 27.7 per 100,000 live births in 1972–1974 to 4.0 in 1992–1994, a decrease of 86%.
- The infant mortality rate for American Indians and Alaska Natives residing in IHS service areas dropped from 22.2 per 1000 live births in 1972–1974 to 8.7 in 1992–1994, a decrease of 61%.
- The leading causes of death for American Indians and Alaska Natives living in IHS service areas were diseases of the heart and malignant neoplasms. Table 8–3 displays the leading causes of death for the entire American Indian and Alaska Native population as well as for all person in the United States for 1996.
- During the years 1992–1994 the IHS age-adjusted death rates for the following causes were considerably higher than those of the entire U.S. population:
  1. Alcoholism—579% greater
  2. Tuberculosis—475% greater
  3. Diabetes mellitus—231% greater

Table 8–3	The 10 Leading Causes of Death for American Indians and Alaska Natives, and for all Persons in the United States 1996

American Indians and Alaska Natives	All Persons
1. Diseases of the heart	1. Diseases of the heart
2. Malignant neoplasms	2. Malignant neoplasms
3. Unintentional injuries	3. Cerebrovascular diseases
4. Diabetes mellitus	4. Chronic obstructive pulmonary diseases
5. Cerebrovascular diseases	5. Unintentional injuries
6. Chronic liver disease and cirrhosis	6. Pneumonia and influenza
7. Pneumonia and influenza	7. Diabetes mellitus
8. Suicide	8. Human immunodeficiency virus infection
9. Chronic obstructive pulmonary diseases	9. Suicide
10. Homicide and legal intervention	10. Chronic liver disease and cirrhosis

From: National Center for Health Statistics. *Health United States 1998 with Socioeconomic Status and Health Chartbook.* (Hyattsville, Md., 1998), pp. 212–213.

4. Accidents—212% greater
5. Suicide—70% greater
6. Pneumonia and influenza—61% greater
7. Homicide—41% greater

MENTAL ILLNESS

The family is often a nuclear family, with strong biological and large extended family networks. Children are taught to respect traditions, and community organizations are growing in strength and numbers. Many American Indians tend to use traditional medicines and healers and are knowledgeable about these resources. People may frequently be treated by a traditional medicine man. The sweat lodge and herbs are frequently used to treat mental symptoms. Several diagnostic techniques include the use of divination, conjuring, and stargazing.

"Ghost sickness" affects some American Indian members of Indian nations. This mental health problem involves a preoccupation with death and the deceased and is associated with witchcraft. Symptoms include bad dreams, weakness, feelings of danger, loss of appetite, and confusion. "Pibloktoq" is a malady that afflicts some members of arctic and subarctic Eskimo communities. It is characterized by abrupt dissociative episodes accompanied by extreme excitement followed by convulsive seizures and coma. (American Psychiatric Association 1994).

Alcoholism is a major mental health problem among American Indians. A comparison of the 10 leading causes of death among American Indians/ Alaska Natives and the general population reveals that unintentional injuries (3), chronic liver disease and cirrhosis (6), suicide (8), and homicide and legal intervention (10) rank higher as causes of death than for the population at large. Each of these causes of death is related both to mental health problems and to alcoholism.

FETAL ALCOHOL SYNDROME

"My son will forever travel through a moonless night with only the roar of the wind for company" (Michael Dorris 1989). This quote reflects on the tragedy of fetal alcohol syndrome, an affliction that affects countless American Indian children. The symptoms include:

- Abnormal growth in height, weight, and/or head circumference
- Central nervous system in behavioral and/or mental health problems
- Appearance with a specific pattern of recognizable deformities

An estimated 70,000 fetal alcohol children are born each year in the United States, many of whom are American Indians. Dorris (1989, 231) further points out that the son of an alcoholic biological father is three times more likely to himself become an abusive drinker.

This problem has grown over time and the impact increases with each generation. Mortality and morbidity rates for American Indians are directly affected by alcohol abuse. Alcohol abuse is the most widespread and severe problem in the American Indian community. It is extremely costly to the people and underlies many of their physical, mental, social, and economic problems, and the problem is growing worse. Hawk Littlejohn, the medicine man of the Cherokee Nation, Eastern band, attributes this problem, from a traditional point of view, to the fact that Native Americans have lost the opportunity to make choices. They can no longer choose how they live or how they practice their medicine and religion. He believes that once people return to a sense of identification within themselves, they begin to rid themselves of this problem of alcoholism. Whatever the solution may be, the problem is indeed immense (Littlejohn 1979).

DOMESTIC VIOLENCE

Another problem related to alcohol abuse in the Native American peoples is domestic violence and the battering of women. A battered woman is one who is physically assaulted by her husband, boyfriend, or some significant other. The assault may range from a push to severe, even permanent, injury, to sexual abuse, to child abuse, and to neglect. Once the pattern of abuse is established, subsequent episodes of abuse tend to get worse. This abuse is not traditional in Native American life but has evolved. True Indian love is based on a tradition of mutual respect and the belief that men and women are part of an ordered universe that should live in peace. In the traditional Native American home, children were raised to respect their parents, and they were not corporally punished. Violence toward women was not practiced. In modern times, however, the sanctions and protections against domestic violence have decreased, and the women are far more vulnerable. Many women are reluctant to admit that they are victims of abuse because they believe that they will be blamed for the assault. Hence, the beatings continue. A number of services are available to women who are victims, such as safe houses and support groups. It is believed that the long-range solution to this problem lies in teaching children—to nurture children and give them self-esteem, to teach boys to love and respect women, and to give girls a sense of worth.

Domestic violence has a profound effect on the community and on the family. A pattern of abuse is easily established. It begins with tension: the female attempts to keep peace, but the male cannot contain himself, a fight erupts, and then the crisis arrives. The couple may make up, only to fight again. Attempts to help must be initiated, or the cycle escalates. The problem is extremely complex. Some of the services available to a household experiencing domestic violence include

1. *Tribal health:* direct services for physical and mental health
2. *Law enforcement:* police protection may be necessary
3. *Legal assistance:* assistance for immediate shelter and emergency food and transportation

In addition to alcohol-related problems, recent studies indicate that incidences of both lung cancer in males and breast cancer in females are increasing.

URBAN PROBLEMS

More than 50% of American Indians live in urban areas; for example, in Seattle there are 15,000 Indians. Although this population is not particularly dense, its rates of diphtheria, tuberculosis, otitis media with subsequent hearing defects, alcohol abuse, inadequate immunization, iron-deficiency anemia, childhood developmental lags, mental health problems (including depression, anxiety, and coping difficulties), and caries and other dental problems are high. As in all dysfunctional families, problems arise that are related to marital difficulties and financial strain, which usually are brought about by unemployment and the lack of education or knowledge of special skills. The tension often is compounded further by alcoholism.

Between 5000 and 6000 Indians live in Boston. They experience the same problems as Native Americans in other cities, yet there is an additional problem. Few non-Indian residents are even aware that there is a Native American community in that city or that it is in desperate need of adequate health and social services.

✹ *Health-Care Provider Services*

Some historical differences in health care relate to geographical locations. Indians living in the eastern part of this country and in most urban areas are *not* covered by the services of the Indian Health Service, services which are available to Native Americans living on reservations in the West. In 1923, tribal government—under the control of the Bureau of Indian Affairs—was begun by the Navajos. Treaties were established by the Navahos with the U.S. government, but in the areas of health and education these treaties were not honored by the United States. Health services on the reservations were inadequate. Consequently, the people were sent to outside institutions for the treatment of illnesses such as tuberculosis and mental health problems. As recently as 1930, the vast Navajo lands had only seven hospitals with 25 beds each. Not until 1955 were Indians finally offered concentrated services with modern physicians. Only since 1965 have more comprehensive services been available to the Navajos.

INDIAN HEALTH SERVICE

The Indian Health Service (IHS) is an agency within the Department of Health and Human Services that was established in 1954 by Public Law 83-568, the Transfer Act. It is responsible for providing Federal health services to American Indians and Alaska Natives. The provision of health services to American Indians and Alaska Natives arose out of the special relationship between the Federal government and Indian Nations that has been given form and substance by numerous treaties, laws, Executive Orders, and Supreme Court decisions. The IHS is the principal health-care provider and advocate for American Indians and Alaska Natives, and its goal is to raise their health status to the highest possible level. The mission of the IHS is to provide a comprehensive health services delivery system for American Indians and Alaska Natives with the opportunity for maximum tribal involvement in developing and managing the programs. The IHS comprises the following 12 regional units:

Aberdeen	Billings	Oklahoma City
Alaska	California	Phoenix
Albuquerque	Nashville	Portland
Bemidji	Navajo	Tucson

The IHS operates 37 hospitals, 61 health centers, 4 school health centers, and 48 health stations in 35 states known as reservation states. The service population is American Indians and Alaska Natives identified to be eligible for IHS services and residing in service areas—geographic areas "on or near" reservations. Reservation states include Arizona, Alaska, Texas, Oklahoma, California, and New Mexico. Figure 8–2 depicts the Indian Health Service Area Offices and the number of service units and facilities operated by IHS and tribes as of October 1, 1996 (U.S. Department of Health and Human Services 1997a, 4–17).

American Indians and Alaska Natives receive a full range of services from the IHS, including preventive care, primary medical care (hospital and ambulatory care), community health, alcoholism programs, rehabilitation services, and secondary medical care. The IHS staff includes practitioners from all sectors of the health-care delivery team including nurses, physicians, pharmacists, and dietitians. The community services provide medics, nurse practitioners, and nurse-midwives. One goal of IHS is to educate American Indians and Alaska Natives to adopt health-promoting lifestyles (U.S. Department of Health and Human Services 1977a).

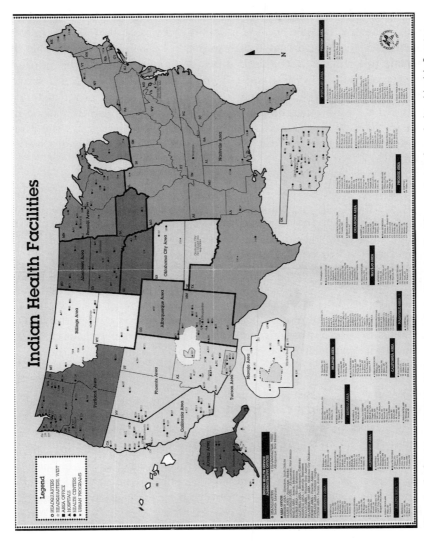

Figure 8-2 Map of IHS facilities and regions. (Reprinted with permission from Indian Health Service. U.S. Department of Health and Human Services. Public Health Service Information Brochure, 1994)

ELIGIBILITY FOR HEALTH CARE

Proposals have been made to redefine eligibility for Indian Health Services that would significantly change the distribution of health-care services. Present regulations stipulate that people are eligible for services if they are of Indian descent and belong to an Indian community served by IHS. No distinction is made concerning the degree of Indian ancestry or specific tribal affiliation as long as the person lives in an area served by IHS. The proposed changes would stipulate that an Indian must (1) be a member or eligible for membership in a federally recognized tribe, (2) be of one quarter or more Indian or Alaska Native ancestry, and (3) reside in a designated health service delivery area. Indian blood quantum is made on the basis of proof of Indian blood by tribal origin, and the proof must be verified by the Bureau of Indian Affairs. The minimal blood quantum level is one-fourth, and the numbers of people with this level or higher are declining (Basherhshur, Steeler, and Murphy 1989).

The ineligibility of Native Americans living on the East Coast to secure such services has caused numerous difficulties for needy Indians.* The providers of health care generally seem to think that Indians should receive health services from the Indian Health Service and try to send them there. Unfortunately, there simply is no Indian Health Service on the East Coast, so Native Americans tend to be shifted around among the regional health-care resources that are available.

Many providers of health-care and social services are not aware that many of the Indians on the East Coast have dual citizenship as a result of the Jay Treaty of 1794, which allows for international citizenship between the United States and Canada, a fact that raises questions about whether Indians can freely cross the border between the United States and Canada and whether those who live in the United States are eligible for welfare or Medicaid.

CULTURAL AND COMMUNICATION PROBLEMS

A factor that inhibits the Indian use of white-dominated health services is a deep, cultural problem: Indians suffer disease when they come into contact with the white health-care provider.† Native Americans feel uneasy because for too many years they have been the victim of haphazard care and disrespectful treatment. All too often conflict arises between what the Native Americans perceive their illness to be and what the physician may diagnose. Native Ameri-

---

*The situation stems from the Indian Renewal Act of 1840 and the Dawes Act of 1887, legislation that disbanded tribes east of the Mississippi and established reservations west of the Mississippi.
†Dr. Red Horse explains the phenomenon of "Indian paranoia" that emerges in a predictable behavior: "It is *not* a sickness but an 'interactive reality' that Native Americans suffer whenever visits to non-Indian clinics are imminent. *Fear* is a variable and often when the fear is too great, help is not sought. For example, if a Native American child has a toothache, the parents may not take the child to the dentist because they fear the dentist's demeaning attitude."

cans, like most people, do not enjoy long waits in clinics, the separation from their families, the unfamiliar, regimented environment of the hospital, or the unfamiliar behavior of the nurses and physicians, who often display demeaning and demanding attitudes. Their response to this treatment varies. Sometimes they remain silent; other times they leave and do not return. Many Native Americans request that if the ailment is not an emergency, they be allowed to see the medicine man first and then receive treatment from the physician. Often when a sick person is afraid of receiving the care of a physician, the medicine man encourages him to go to the hospital.

Health-care providers must be aware of several factors when they communicate with Native Americans. One of them is recognition of the importance of nonverbal communication. Often Native Americans observe the provider and say very little. The patient may expect the provider to deduce the problem through instinct rather than by the extensive use of questions during history taking. In part, this derives from the belief that direct quoting is intrusive on individual privacy. When examining a Native American with an obvious cough, the provider might be well advised to use a declarative statement— "You have a cough that keeps you awake at night"—and then allow time for the client to respond to the statement.

It is Indian practice to converse in a very low tone of voice. It is expected that the listener will pay attention and listen carefully in order to hear what is being said. It is considered impolite to say, "Huh?" "I beg your pardon," or to give any indication that the communication was not heard. Therefore, an effort should be made to speak with clients in a quiet setting where they will be heard more easily.

Note taking is taboo. Indian history has been passed through generations by means of verbal story telling. Native Americans are sensitive about note taking while they are speaking. When one is taking a history or interviewing, it may be preferable to use memory skills rather than to record notes. This more conversational approach may encourage greater openness between the client and the provider.

Another factor to be considered is differing perceptions of time between the Native American client and the provider. Life on the reservation is not governed by the clock but by the dictates of need. When an Indian moves from the reservation to an urban area, this cultural conflict concerning time often exhibits itself as lateness for specific appointments. One solution would be the use of walk-in clinics.

AMERICAN INDIAN HEALTH-CARE MANPOWER

The number of Native Americans enrolled in most health programs in selected health professions is low. Tables 8–4 and 8–5 give the relative enrollment compared with total program enrollment and non-Hispanic white enrollment. Efforts must be made to recruit, maintain, and graduate more American Indians into the health professions.

| *Table 8–4* | **American Indian Enrollment in Selected Health Professions Schools, 1995–1996** |

	Total Program Enrollment	American Indian Enrollment
Allopathic medicine	66,970	501
Osteopathic medicine	8,475	85
Podiatry	2,312	12
Dentistry	16,374	73
Optometry	5,178	22
Pharmacy	33,205	151
Registered nursing	261,219	1,900

From: National Center for Health Statistics. *Health United States 1998 with Socioeconomic Status and Health Chartbook.* (Hyattsville, Md., 1998), pp. 330–331.

| *Table 8–5* | **Percentage of American Indian Enrollment in Selected Health Professions Schools Compared with Non-Hispanic White, 1995–1996 Enrollment** |

Profession	Non-Hispanic White (%)	American Indian (%)
Allopathic medicine	66.6	0.7
Osteopathic medicine	80.3	1.0
Podiatry	77.2	0.5
Dentistry	68.0	0.4
Optometry	75.4	0.4
Pharmacy	71.9	0.5
Registered nurses	82.4	0.7

From: National Center for Health Statistics. *Health, United States, 1998, with Socioeconomic Status and Health Chartbook.* (Hyattsville, Md., 1998), pp. 330–331.

❋ *References*

American Indian Women of Minnesota, Inc n.d. Battered Women—Definition. Through a grant sponsored by the Department of Corrections, Minnesota State Task Force on Battered Women, Minnesota Council of Churches and the American Lutheran Church.

———. 1984. The Dakota View of Domestic Violence. *The Circle Newspaper of the Boston Indian Council* (February/March): 8–10.

American Psychiatric Association. 1994. *Diagnostic and Statistical Manual of Mental Disorders,* 4th ed. Washington, D.C.

Basherhshur, R., Steeler, W., and Murphy, T. 1989. On Changing Indian Eligibility or Health Care. *American Journal of Public Health* 77 (May): 690–693.

Bilagody, H. 1969. An American Indian Looks at Health Care. In *The Ninth Annual Training Institute for Psychiatrist-Teachers of Practicing Physicians,* edited by R. Feldman and D. Buch. Boulder, Colo.: WICHE, No. 3A30.

Boyd, D. 1974. *Rolling Thunder*. New York: Random House. 1974.

Brown, D. 1970. *Bury My Heart at Wounded Knee*. New York: Holt.

Deloria, V. Jr. 1969. *Custer Died for Your Sins*. New York: Avon Books.

———. 1974. *Behind the Trail of Broken Treaties*. New York: Delacorte.

Dorris, M. 1989. *The Broken Cord*. New York: Harper & Row.

Fortney, A. J. 1977. Has White Man's Lease Expired? *Boston Sunday Globe* (23 January).

Kluckhohn, C., and Leighton, D. 1962. *The Navaho*, rev. ed. Garden City, NY: Doubleday.

Knox, M. E., and Adams, L. 1988. Traditional Health Practices of the Oneida Indian. Research report. College of Nursing, University of Wisconsin at Oshkosh.

Leek, S. 1975. *Herbs: Medicine and Mysticism*. Chicago: Henry Regnery.

Littlejohn, H. 1979. Interview. Boston State College, Boston, Mass. 9 June.

National Center for Health Statistics. 1998. *Health, United States, 1998, with Socioeconomic Status and Health Chartbook*. Hyattsville, Md.

Primeaux, H. 1977. American Indian Health Care Practices: A Cross-Cultural Perspective. *Nursing Clinics of North America* 12(1) (March): 57.

Spector, R. 1992. Culture, Ethnicity, and Nursing. In *Fundamentals of Nursing*, 3d ed., edited by P. Potter, and A. Perry. St. Louis: Mosby-Year Book.

U.S. Department of Health and Human Services. 1992. *Healthy People 2000. National Health Promotion and Disease Prevention Objectives—Full Report with Commentary*. Boston: Jones and Bartlett.

———. 1997a. *Comprehensive Health Care Program for American Indians and Alaska Natives*. Rockville, Md: Public Health Service, Indian Health Service.

———1997b. Regional Differences in Indian Health, Rockville, Md: Public Health Service, Indian Health Service.

———. 1997c. *Trends in Indian Health*. Rockville, Md: Public Health Service, Indian Health Service.

———. 1998. *Health United States 1998 with Socioeconomic Status and Health Chartbook*. Hyattsville, Md: Centers for Disease Control and Prevention.

Wyman, L. C. 1966. Navaho Diagnosticians. In *Medical Care*, edited by W. R. Scott and E. H. Volkhart. New York: Wiley.

Zuckoff, M. 1995. More and More Claiming American Indian Heritage. *Boston Globe*. 18 April.

*Figure 8–1 from page 175

From left to right—top to bottom: This chapter-opening quilt panel of HEALTH-related images depicts objects people of North American Indian heritage may use to protect, maintain, and/or restore their physical, mental, or spiritual HEALTH. The **storyteller** represents the art of storytelling, which is a fundamental way by which the traditions are handed down from one generation to the next in the form of sacred stories. The **basket,** woven by a MicMac woman, depicts the art of basket weaving, which is an essential art in American Indian life. The tiny bead-crafted **cradle board** from the MicMac Nation not only represents a way of carrying on the craft of beading but also demonstrates the way a newborn baby is cared for and carried by the mother. The **beaded necklace** is from the Cherokee Nation—Real People. The beads represent tears of sorrow, grief, and hopelessness; the corn seeds look like tears and are the color of sorrow. The necklace is worn by Cherokee women as a reminder of the Trail of Tears. The **clay medicine bowl** of the American Indians in New Mexico has sacred corn meal placed in it and a small bear amulet; it is placed in a sacred part of the home to protect the home. The **bear** is a sacred animal to American Indians, as it is symbolic of the power of nature and the healing in nature. **Sweet grass** from the American Indian Sioux Nation is burned, and the smoke is used to purify a room or home. The **medicine bag** from the Acama Pueblo in New Mexico is used to hold herbs used in restoring health. The **baby net** is from the Acho Dene Nation in Canada. Traditional lore says that if you keep this baby net near your baby, it will filter out illness and keep the baby well.

Chapter 9

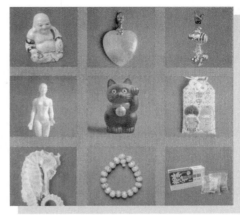

HEALTH and Illness in the Asian/Pacific Islander American Community

"But when she arrived in the new country, the immigration officials pulled her swan away from her leaving the woman fluttering her arms and with only one swan feather for a memory."

—Amy Tan

The more than 11 million people who constitute the Asian and Pacific Islander communities are the nation's third largest emerging majority group. This group is characterized by its diversity: more than 30 different languages are spoken and there are a similar number of cultures (Martin 1992). The National Center for Health Statistics is now using the following categories to code this population:

Coded prior to 1992	Expanded coding beginning with 1992
Chinese	Vietnamese
Japanese	Asian Indian
Hawaiian	Korean
Filipino	Samoan
Other API	Guamanian
	Remaining API

This chapter focuses on the traditional health and illness beliefs and practices of the Chinese Americans because those of many of the other Asians/Pacific Islanders are derived in part from the Chinese tradition.

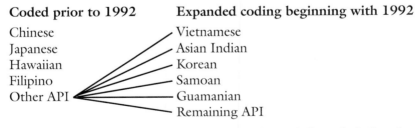

Figure 9–1 (From left to right, top to bottom) Figure of Buddha, jade, diashi (omanori), acupuncture figurine, cat figurine, amulet, sea horse, beaded bracelet, essence of tienchi flowers. *(For more information on each picture see explanation at the end of chapter.*)*

🌸 *Background*

Chinese immigration to the United States began over 100 years ago. In 1850 there were only 1000 Chinese inhabitants in this country; in 1880 there were well over 100,000. This rapid increase occurred in part because of the discovery of gold in California and in part because of the need for cheap labor to build the transcontinental railroads. The immigrants were laborers who met the needs of the dominant society. Like many early immigrant groups, they came here intending only to stay as temporary workers. Mainly men came. They clung closely to their customs and beliefs and stayed together in their own communities. The hopes that many had for a better life when they came to the United States did not materialize. Subsequently, many of the workers and their kin returned to China before 1930. Part of the disharmony and disenchantment occurred because these immigrants were not white and did not have the same culture and habits as whites. For these reasons, they were not welcomed, and many jobs were not open to them. For example, Chinese immigrant workers were excluded from many mining, construction, and other hard-labor jobs even though the transcontinental railroad was constructed mainly by Chinese laborers. Between 1880 and 1930, the Chinese population declined by nearly 20%. One factor that helped perpetuate this decline in population was a series of exclusion acts halting further immigration. The people who remained behind were relegated to menial jobs, such as cooking and dishwashing. The Chinese workers first took these jobs in the West and later moved eastward throughout the United States. They tended to move to cities where they were allowed to let their entrepreneurial talents surface—their main pursuits included running small laundries, food shops, and restaurants.

The people settled in tightly knit groups in urban neighborhoods that took the name "Chinatown." Here they were able to maintain the ancient traditions of their homeland. They were hard workers, and in spite of the dull, menial jobs usually available to them, they were able to survive.

Both U.S. immigration laws and political problems in China had an effect on the nature of today's Chinese population. When the exclusion acts were passed, many men were left alone in this country without the possibility that their families would join them. For this reason, a great majority of the men spent many years alone. In addition, the political oppression experienced by the Chinese in the United States was compounded when, at a time immigration laws were relaxed here after World War II, people were unable to return to or leave China because of that country's restrictive new regulations. By 1965, however, a large number of refugees who had relatives here were able to come to this country. They settled in the Chinatowns of America, causing the population of these areas to swell. The rate of increase since 1965 has been 10% per year.

❧ *Traditional Definitions of* HEALTH *and Illness*

[handwritten: preventive emphasis]

Chinese medicine teaches that health is a state of spiritual and physical harmony with nature. In ancient China, the task of the physician was to prevent illness. A first-class physician not only cured an illness but could also prevent disease from occurring. A second-class physician had to wait for patients to become ill before they could be treated. The physician was paid by the patient while the patient was healthy. When illness occurred, payments stopped. Indeed, not only was the physician not paid for his services when the patient became ill, but he also had to provide and pay for the needed medicine (Mann 1972, 222).

To understand the Chinese philosophy of health and illness, it is necessary to look back at the age-old philosophies from which more current ideas have evolved. The foundation rests in the religion and philosophy of Taoism. Taoism originated with a man named Lao-Tzu, who is believed to have been born about 604 B.C. The word *Tao* has several meanings: way, path, or discourse. On the spiritual level, it is the way of ultimate reality. It is the way of all nature, the primeval law that regulates all heavenly and earthly matters. To live according to the Tao, one must adapt oneself to the order of nature. Chinese medical works revere the ancient sages who knew the way and "led their lives in *Tao*" (Smith 1958, 175–192).

The Chinese view the universe as a vast, indivisible entity, and each being has a definite function within it. No one thing can exist without the existence of the others. Each is linked in a chain that consists of concepts related to each other in harmonious balance. Violating this harmony is like hurling chaos, wars, and catastrophes on humankind—the end result of which is illness. Individuals must adjust themselves wholly within the environment. Five elements—wood, fire, earth, metal, and water—constitute the guiding principles of humankind's surroundings. These elements can both create and destroy each other. For example, "wood creates fire," "two pieces of wood rubbed together produce a spark," "wood destroys earth," "the tree sucks strength from the earth." The guiding principles arise from this "correspondences" theory of the cosmos (Wallnöfer and von Rattauscher 1972, 12–16, 19–21). Tables 9–1 and 9–2 highlight common elements of Asian/Pacific Island cultures and give examples of cultural phenomena affecting health care.

For a person to remain healthy, his or her actions must conform to the mobile cycle of the correspondences. The exact directions for achieving this were written in such works as the *Lu Chih Ch'un Ch'iu* (Spring and Autumn Annals) written by Lu Pu Wei, who died circa 230 B.C.

The *holistic concept*, as explained by Dr. P. K. Chan (1988), is an important idea of traditional Chinese medicine in preventing and treating diseases. It has two main components:

1. A human body is regarded as an integral organism, with special emphasis on the harmonic and integral interrelationship between the viscera

| Table 9-1 | Highlights of Common Elements of Asian Cultures |

The teachings of Asian religions, including Confucianism and Buddhism, are complementary and have played a major role in the shaping of the cultural values in Asia.

Buddhism teaches:

- Harmony/nonconfrontation—(silence as a virtue)
- Respect for life
- Moderation in behavior, self-discipline, patience, humility, modesty, friendliness, self-lessness, dedication, and loyalty to others
- Individualism devalued

Confucianism teaches:

- Achievement of harmony through observing the five basic relationships of society
  1. Ruler and ruled
  2. Father and son
  3. Husband and wife
  4. Older and younger brother
  5. Between friends
- Hierarchical roles, social class system, clearly defined behavioral code
- Importance of family
- Filial piety and respect for elders
- High regard for education and learning

Taoism teaches:

- Harmony between humans and nature
- Nature is benign because *yin* (evil) and *yang* (good) are in balance and harmony.
- Happiness and a long life
- Charity, simplicity, patience, avoidance of confrontation and an indirect approach to problems

Shamanism teaches:

- Emphasis on nature
- Everything in nature is endowed with a spirit

From: Romo, R. G. "Hispanic Health Traditions and Issues. Presented at the Minnesota Health Educators Conference, *Health Education: Expanding Our Horizons,* May 3, 1995. Reprinted with permission.

and the superficial structures in these close physiological connections, and their mutual pathological connection. In Chinese medicine, the local pathological changes always are considered in conjunction with other tissues and organs of the entire body, instead of considered alone.

2. Special attention is paid to the integration of the human body with the external environment. The onset, evolution, and change of disease are considered in conjunction with the geographic, social, and other environmental factors.

Table 9–2	**Examples of Cultural Phenomena Affecting Health Care Among Americans of Asian/Pacific Islander Heritage**
Nations of Origin:	China, Japan, Hawaii, the Philippines, Vietnam, Asian India, Korea, Samoa, Guam, and the remaining Asian/Pacific islands
Environmental Control:	Traditional health and illness beliefs may continue to be observed by "traditional" people
Biological Variations:	Hypertension
	Liver cancer
	Stomach cancer
	Coccidioidomycosis
	Lactose intolerance
	Thalassemia
Social Organization:	Family—hierarchical structure, loyalty
	Large, extended family networks
	Devotion to tradition
	Many religions, including Taoism, Buddhism, Islam, and Christianity
	Community social organizations
Communication:	National language preference
	Dialects, written characters
	Use of silence
	Nonverbal and contextual cueing
Space:	Noncontact people
Time Orientation:	Present

Adapted from: Spector, R. "Culture, Ethnicity, and Nursing. In *Fundamentals of Nursing,* ed. P. Potter and A. Perry. St. Louis: Mosby-Year Book, 1992), p. 101. Reprinted with permission.

Four thousand years before the English physician William Harvey described the circulatory system in 1628, *Huang-ti Nei Ching* (Yellow Emperor's Book of Internal Medicine) was written. This is the first known volume that describes the circulation of blood. It described the oxygen-carrying powers of blood and defined the two basic world principles: *yin* and *yang,* powers that regulate the universe. *Yang* represents the male, positive energy that produces light, warmth, and fullness. *Yin* represents the female, negative energy—the force of darkness, cold, and emptiness. Yin and yang exert power not only over the universe but also over human beings.

Yin and yang were further explained by Dr. Chan as having been originally a philosophical theory in ancient China. Later, the theory was incorporated into Chinese medicine. The theory holds that "everything in the Universe contains two aspects—yin and yang, which are in opposition and also in unison. Hence, matters are impelled to develop and change." In traditional Chinese medicine, the phenomena are further explained as follows:

- Matters that are dynamic, external, upward, ascending, and brilliant belong to yang.

- Those that are static, internal, downward, descending, dull, regressive, and hypoactive are yin.
- Yin flourishing and yang vivified steadily is the state of health. Yin and yang regulate themselves in the basic principle to promote the normal activities of life.
- Illness is the disharmony of yin and yang, a disharmony that leads to pathological changes, with excesses of one and deficiencies of the other, disturbances of vital energy and blood, malfunctioning of the viscera, and so forth (Chan 1988).

The various parts of the human body correspond to the dualistic principles of yin and yang. The inside of the body is yin; the surface of the body is yang. The front part of the body is yin; the back is yang. The five *ts'ang* viscera—liver, heart, spleen, lungs, and kidney—are yang; the six *fu* structures—gallbladder, stomach, large intestine, small intestine, bladder, and "warmer"—are yin. (The "warmer" is now believed to be the lymph system.) The diseases of winter and spring are yin; those of summer and fall are yang. The pulses are controlled by yin and yang. If yin is too strong, the person is nervous and apprehensive and catches colds easily. If the individual does not balance yin and yang properly, his or her life will be short. Half of the yin forces are depleted by age 40, at 40 the body is sluggish, and at 60 the yin is totally depleted, at which time the body deteriorates. Yin stores the vital strength of life. Yang protects the body from outside forces, and it too must be carefully maintained. If yang is not cared for, the viscera are thrown into disorder, and circulation ceases. Yin and yang cannot be injured by evil influences. When yin and yang are sound, the person lives in peaceful interaction with mind and body in proper order (Wallnöfer and von Rattauscher 1972).

Chinese medicine has a long history. The Emperor Shen Nung, who died in 2697 B.C. was known as the patron god of agriculture. He was given this title because of the 70 experiments he performed on himself by swallowing a different plant every day and studying the effects. During this period of self-experimentation, Nung discovered many poisonous herbs and rendered them harmless by the use of antidotes, which he also discovered. His patron element was fire, for which he was known as the Red Emperor. The Emperor Shen Nung was followed by Huang-ti, whose patron element was earth. Huang-ti was known as the Yellow Emperor and ruled from 2697 B.C. to 2595 B.C. The greater part of his life was devoted to the study of medicine. Many people ascribe to him the recording of the *Nei Ching,* the book that embraces the entire realm of Chinese medical knowledge. The treatments described in the *Nei Ching*—which became characteristic of Chinese medical practice—are almost totally aimed at reestablishing balances that are lost within the body when illness occurs. Disrupted harmonies are regarded as the sole cause of disease. Surgery was rarely resorted to, and when it was, it was used primarily to remove malignant tumors. The *Nei Ching* is a dialogue between Huang-ti and his minister, Ch'i Po. It begins with the concept of the Tao and the cosmological patterns of the universe and goes on to describe the powers of the yin and yang. This learned treatise discusses in great detail the therapy of the pulses and how a diagnosis can be made on the basis of alterations in the pulse beat. It also describes various kinds of fevers and the use of acupuncture (Wallnöfer and von Rattauscher 1972, 26–28).

The Chinese view their bodies as a gift given to them by their parents and forebears. A person's body is not his or her personal property. It must be cared for and well maintained. Confucius taught that "only those shall be truly revered who at the end of their lives will return their physical bodies whole and sound."

The body is composed of five solid organs *(ts'ang)*, which collect and store secretions, and five hollow organs *(fu)*, which excrete. The heart and liver are regarded as the noble organs. The head is the storage chamber for knowledge, the back is the home of the chest, the loins store the kidneys, the knees store the muscles, and the bones store the marrow.

The Chinese view the functions of the various organs as comparable to the functions of persons in positions of power and responsibility in the government. For example, the heart is the ruler over all other civil servants, the lungs are the administrators, the liver is the general who initiates all the strategic actions, and the gallbladder is the decision maker.

The organs have a complex relationship that maintains the balance and harmony of the body. Each organ is associated with a color. For example, the heart—which works in accordance with the pulse, controls the kidneys, and harmonizes with bitter flavors—is red. In addition, the organs have what is referred to as an "aura," the meaning of which, in the medical context, is health. The aura is determined by the color of the organ. In the balanced, healthy body, the colors look fresh and shiny.

Disease is caused by an upset in the balance of yin and yang. The weather, too, has an effect on the body's balance and the body's relationship to yin and yang. For example, heat can be injurious to the heart, and cold is injurious to the lungs. Overexertion is harmful to the body. Prolonged sitting is harmful to the flesh and spine, and prolonged lying in bed can be harmful to the lungs.

Disease is diagnosed by the Chinese physician through inspection and palpation. During inspection, the Chinese physician looks at the tongue (glossoscopy), listens and smells (osphretics), and asks questions (anamnesis). During palpation, the physician feels the pulse (sphygmopalpation).

The Chinese believe that there are many different pulse types, which are all grouped together and must be felt with the three middle fingers. The pulse is considered the storehouse of the blood, and a person with a strong, regular pulse is considered to be in good health. By the nature of the pulse, the physician is able to determine various illnesses. For example, if the pulse is weak and skips beats, the person may have a cardiac problem. If the pulse is too strong, the person's body is distended (Wallnöfer and von Rottauscher 1972).

There are six different pulses, three in each hand. Each pulse is specifically related to various organs, and each pulse has its own characteristics. According to ancient Chinese sources, there are 15 ways of characterizing the pulses. Each of these descriptions accurately determines the diagnosis. There are seven *piao* pulses (superficial) and eight *li* pulses (sunken). An example of an illness that manifests with a *piao* pulse is headache; anxiety manifests with a *li* pulse. The pulses also take on a specific nature with various conditions. For example, specific pulses are associated with epilepsy, pregnancy, and the time just before death.

The Chinese physician is aided in making a diagnosis by the appearance of the patient's tongue. More than 100 conditions can be determined by glossoscopic examination. The color of the tongue and the part of the tongue that does not appear normal are the essential clues to the diagnosis.

Breast cancer has been known to the Chinese since early times. "The disease begins with a knot in the breast, the size of a bean, and gradually swells to the size of an egg. After seven or eight months it perforates. When it has perforated, it is very difficult to cure" (Wallnöfer and von Rottauscher 1972).

❀ *Traditional Methods of* HEALTH *Maintenance and Protection*

The Chinese often prepare amulets to prevent evil spirits. These amulets consist of a charm with an idol or Chinese character painted in red or black ink and written on a strip of yellow paper. These amulets are hung over a door or pasted on a curtain or wall, worn in the hair, or placed in a red bag and pinned on clothing. The paper may be burned and the ashes mixed in hot tea and swallowed to ward off evil. Jade is believed to be the most precious of all stones because it is seen as the giver of children, health, immortality, wisdom, power, victory, growth, and food. Jade charms are worn to bring health, and should they turn dull or break, the wearer will surely meet misfortune. The charm prevents harm and accidents. Children are kept safe with jade charms, and adults are made pure, just, humane, and intelligent by wearing them (Morgan [1942] 1972, 133–134).

❀ *Traditional Methods of* HEALTH *Restoration*

TRADITIONAL HEALERS

The physician was the primary healer in Chinese medicine. Physicians who had to treat women encountered numerous difficulties because men were not allowed to touch directly women who were not family members. Thus, a diagnosis might be made through a ribbon that was attached to the woman's wrist. As an alternative to demonstrating areas of pain or discomfort on a woman's body, an alabaster figure was substituted. The area of pain was pointed out on the figurine (Dolan 1973, 30).

Not much is known about women doctors except that they did exist. Women were known to possess a large store of medical talent. There were also midwives and female shamans. The female shamans possessed gifts of prophecy. They danced themselves into ecstatic trances and had a profound effect on the people around them. As the knowledge that these women possessed was neither known nor understood by the general population, they were feared rather than respected. They were said to know all there was to know about life, death, and birth.

CHINESE PEDIATRICS

Babies are breastfed because neither cows' milk nor goats' milk is acceptable to the Chinese. Sometimes children are nursed for as long as four or five years.

Since early time the Chinese have known about and practiced immunization against smallpox. A child was inoculated with the live virus from the crust of a pustule from a smallpox victim. The crust was ground into a powder, and this powder was subsequently blown into the nose of the healthy child through the lumen of a small tube. If the child was healthy, he did not generally develop a full-blown case of smallpox but instead acquired immunity to this dreaded disease (Wallnöfer and von Rottauscher).

ACUPUNCTURE

Acupuncture is an ancient Chinese practice of puncturing the body to cure disease or relieve pain. The body is punctured with special metal needles at points that are precisely predetermined for the treatment of specific symptoms. According to one source, the earliest use of this method was recorded between 106 B.C. and A.D. 200. According to other sources, however, it was used even earlier. This treatment modality stems from diagnostic procedures described earlier. The most important aspect of the practice of acupuncture is the acquired skill and ability to know precisely where to puncture the skin. Nine needles are used in acupuncture, each with a specific purpose. The following is a list of the needles and their purposes (Wallnöfer and von Rottauscher).

- Superficial pricking: arrowhead needle
- Massaging: round needle
- Knocking or pressing: blunt needle
- Venous pricking: sharp three-edged needle
- Evacuating pus: swordlike needle
- Rapid pricking: sharp, round needle
- Puncturing thick muscle: sharp, round needle
- Puncturing thick muscle: long needle
- Treating arthritis: large needle
- Most extensively used: filiform needle

The specific points of the body into which the needles are inserted are known as *meridians*. Acupuncture is based on the concept that certain meridians extend internally throughout the body in a fixed network. There are 365 points on the skin where these lines emerge. Since all the networks merge and have their outlets on the skin, the way to treat internal problems is to puncture the meridians, which are also categorically identified in terms of yin and yang, as are the diseases. The treatment goal is to restore the balance of yin and yang (Wallnöfer and von Rottauscher). The practice of this art is far too complex to explain in great detail in these pages.

Readers may find it interesting to visit acupuncture clinics in their area. After the therapist carefully explains the art and science of acupuncture, one may be able to grasp the fundamental concepts of this ancient treatment. The practice of acupuncture is based in antiquity, yet it took a long time for it to be accepted as a legitimate method of healing by practitioners of the Western medical system. Currently, numerous acupuncture clinics attract a fair number of non-Asians, and acupuncture is being used as a method of anesthesia in some hospitals.

MOXIBUSTION

Moxibustion has been practiced for as long as acupuncture. Its purpose, too, is to restore the proper balance of yin and yang. Moxibustion is based on the therapeutic value of heat, whereas acupuncture is a cold treatment. Acupuncture is used mainly in diseases in which there is an excess of yang, and moxibustion is used in diseases in which there is an excess of yin. Moxibustion is performed by heating pulverized wormwood and applying this concoction directly to the skin over certain specific meridians. Great caution must be used in this application because it cannot be applied to all the meridians that are used for acupuncture. Moxibustion is believed to be most useful during the period of labor and delivery, if applied properly.

Other important traditional HEALTH restoring practices are cupping, bleeding, and massage (*Tui Na*).

- Cupping, as seen in Figures 9–2 a and b involves creating a vacuum in a small glass by burning the oxygen out of it, then promptly placing the glass on the person's skin surface. Cupping draws blood and lymph to the body's surface that is under the cup. This increases the local circulation. The purpose for doing this is to remove cold and damp "evils" from the body and/or to assist blood circulation. The procedure is frequently used to treat lung congestion.
- Bleeding, often done with the use of leeches, is performed to "remove heat from the body." Only small amounts of blood are removed.
- Massage, *Tui Na*, "pushing and pulling" is a complex system of massage or manual acupuncture point stimulation that is used on orthopedic and neurological conditions (Ergil 1996, 208–209).

HERBAL REMEDIES

Medicinal herbs were used widely in the practice of ancient Chinese healing. Many of these herbs are available and in use today.

Herbology is an interesting subject. The gathering season of an herb was important for its effect. It was believed that some herbs were better if gathered at night and that others were more effective if gathered at dawn. The ancient sages understood quite well the dynamics of growth. It is known today that a plant may not be effective if the dew has been allowed to dry on its leaves. The herbalist believes that the ginseng root must be harvested only at midnight in a full moon if it is to have therapeutic value. Ginseng's therapeutic value is due to its nonspecific action. The herb, which is derived from the root of a plant that resembles a man,* is recommended for use in more than two dozen ailments, including anemia, colics, depression, indigestion, impotence, and rheumatism (Wallnöfer and von Rottauscher). It has maintained its reputation for centuries and continues to be a highly valued and widely used substance.

To release all the therapeutic properties of ginseng and to prepare it properly are of paramount importance. Ginseng must not be prepared in anything made of metal because it is believed that some of the necessary constituents are leeched out by the action of the metal. It must be stored in crockery. It is boiled in water until only a sediment remains. This sediment is pressed into a crock and stored. Some of the specific uses of ginseng are (Wallnöfer and von Rottauscher 1972):

- *To stimulate digestion*—Rub ginseng to a powder, mix with the white of an egg, and take three times per day.
- *As a sedative*—Prepare a light broth of ginseng and bamboo leaves.
- *For faintness after childbirth*—Administer a strong brew of ginseng several times a day.
- *As a restorative for frail children*—Give a dash of raw, minced ginseng several times per day.

There are many Chinese medicinal herbs, but none is so famous as ginseng.

I had the opportunity to visit, with one of my Asian American students, an import–export store in Boston's Chinatown where they sell Chinese herbs—if one has the proper prescriptions. The front of the store is a gift shop that attracts tourists. A room in the back is separated from the rest of the store. We were allowed to enter this room when the student explained to the proprietor, in Chinese, that I was her teacher and that she had brought me to the store to purchase herbs. We stayed there for quite a long time, observing the people who came in with prescriptions. The man carefully weighed different herbs, mixed them together, and dispensed them. We asked to purchase some of the herbs that he took from the drawers lining the entire wall behind him. He refused to sell us anything except some of the preparations that were on the counter because a prescription was necessary to purchase any of the herbal compounds that he prepared. Undaunted, we purchased a wide variety of herbs that could be used for indigestion, in addition to ointments and liniments used for sore muscles and sprains.

In addition to herbs and plants, the Chinese use other products with medicinal and healing properties. Some of these products were also used in an-

*Early Chinese healers believed that if the name of a plant resembled the disease in question, the plant would be effective in the treatment of the disease.

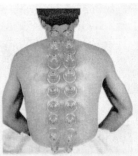

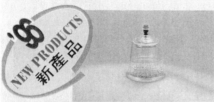
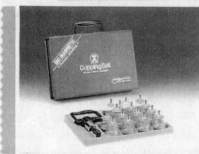
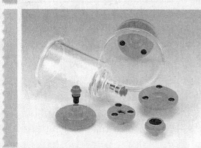

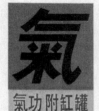

Figure 9-2a Cupping.

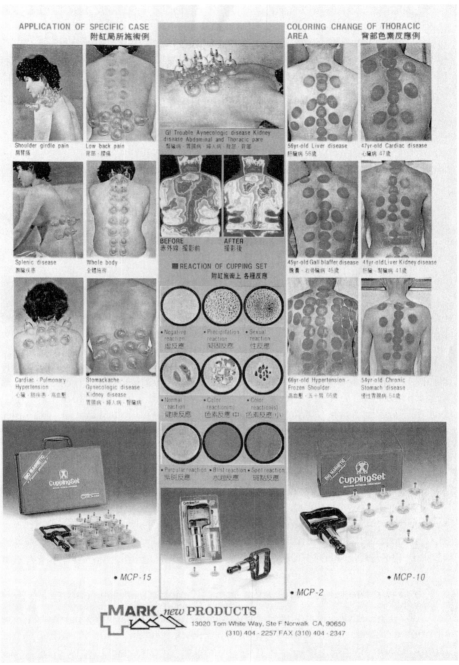

Figure 9–2b Cupping.

cient Europe and are still used today. For example, in China, boys' urine was used to cure lung diseases, soothe inflamed throats, and dissolve blood clots in pregnant women. In Europe, it was used during the two world wars as emergency treatment for open wounds. Urea is still used today as a treatment that promotes the healing of wounds. Other popular Chinese remedies include

- *Deer antlers*—Used to strengthen bones, increase a man's potency, and dispel nightmares
- *Lime calcium*—Used to clear excessive mucus
- *Quicksilver*—Used externally to treat venereal diseases
- *Rhinoceros horns*—Highly effective when applied to pus boils; an antitoxin for snakebites
- *Turtle shells*—Used to stimulate weak kidneys and to remove gallstones
- *Snake flesh*—Eaten as a delicacy to keep eyes healthy and vision clear
- *Seahorses*—Pulverized and used to treat gout

❧ *Current Health Problems*

In many instances, people who were born in the United States into families established here for generations are largely indistinguishable from the general population in their health-care beliefs. Other groups, however, especially new immigrants, differ from the general population on many social and health-related issues. National data do not cover this population because it is relatively small; however, it is possible to determine group morbidity and mortality rates at state statistical levels. Most of the studies are conducted in California, which has the largest Asian/Pacific Islander population. The following are examples of the findings (U.S. Department of Health and Human Services 1992, 36):

- The breast cancer incidence for Native Hawaiian women is 111 per 100,000 women compared with 86 per 100,000 white women.
- The lung cancer rate is 18% higher among Southeast Asian men than for the white men.
- The liver cancer rate is more than 12 times higher among Southeast Asians than within the white population.
- The incidence of tuberculosis is 40 times higher among Southeast Asians than for the total population.
- There are higher rates of hepatitis B among Southeast Asians.

Poor health is found among the residents of Chinatowns partly because of poor working conditions. Many people work long hours in restaurants and laundries and receive the lowest possible wages for their hard work. Many cannot afford even minimal, let alone preventive, health care (Li et al. 1972).

Americans of Asian and Pacific Island heritage experience unique barriers, including linguistic and cultural differences, when they try to access the unfamiliar health care system (U.S. Department of Health and Human Services 1992, 36).

Language difficulties and adherence to native Chinese culture compound problems already associated with poverty, crowding, and poor health. Many people still prefer the traditional forms of Chinese medicine and seek help from Chinatown "physicians" who treat them with traditional herbs and other methods. Often, Asian people do not seek help from the Western system at all. Others use Chinese methods in conjunction with Western methods of health care, although the Chinese find many aspects of Western medicine distasteful. For example, they cannot understand why so many diagnostic tests, some of which are painful, are necessary. They do, however, accept the practice of immunization and the use of X-rays.

They are most upset by the practice of drawing blood. Chinese people cannot understand why the often frequent taking of blood samples considered routine in Western medicine are necessary. Blood is seen as the source of life for the entire body, and they believe that it is not regenerated. The Asian reluctance to have blood drawn for diagnostic tests may have its roots in the revered teachings of Confucius. The Chinese people also believe that a good physician should be able to make a diagnosis simply by examining a person. Consequently, they do not react well to the often painful procedures used in Western diagnostic workups. Some people—because of their distaste for this procedure—leave the Western system rather than tolerate the pain. The Chinese have deep respect for their bodies and believe that it is best to die with their bodies intact. For this reason, many people refuse surgery or consent to it only under the most dire circumstances. This reluctance to undergo intrusive surgical procedures has deep implications for those concerned with providing health care to Asian Americans.

The hospital is an alien place to the Chinese. Not only are the customs and practices strange but also the patients often are isolated from the rest of their people, which enhances the language barrier and feelings of helplessness. Something as basic as food creates another problem. Hospital food is strange to Asian patients and is served in an unfamiliar manner. The typical Chinese patient rarely complains about what bothers him or her. Often the only indication that there may be a problem is an untouched food tray and the silent withdrawal of the patient. Unfortunately, the silence may be regarded by the nurses as reflecting good, complacent behavior, and the health-care team exerts little energy to go beyond the assumption. The Chinese patient who says little and complies with all treatment is seen as stoic, and there is little awareness that deep problems may underlie this "exemplary" behavior. Ignorance on the part of health-care workers may cause the patient a great deal of suffering.

Much action has been taken in recent years to make Western health care more available and appealing to the Chinese. In Boston, for example, there is a health clinic staffed primarily by Chinese-speaking nurses and physicians who work as paid employees and as volunteers. Most of the common health-related pamphlets have been translated into Chinese and are distributed to the patients. Booklets on such topics as breast self-examination and smoking cessation are available. Since the language spoken in the clinic is mandarin Chinese, the problem of interpreters has been largely eliminated. The care is personal, and the patients are made to feel comfortable. Unnecessary and painful tests are avoided as much as possible. In addition, the clinic, which is open for long hours, provides social services and employment placements and is quite popular with the community. Although it began as a parttime, storefront operation, the clinic is now housed in its own building.

Table 9–3 compares the 10 leading causes of death among Asian/Pacific Islanders with those of the general population.

The following is a synopsis of cultural beliefs regarding mental health and illness, possible causes of mental illness, and methods of preventing mental illness among people of Asian/Pacific Island origin. Little knowledge or skills in mental health therapy are seen in the Asian communities, as mental illness is much ignored in medical classics. Two points must be noted: the importance placed on the family in caring for the mentally ill and the tendency to identify mental illness in somatic terms. There is a tremendous amount of stigma attached to mental illness. Asian patients tend to come to the attention of mental health workers late in the course of their illness, and they come with a feeling of hopelessness (Lin 1982, 69–73).

One example of cross-cultural therapy is the Japanese practice of Morita therapy. This 70-year-old treatment originated from a treatment for *shinkeishitsu,* a form of compulsive neurosis with aspects of neurasthenia. The patient is separated from the family for 1 to 2 weeks and taught that one's feelings are the same as the Japanese sky and instantly changeable. One cannot be responsible for how one feels, only for what one does. At the end of therapy, the patient focuses on what is being done and less on their inner feelings, symptoms, concerns, or obsessive thoughts (Yamamoto 1982, 50). Table 9–4 provides examples of cultural-bound mental health syndromes.

A resource list of selected health-related organizations for the Asian/Pacific Islander communities may be found in Appendix VIII.

Table 9–3 | **The 10 Leading Causes of Death for Asian/Pacific Islanders and for All Persons, 1996**

Asian/Pacific Islanders	All Persons
1. Diseases of the heart	Diseases of the heart
2. Malignant neoplasms	Malignant neoplasms
3. Cerebrovascular diseases	Cerebrovascular diseases
4. Unintentional injuries	Chronic obstructive pulmonary diseases
5. Pneumonia and influenza	Unintentional injuries
6. Chronic obstructive pulmonary diseases	Pneumonia and influenza
7. Diabetes mellitus	Diabetes mellitus
8. Suicide	Human immunodeficiency virus infection
9. Homicide and legal intervention	Suicide
10. Nephritis, nephrotic syndrome, and nephrosis	Chronic liver disease and cirrhosis

From: National Center for Health Statistics. *Health United States 1998 with Socioeconomic Status and Health Chartbook.* (Hyattsville, Md., 1998), pp. 212–213.

| *Table 9–4* | Culture-Bound Mental HEALTH Syndromes |

Traditional Malady	Symptoms	Regions Located
Hwa-byung or wool-hwa-byung	"Anger syndrome" attributed to the suppression of anger; insomnia, fatigue, fear of impending death, indigestion anorexia, and dyspnea	Korea
Koro	Sudden and intense anxiety that causes the penis (or, in females, the vulva and nipples) to recede into the body and cause death	South and east Asia with many names, such as *shuk yang, shook yong,* or *suo yang* in China
Qi-gong psychotic reaction	Dissociative, paranoid, or other psychotic or nonpsychotic symptoms	China
Taijin kyofusho	An individual's intense fear that their body, its parts, or its functions, are offensive to others	Japan

From: American Psychiatric Association. 1994. *Diagnostic and Statistical Manual of Mental Disorders,* 4th ed. Washington DC.

ASIAN AMERICAN HEALTH MANPOWER

Asian Americans, a group that constituted 3.7% of the overall United States population in the 1990 census are for the most part well represented in the health professions, as illustrated in Tables 9–5 and 9–6. Today, persons who desire to be physicians in China have the option of studying either Chinese or Western medicine. If they select Western medicine, a limited amount of Chinese medicine is also taught. As Chinese traditional medicine is becoming better recognized and better understood in the United States more doors are being opened to those who prefer or understand this mode of treatment.

| *Table 9–5* | Asian Enrollment in Selected Health Professions Schools. 1995–1996 |

	Total Program Enrollment	Asian Enrollment
Allopathic medicine	66,970	11,352
Osteopathic medicine	8,475	933
Podiatry	2,312	303
Dentistry	16,374	3,433
Optometry	5,178	937
Pharmacy	33,205	5,695
Registered nursing	261,219	10,444

From: National Center for Health Statistics. *Health, United States, 1998, with Socioeconomic Status and Health Chartbook.* (Hyattsville, Md., 1998), pp. 330–331.

Table 9–6 | **Percentage of Asians Enrolled in Selected Health Professions Schools Compared with Non-Hispanic Whites, 1995–96**

Profession	Non-Hispanic White (%)	Asian (%)
Allopathic medicine	66.6	17.0
Osteopathic medicine	80.3	11.0
Podiatry	77.2	13.1
Dentistry	68.0	21.0
Optometry	75.4	18.1
Pharmacy	71.9	17.2
Registered nurses	82.4	4.0

From: National Center for Health Statistics. *Health, United States, 1998, with Socioeconomic Status and Health Chartbook.* (Hyattsville, Md., 1998), pp. 330–331.

❧ References

American Psychiatric Association. 1994. *Diagnostic and Statistical Manual of Mental Disorders,* 4th ed. Washington, D.C.

Chan, Dr. P. K. Herb Specialist, Interview by author. New York City, 3 August 1988. Dr. Chan prepared a supplemental written statement in Chinese and English for inclusion in this text.

Dolan, J. 1973. *Nursing in Society: A Historical Perspective.* Philadelphia: W. B. Saunders.

Ergil, K. V. 1996. China's Traditional Medicine. In *Fundamentals of Complementary and Alternative Medicine.* Edited by M. S. Micozzi. New York: Churchill Livingstone.

Li, F. P., Schlief, N. G., Chang, C., J., et al. 1972. Health Care for the Chinese Community in Boston. *American Journal of Public Health* (April): 537.

Lin, K. M. 1982. Cultural Aspects in Mental Health for Asian Americans. In *Cross-Cultural Psychiatry.* Edited by A. Gaw. Boston: John Wright.

Mann, F. 1972. *Acupuncture.* New York: Vintage Books.

Martin, J. A. 1995. Birth Characteristics for Asian or Pacific Islander Subgroups, 1992. *Monthly Vital Statistics Report, National Center for Health Statistics* 43(10):1.

Morgan, H. T. [1942] 1972. *Chinese Symbols and Superstitions.* Detroit: Gale Research. Reprint, S. Pasadena, Calif.: Ione Perkins.

National Center for Health Statistics. 1998. *Health United States 1998 with Socioeconomic Status and Health Chartbook.* Hyattsville, Md.

Romo, R. G. 1995. "Hispanic Health Traditions and Issues." Paper presented at the Minnesota Health Educators Conference, *Health Education: Expanding Our Horizons,* May 3.

Smith, H. 1958. *The Religions of Man.* New York: Harper and Row.

Spector, R. 1992. Culture, Ethnicity, and Nursing. In *Fundamentals of Nursing,* edited by P. Potter and A. Perry. St. Louis: Mosby-Year Book.

U.S. Department of Health and Human Services. 1992. *Healthy People 2000 National Health Promotion and Disease Prevention Objectives—Full Report with Commentary.* Boston: Jones and Bartlett, 36.

Wallnöfer, H., and von Rottauscher. A. 1972. *Chinese Folk Medicine.* Translated by M. Palmedo. New York: American Library.

Yamamoto, J. 1982. Japanese Americans. In *Cross-Cultural Psychiatry.* Edited by A. Gaw. Boston: John Wright.

*Figure 9–1 from page 195

From left to right—top to bottom: The chapter-opening quilt panel depicts images of objects and substances people of Asian origins may use to protect, maintain, and/or restore HEALTH. **Buddha,** from China, is a powerful religious symbol. It is placed in homes that have shrines, with the Buddha as the central figure and where incense is burned. Fruit and other foods may be offered to the Buddha or to the souls of dead relatives. It serves to maintain, protect, and restore HEALTH. **Jade,** from China, is believed to be the most precious of all stones. It is the giver of children, health, immortality, and wisdom. Jade charms are worn to bring health—to prevent harm and accidents—and serve in these ways to protect HEALTH. The **daishi (omanori),** from Japan, is an amulet hung in the car and is believed to protect the driver and passengers and ensure safe driving. It may also be hung in the home or in one's place of business for protection of HEALTH. The **acupuncture figurine,** from China, is a statue of a woman. It depicts the location of the meridians and is used for the location of points for the insertion of acupuncture needles or for moxibustion. **Cat** figurine, from Japan, is placed in the home for good luck and HEALTH protection. An **amulet,** from Japan, is pinned on a person's undergarments and worn for HEALTH protection from evil spirits. The **sea horse,** is a HEALTH restoration item, from China. This sea creature is ground into a powder, cooked as a tea, and the liquid is used externally as a soothing compress to treat gout. A **beaded bracelet** with inscriptions from the Tao is placed on a baby's or child's wrist for HEALTH protection. **Essence of tienchi flowers** are an herbal remedy from China. This product retains the fragrance of the original flowers and, once brewed, is a refreshing beverage. It has several therapeutic uses, both external and internal, including treating facial pimples of puberty, dizziness, nausea, hot temper, heat on the palms, and teeth grinding.

Chapter 10

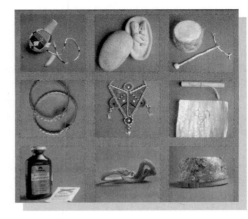

HEALTH and Illness in Black American Communities

*. . . some people don't understand that it is the nature of the
eye to have seen forever, and the nature of the mind to recall
anything that was ever known.*

—Alice Walker

Black or African Americans are the nations largest emerging majority population, constituting an estimated 12.1% of the population of the United States in
1998 (Bureau of the Census 1999). Most members of the present black American community have their roots in Africa, and the majority descend from people who were brought here as slaves from the west coast of Africa (Bullough
and Bullough 1972, 39–41). The largest importation of slaves occurred during
the seventeenth century, which means that black people have been living in the
United States for many generations. Today, a number of blacks have immigrated to the United States voluntarily—from African countries, the West Indian islands, the Dominican Republic, Haiti, and Jamaica.

Black Americans live in all regions of the country and are represented in
every socioeconomic group; however, one-third of the group lives in poverty,
a rate three times that of the white population. Over half of black Americans
live in urban areas surrounded by the symptoms of poverty—crowded and inadequate housing, poor schools, and high crime rates (U.S. Department of
Health and Human Services 1992, 32). For example, Kotlowitz (1995) de-

The author especially acknowledges those students who, over several years, have provided much of the data
for this chapter.

Figure 10–1 (From left to right, top to bottom) Beaded gourd, egg with mating couple, drum,
silver bangle bracelets, beaded breastplate, talisman, rectified turpentine with sugar, dried
snake, hat. *(For more information on each picture see explanation at the end of chapter.*)*

scribes the Henry Horner Homes in Chicago as "16 high-rise buildings which stretch over eight blocks and at last census count housed 6000 people, 4000 of whom are children." He goes on to present two facts about public housing: "Public housing served as a bulwark to segregation and as a kind of anchor for impoverished neighborhoods." and "It was built on the cheap—the walls are a naked cinder block with heating pipes snaking through the apartment; instead of closets, there are eight-inch indentations in the walls without doors; and the heating system so storms out of control in the winter that it is 85 degrees."

❀ *Background*

According to some sources, the first black people to enter this country arrived a year earlier than the Pilgrims, in 1619. Other sources claim that blacks arrived with Columbus in the fifteenth century (Bullough and Bullough 1972, 39–41). In any event, the first blacks who came to the North American continent did not come as slaves, but between 1619 and 1860, more than 4 million people were transported here as slaves. One need read only a sampling of the many accounts of slavery to appreciate the tremendous hardships that the captured and enslaved people experienced during that time. Not only was the daily life of the slave very difficult, but the experience of being captured, shackled, and transported in steerage was devastating. Many of those captured in Africa died before they arrived here. The strongest and healthiest people were snatched from their homes by slave dealers and transported en masse in the holds of ships to the North American continent. In general, black captives were not taken care of or recognized as human beings and treated accordingly. Once here, they were sold and placed on plantations and in homes all over the country—it was only later that the practice was confined to the South. Families were separated; children were wrenched from their parents and sold to other buyers. Some slave owners bred their slaves much like farmers breed cattle today, purchasing men to serve as studs, and judging women based on whether they would produce the desired stock with a particular man (Haley 1976). Yet, in the midst of all this inhuman and inhumane treatment, the black family grew and survived. Gutman (1976) in his careful documentation of plantation and family records traces the history of the black family from 1750 to 1925 and points out the existence of families and family or kinship ties before and after the Civil War, dispelling many of the myths about the black family and its structure. Despite overwhelming hardships and enforced separations, the people managed in most circumstances to maintain both a family and community awareness.

Ostensibly, the Civil War ended slavery, but in many ways, it did not emancipate blacks. Daily life after the war was fraught with tremendous difficulty, and black people—according to custom—were stripped of their civil rights. In the South, black people were overtly segregated, most living in conditions of extreme hardship and poverty. Those who migrated to the North over the years were subject to all the problems of fragmented urban life: poverty, racism, and covert segregation (Bullough and Bullough 1972, 43; Kain 1969, 1–30).

Box 10–1 *Highlights of the Civil Rights Movement*

1955	Rosa Parks refuses to give up her seat on a bus in Montgomery, Alabama, and the bus boycott in Alabama begins
1956	*Brown v. the Board of Education* marks the beginning of the desegregation of public schools
1959	Sit-ins at lunch counters
1961	Segregation of interstate bus terminals ruled unconstitutional
1962	Civil Rights Movement formally organized
1963	March on Washington led by Dr. Martin Luther King Jr.
1964	Civil Rights Act passed
1965	Malcolm X and Dr. Martin Luther King Jr. assassinated
1965–1968	Over 100 race riots in American cities
1991	Beating of Rodney King
1992	Major race riots in Los Angeles
1995	Million Man March

The historic problems of the black community need to be appreciated by the health-care provider who attempts to juxtapose modern practices and traditional health and illness beliefs. In addition, health-care providers must be aware of the ongoing and historical events in the struggle for civil rights that affect people's lives. Box 10–1 highlights several events in the history of this struggle.

❧ *Traditional Definitions of* HEALTH *and Illness*

According to Jacques 1976 the traditional definition of health stems from the African belief about life and the nature of being. To the African, life was a process rather than a state. The nature of a person was viewed in terms of energy force rather than matter. All things, whether living or dead, were believed to influence one another. Therefore, one had the power to influence one's destiny and that of others through the use of *behavior,* whether proper or otherwise, as well as through *knowledge* of the person and the world. When one possessed health, one was in harmony with nature; illness was a state of disharmony. Traditional black belief regarding HEALTH did not separate the mind, body, and spirit.

Disharmony, that is, illness, was attributed to a number of sources, primarily demons and evil spirits. These spirits were generally believed to act of their own accord, and the goal of treatment was to remove them from the body of the ill person. Several methods were employed to attain this result, in addition to voodoo, which is discussed in the next section. The traditional healers, usually women, possessed extensive knowledge regarding the use of herbs and roots in the treatment of illness. Apparently, an early form of small-pox immunization was used by slaves. Women practiced inoculation by scraping a piece of cowpox crust into a place on a child's arm. These children appeared to have a far lower incidence of smallpox than those who did not receive the immunization.

The old and the young were cared for by all members of the community. The elderly were held in high esteem because African people believed that the living of a long life indicated that a person had the opportunity to acquire much wisdom and knowledge. Death was described as the passing from one realm of life to another (Jacques 1976, 117) or as a passage from the evils of this world to another state. The funeral was often celebrated as a joyous occasion, with a party after the burial. Children were passed over the body of the deceased so that the dead person could carry any potential illness of the child away with him.

Many of the preventive and treatment practices of black people have their roots in Africa but have been merged with the approaches of Native Americans to whom the blacks were exposed and with the attitudes of whites among whom they lived and served. Then as today, illness was treated in a combination of ways. Methods found to be most useful were handed down through the generations.

HEALTH TRADITIONS

The following sections describe practices employed to maintain and protect HEALTH and to treat various types of maladies to restore HEALTH. This discussion cannot encompass all the types of care given to and by the members of the black community but instead presents a sample of the richness of the traditional HEALTH practices that have survived over the years.

HEALTH MAINTENANCE AND PROTECTION

Essentially, HEALTH is maintained with proper diet—that is, eating three nutritious meals a day, including a hot breakfast. Rest and a clean environment also are important. Laxatives were and are used to keep the system "running" or "open."

Asafetida—rotten flesh that looks like a dried-out sponge—is worn around the neck to prevent the contraction of contagious diseases. Cod-liver oil is taken to prevent colds. A sulfur and molasses preparation is used in the spring because it is believed that at the start of a new season people are more susceptible to illness. This preparation is rubbed up and down the back, not taken internally. A physician is not consulted routinely and is not generally regarded as the person to whom one goes for the prevention of disease.

Copper or silver bracelets may be worn around the wrist from the time a woman is a baby or young child. These bracelets are believed to protect the wearer as she grows. If for any reason these bracelets are removed, harm befalls the owner. In addition to granting protection, these bracelets indicate when the wearer is about to become ill: the skin around the bracelet turns black, alerting the woman to take precaution against the impending illness.

These precautions consist of getting extra rest, praying more frequently, and eating a more nutritious diet.

HEALTH RESTORATION

The most common method of treating illness is prayer. The laying on of hands is described quite frequently. Rooting, a practice derived from voodoo, also is mentioned. In rooting, a person (usually a woman) is consulted as to the source of a given illness, and she then prescribes the appropriate treatment. Magic rituals often are employed (Davis 1998).

The following home remedies have been reported by some black people as being successful in the treatment of disease.

1. Sugar and turpentine are mixed together and taken by mouth to get rid of worms. This combination can also be used to cure a backache when rubbed on the skin from the navel to the back.
2. Numerous types of poultices are employed to fight infection and inflammation. The poultices are placed on the part of the body that is painful or infected to draw out the cause of the affliction.

   One type of poultice is made of potatoes. The potatoes are sliced or grated and placed in a bag, which is placed on the affected area of the body. The potatoes turn black, and as this occurs, the disease goes away. It is believed that as these potatoes spoil, they produce a penicillin mold that is able to destroy the infectious organism. Another type of poultice is prepared from cornmeal and peach leaves that are cooked together and placed either in a bag or in a piece of flannel cloth. The cornmeal ferments and combines with an enzyme in the peach leaves to produce an antiseptic that destroys the bacteria and hastens the healing process. A third poultice, made with onions, is used to heal infections, and a flaxseed poultice is used to treat earaches.
3. Herbs from the woods are used in many ways. Herb teas are prepared—for example, from goldenrod root—to treat pain and reduce fevers. Sassafras tea frequently is used to treat colds. Other herbs that are boiled to make a tea include the root or leaf of rabbit tobacco.
4. Bluestone, a mineral found in the ground, is used as medicine for open wounds. The stone is crushed into a powder and sprinkled on the affected area. It prevents inflammation and is also used to treat poison ivy.
5. To treat a "crick" in the neck, two pieces of silverware are crossed over the painful area in the form of an X.
6. Nine drops of turpentine nine days after intercourse act as a contraceptive.
7. Cuts and wounds can be treated with sour or spoiled milk that is placed on stale bread, wrapped in a cloth, and placed on the wound.
8. Salt and pork (salt pork) placed on a rag also can be used to treat cuts and wounds.

9. A sprained ankle can be treated by placing clay in a dark leaf and wrapping it around the ankle.
10. A remedy for treating colds is hot lemon water with honey.
11. When congestion is present in the chest and the person is coughing, the chest is rubbed with hot camphorated oil and wrapped with warm flannel.
12. An expectorant for colds consists of chopped raw garlic, chopped onion, fresh parsley, and a little water, all mixed in a blender.
13. Hot toddies are used to treat colds and congestion. These drinks consist of hot tea with honey, lemon, peppermint, and a dash of brandy or whatever alcoholic beverage the person likes and is available. Vicks Vaporub also is swallowed.
14. A fever can be broken by placing raw onions on the feet and wrapping them in warm blankets.
15. Boils are treated by cracking a raw egg, peeling the white skin off the inside of the shell, and placing it on the boil. This brings the boil to a head.
16. Garlic can be placed on the ill person or in the room to remove the "evil spirits" that have caused the illness.

FOLK MEDICINE

In the black community, folk medicine previously practiced in Africa is still employed. The methods have been tried and tested and are still relied on. Healers or voodoo practitioners make no class or status distinctions among their clients, treating everyone fairly and honestly. This tradition of equality of care and perceived effectiveness accounts for the faith placed in the practices of the healer and in other methods. In fact, the home remedies used by some members of the black community have been employed for many generations. Another reason for their ongoing use is that hospitals are distant from people who live in rural areas. By the time they might get to the hospital they would be dead. Yet many of the people who continue to use these remedies live in urban areas close to hospitals—sometimes even world-renowned hospitals. Nonetheless, the use of folk medicine persists, and many people avoid the local hospital except in extreme emergencies.

❋ Traditional Methods of Healing

VOODOO OR VOUDOU

Voodoo, or American Voudou, is a belief system often alluded to but rarely described in any detail (Davis 1998). At various times, patients may mention terms, such as "fix," "hex," or "spell." It is not clear whether voodoo is *fully* practiced today, but there is some evidence in the literature that there are people who still believe and practice it to some extent (Wintrob 1972). It also has been reported that many black people continue to fear voodoo and believe that when they become ill they have been "fixed." Voodoo involves two forms of magic: white magic, described as harmless, and black magic, which is quite dangerous. Belief in magic is, of course, ancient (Hughes and Bontemps 1958, 184–185).

Voodoo came to this country about 1724, with the arrival of slaves from the West African coast, who had been sold initially in the West Indies. The people who brought voodoo with them were "snake worshippers." *Vodu*, the name of their god, became with the passage of time *voodoo* (also *hoodoo*), an all-embracing term that included the god, the sect, the members of the sect, the priests and priestesses, the rites and practices, and the teaching (Tallant 1946, 19).

Tallant goes on to explain that the sect spread rapidly from the West Indies. In 1782 the governor of Louisiana prohibited the importation of slaves from Martinique because of their practice in voodooism. (Despite the fact that gatherings of slaves were forbidden in Louisiana, small groups persisted in practicing voodoo.) In 1803 the importation of slaves to Louisiana from the West Indies was finally allowed, and with them came a strong influence of voodoo. The practice entailed a large number of rituals and procedures. The ceremonies were held with large numbers of people, usually at night and in the open country. "Sacrifice and the drinking of blood were integral parts of all the voodoo ceremonies." There were those who believed that this blood was from children. However, it was most commonly thought to be the blood of a cat or young goat. Such behavior evolved from primitive African rites, to which Christian rituals were added to form the ceremonies that exist today. Leaders of the voodoo sect tended to be women, and stories abound in New Orleans about the workings of the sect and the women who ruled it—such as Marie Laveau.

In 1850 the practice of voodoo reached its height in New Orleans. At that time, the beliefs and practices of voodoo were closely related to beliefs about health and illness. For example, many illnesses were attributed to a "fix" that was placed on one person out of anger. *Gris-gris,* the symbols of voodoo, were used to prevent illness or to give illness to others. Some examples of commonly used gris-gris follow (Tallant 1946, 226):

1. Good gris-gris. Powders and oils that are highly and pleasantly scented. The following are examples of good gris-gris: love powder, colored and scented with perfume; love oil, olive oil to which gardenia perfume has been added; luck water, ordinary water that is purchased in many shades (red is for success in love, yellow for success in money matters, blue for protection and friends).
2. Bad gris-gris. Oils and powders that have a vile odor. The following are examples of bad gris-gris: anger powder, war powder, and moving powder, which are composed of soil, gunpowder, and black pepper, respectively.
3. Flying devil oil is olive oil that has red coloring and cayenne pepper added to it.
4. Black cat oil is machine oil.

In addition to these oils and powders, a variety of colored candles are used, the color of the candle symbolizing the intention. For example, white symbolizes peace, red victory, pink love, yellow driving off enemies, brown attracting money, and black doing evil work and bringing bad luck (Tallant 1946, 226).

The following story exhibits the profound influence that belief in voodoo can have on a person. It was reported in Baltimore, Maryland, in 1967.

> The patient was a young, married black woman who was admitted to the hospital for evaluation of chest pain, syncope, and dyspnea. Her past history was one of good health. However, she had gained over 50 pounds in the past year and was given to eating Argo starch. She began to have symptoms 1 month before she was admitted. Her condition grew worse once in the hospital, and she was treated for heart failure and also for pulmonary embolism. She revealed that she had a serious problem. She had been born on Friday, the thirteenth, in the Okefenokee Swamp and was delivered by a midwife who delivered three children that day. The midwife told the mothers that the children were hexed and that the first would die before her 16th birthday, the second before her 21st birthday, and the third (the patient) before her 23rd birthday. The first girl was a passenger in a car involved in a fatal crash the day before her 16th birthday, the second girl was celebrating her 21st birthday in a saloon when a stray bullet hit and killed her. This patient also believed she was doomed. She, too, died—on August 12—a day before her 23rd birthday (Webb 1971, 1–3).

There are a number of Catholic saints or relics to whom or to which the practitioners of voodoo attribute special powers. Portraits of Saint Michael, who makes possible the conquest of enemies, Saint Anthony de Padua, who brings luck, Saint Mary Magdalene, who is popular with women who are in love, the Virgin Mary, whose presence in the home prevents illness, and the Sacred Heart of Jesus, which cures organic illness may be prominently displayed in the home of people who believe in voodoo (Tallant 1946, 228). These gris-gris are available today and can be purchased in stores in many American cities.

OTHER PRACTICES

Many blacks believe in the power of some people to heal and help others, and there are many reports of numerous healers among the communities. This reliance on healers reflects the deep religious faith of the people. (Maya Angelou vividly describes this phenomenon in her book *I Know Why the Caged Bird Sings*.) For example, many blacks followed the Pentecostal movement long before its present more general popularity. Similarly, people often went to tent meetings and had an all-consuming belief in the healing powers of religion.

Another practice takes on significance when one appreciates its historical background: the eating of Argo starch. "Geophagy," or eating clay and dirt, occurred among the slaves, who brought the practice to this country from Africa. In *Roots*, Haley mentions that pregnant women were given clay because it was believed to be beneficial to both the mother and the unborn child (Haley 1976, 32). In fact, red clays are rich in iron. When clay was not available, dirt was substituted. In more modern times, when people were no longer living on farms and no longer had access to clay and dirt, Argo starch became the substitute (Dunstin 1969).

> It was my fortune, or misfortune to be born into a family that practiced geophagy (earth eating) and pica (eating Argo laundry starch). Even before I became pregnant I showed an interest in eating starch. It was sweet and dry, and I could take it or leave it. After I became pregnant, I found I wanted not only starch, but bread, grits, and potatoes. I found I craved starchy substances. I stuck to starchy substances and dropped the Argo because it made me feel sluggish and heavy.*

It is believed that anemia arose from this practice of substituting non–iron-rich clays or starch for red clays that contain iron. Table 10–1 illustrates examples of cultural phenomena that affect health care among black or African Americans.

Table 10–1 **Examples of Cultural Phenomena Affecting Health Care Among Black Americans**

Nations of origin:	Many West African countries (as slaves)
	West Indian Islands
	Dominican Republic
	Haiti
	Jamaica
Environmental control:	Traditional health and illness beliefs may continue to be observed by "traditional" people
Biological variations:	Sickle-cell anemia
	Hypertension
	Cancer of the esophagus
	Stomach cancer
	Coccidioidomycosis
	Lactose intolerance
Social organization:	Family: many single-parent households headed by females
	Large, extended family networks
	Strong church affiliations within community
	Community social organizations
Communication:	National languages
	Dialect: Pidgin
	French, Spanish, Creole
Space:	Close personal space
Time orientation:	Present over future

Adapted from: Spector, R. "Culture, Ethnicity, and Nursing," in *Fundamentals of Nursing,* 3d ed., ed. P. Potter and A. Perry. (St. Louis: Mosby-Year Book, 1992), p. 101. Reprinted with permission.

---

*This experience was reported by a student, who consented to having her description included in this book.

BLACK MUSLIMS[†]

Many members of the black community are practicing Muslims. Religious beliefs are an important part of the Muslim lifestyle, and health-care providers should be familiar with them. Islamic dietary restrictions consist of eating a strictly kosher diet, and a newly admitted patient who refuses to eat should be asked if the hospital's ordinary diet interferes with his or her religious beliefs. *Kosher* means not eating pork or any pork products (such as nonbeef hamburger and ham) or any "soul foods" (such as black-eyed beans, kidney beans, ham hocks, bacon, or pork chops). Muslims consider such foods to be filthy and are taught that a "person is what he eats."

Islamic law teaches that certain foods affect the way a person thinks and acts. Therefore, one's diet should consist of food that has a clean, positive effect. Beans, such as black-eyed, kidney, and lima, are avoided because they are hard to digest and are meant for animal (not human) consumption. Muslims do not drink alcohol because they feel that it dulls the senses and causes illness.

Muslims fast for a 30-day period during the year (fast of Ramadan), at which time they consume no meat of land animals and eat only one meal per day, in the evening. Nothing is taken by mouth from 5:00 A.M. until sundown, although ill Muslims, small children, and pregnant women are exempt from this rule.

The Muslim lifestyle is strictly regulated. According to those who have practiced the religion for many generations, this stems in part from the need for self-discipline, which many black people have not had because of living conditions associated with urban decay and family disintegration. Muslims believe in self-help and assist in uplifting each other. The Muslim lifestyle is not so rigid that the people do not have good times. Good times, however, are tempered with the realization that too much indulgence in sport and play can present problems. To Muslims, life is precious: If they need a transfusion to live, they will accept it. Because of their avoidance of pork or pork products, however, it is important to understand that a diabetic Muslim will refuse to take insulin that has a pork base. If the insulin is manufactured from the pancreas of a pig, it is considered unclean and will not be accepted.

Many Muslim subsects differ in their practice and philosophy of Islam. Members of some sects dress in distinctive clothing—for example, the women wear long skirts and a covering on the head at all times. Other sects are less strict about dress. Some adherents do not follow the kosher diet and are allowed to smoke and drink alcoholic beverages in moderation. In some sects, men practice polygamy and have a number of concubines.

[†]This material is adapted from a paper prepared by a student who is a practicing Muslim, who wanted to share her beliefs. She concluded: "I hope this will help a bit in understanding a Muslim who may be a patient."

❧ *Current Health-Care Problems*

HEALTH DIFFERENCES BETWEEN BLACK AND WHITE POPULATIONS

Morbidity. The available data demonstrate a low use of health services by blacks and lower incidences of diseases. This is misleading, however, and can be attributed to such factors as the lack of access to the health services, low income, and a tendency to self-treat illness and to wait until symptoms are so severe that a doctor must be seen. When statistical adjustments are made for age, blacks exceed whites in the average number of days spent on bedrest and the number of days in restricted activity. In addition, blacks have a greater incidence of tooth decay than whites and have greater periodontal disease. Adolescent pregnancy is a major concern with the population. The risk of infant mortality and low birth weight are also greater in the community as is the rate of low birth weight babies. A greater percentage of blacks suffer with mental illness than the relative proportion of blacks in the overall population would predict. In 1989, 703,000 adults with serious mental illness received government disability payment for their mental disorder. Of this population, 20.5% were white and 43.8% were black (Manderschield and Sonnenschein 1992, 262).

Sickle-Cell Anemia. The sickling of red blood cells is a genetically inherited trait that is hypothesized to have originally been an African adaptation to fight malaria. This condition occurs only in blacks and causes the normal disklike red blood cell to assume a sickle shape. Sickling results in hemolysis and thrombosis of red blood cells because these deformed cells do not flow properly through the blood vessels. Sickle-cell disease comprises the following blood characteristics:

1. The presence of two hemoglobin-S genes *(Hb SS)*
2. The presence of the hemoglobin-S gene with another abnormal hemoglobin gene (*Hb SC, Hb SD,* etc.)
3. The presence of the hemoglobin-S gene with a different abnormality in hemoglobin synthesis

Some people (carriers) have the sickle-cell trait (*HbSS, HbSC,* or others) but do not experience symptoms of the disease.

The clinical manifestations of sickle-cell disease include hemolysis, anemia, and states of sickle-cell crises in which severe pain occurs in the areas of the body where the thrombosed red cells are located. The cells also tend to clump in abdominal organs, such as the liver and the spleen. At present, statistics indicate that only 50% of children with sickle-cell disease live to adulthood. Some children die before the age of 20, and some suffer complications during their lifetime that are chronic and irreversable.

It is possible to detect the sickle-cell trait in healthy adults and to provide genetic counseling about their risk of bearing children with the disease. However, for many people, this is not an option (Bullock and Jilly 1975, 234–272). The cost of genetic counseling, for example, may be prohibitive.

Mortality.   Blacks born in 1996 in the United States will live, on average, 6.6 fewer years than whites. The life expectancy for whites is 76.8 years; for blacks, it is 70.2.

The leading chronic diseases that are causes of death for African Americans are the same as those for whites, but the rates are greater. For example,

- Black men die from strokes at almost twice the rate of men in the white population. Stroke mortality is higher for the black population. In 1996 the age-adjusted death rate for stroke was 80% higher than for whites. (National Center for Health Statistics 1998, 11).
- Coronary heart disease death rates are higher for Black American women than for white women.
- Black men experience a higher risk of cancer than white men do.
- Diabetes is 33% more common among Black Americans than among whites.
- Black American babies are twice as likely as white babies to die before their first birthday.
- Homicide is the most frequent cause of death for Black American men between the ages of 15 and 34. The homicide rate for those between ages 25 and 34 is seven times that for whites.
- The rate of AIDS among Black American men generally is more than triple that for white men. Among women and children the gap is even wider (Department of Health and Human Services 1993, 44).

Table 10–2 lists the 10 leading causes of death for Black Americans and compares them with the causes of death for the general population in 1996.

Table 10–2 **The 10 Leading Causes of Death for Black Americans and for all Persons, 1996**

Black Americans	All Persons
1. Diseases of the heart	1. Diseases of the heart
2. Malignant neoplasms	2. Malignant neoplasms
3. Cerebrovascular diseases	3. Cerebrovascular diseases
4. Human immunodeficiency virus infection	4. Chronic obstructive pulmonary diseases
5. Unintentional injuries	5. Unintentional injuries
6. Diabetes mellitus	6. Pneumonia and influenza
7. Homicide and legal intervention	7. Diabetes mellitus
8. Pneumonia and influenza	8. Human immunodeficiency virus infection
9. Chronic obstructive pulmonary diseases	9. Suicide
10. Certain conditions originating in the perinatal period	10. Chronic liver disease and cirrhosis

From: National Center for Health Statistics. *Health, United States, 1998, with Socioeconomic Status and Health Chartbook.* (Hyattsville, Md., 1998), p. 212.

Table 10–3 further compares selected health problems and their manifestations in the white and black communities.

MENTAL HEALTH TRADITIONS

The family often has a matriarchal structure, and there are many single-parent households headed by females but there are strong and large extended family networks. There is a continuation of tradition and a strong church affiliation within the families and community. Members of the community may be treated by a traditional voodoo priest or the "Old Lady" ("granny" or "Mrs. Markus") or other traditional healers, and herbs are frequently used to treat mental symptoms. Several diagnostic techniques include the use of Biblical phrases and/or material from old folk medical books, observation, and/or entering the spirit of the client. The therapeutic measures included various rituals such as the reading of bones, wearing special garments, or some rituals from voodoo (Spurlock 1982, 173). Table 10–4 lists selected folk mental illness syndromes observed among blacks.

BLACKS AND THE HEALTH-CARE SYSTEM

To the black person, receiving health care is all too often a degrading and humiliating experience. In many settings, black patients continue to be viewed as beneath the white health-care giver. Quite often the insult is a subtle part of *experiencing* the health-care system. The insult may be intentional or unintentional. An intentional insult is, of course, a blatant remark or mistreatment. An unintentional insult is more difficult to define. A health-care provider may not *intend* to demean a person, yet an action or tone of voice may be interpreted as insulting. The provider may have some covert, underlying fears or difficulties in relating to blacks, but the patient quite often senses the difficulty. An unintentional insult may occur because the provider is not fully aware of the client's background and is unable to comprehend many of the client's beliefs and practices. The client, for example, may be afraid of the impending medical procedures and the possibility of misdiagnosis or mistreatment. It is not a secret among the people of the black community that those who receive care in public clinics and hospitals—and even in clinics of private institutions—are the "material" on whom students practice and on whom medical research is done.

Some blacks fear or resent health clinics. When they have a clinic appointment, they usually lose a day's work because they have to be at the clinic at an early hour and often spend many hours waiting to be seen by a physician. They often receive inadequate care, are told what their problem is in incomprehensible medical jargon, and are not given an identity, being seen rather as a body segment ("the appendix in treatment room A"). Such an experience creates a tremendous feeling of powerlessness and alienation from the system. In some parts of the country, segregation and racism are overt. There continue to be reports of hospitals that refuse admission to black patients. In one case, a black woman in labor was not admitted to a hospital because she had not "paid the bill from the last baby." There was not enough time to get her to an-

| *Table 10–3* | Comparison of Selected Health Problems in White and Black Americans |

Problem	Black Morbidity/Mortality Compared with White Morbidity/Mortality
Cardiovascular disease	Age-adjusted death rates for all causes were 60% higher in black men than in white men; 56% higher in black women than in white women.
Coronary artery disease (CHD)	CHD mortality rates in 1984 were similar among black and white men; women's rates are higher in blacks.
Cerebrovascular disease	Stroke is the single disease entity that accounts for most of the excess black mortality compared with whites.
Hypertension (HBP)	In blacks, HBP develops at a younger age and is more severe than in whites.
End-stage renal disease (ESRD)	Blacks are disproportionately represented in the total ESRD pool and in the number of new people who develop this problem each year. Currently, 25% of ESRD patients have functioning kidney transplants (30% of whites with ESRD and 13% of blacks have functioning transplants; 51% of whites are treated with dialysis, 74% of blacks.
Cancer	In 1989, the age-adjusted cancer incidence rate was 401.2/100,000 for blacks; 379.5 for whites. In 1990, the mortality rate was 182/100,000 for blacks compared with 131.5 for whites. The five-year survival rate for cancer in blacks diagnosed from 1983 to 1988 was about 38.3% and for whites, 53.5%.
Chronic obstructive pulmonary disease (COPD)	Between 1979 and 1990 the age-adjusted COPD mortality rate for blacks rose 52.3% and for whites, 34.9%. Studies have shown the adverse effects of pollution on the respiratory tract; blacks (59.7%) were more likely than whites (27%) to live in central cities where exposure to air pollution is greater.
Sickle-cell disease (SCD)	The group of genetic disorders known as SCD is the most common genetic disorder within the black population; the incidence is 1 in every 500 live black births.
Ophthalmology	The findings of numerous surveys indicate significantly higher incidences of blindness and visual impairment in blacks compared with whites.

(continued)

other hospital, and she was forced to deliver in an ambulance. In light of this type of treatment, it is no wonder that some black people prefer to use time-tested home remedies rather than be exposed to the humiliating experiences of hospitalization.

Another reason for the ongoing use of home remedies is poverty. Indigent people cannot afford the high costs of American health care. Quite often—even with the help of Medicaid and Medicare—the hidden costs of acquiring health services, such as transportation and child care, are a heavy bur-

Table 10–3 Comparison of Selected Health Problems in White and Black Americans—Continued

Problem	Black Morbidity/Mortality Compared with White Morbidity/Mortality
AIDS	The HIV/AIDS epidemic and other sexually transmitted diseases threaten to decimate the black community. In AIDS cases among blacks, 78% have occurred in men, 19% in adult women, and 3% in children younger than 13 years. HIV-positive rates of 3.9/1000 have been reported in black military recruits, compared with 0.9/1000 in whites.
Sexually transmitted diseases (STDs)	There is a high incidence of STDs in the black community; for example, there has been a rapid increase of infectious primary and secondary syphilis among blacks since 1985.
Intentional injuries: homicide and suicides	*Homicide:* In recent years the homicide rate among blacks has exceeded that for all racial groups in the United States and may rank highest in the world. *Suicide:* Generally the suicide rate is lower in the black community than in the white community, but young black males, who experience high rates of interpersonal violence, have a relatively high rate of suicide.
Unintentional injuries	Among black Americans, injuries were responsible for more deaths than any other cause in 1989; these included motor vehicle accidents (16.88/100,000), fires and burns (5.52), and drownings (4.22).
Chemical use	In general, alcohol and tobacco are the most used and abused substances in this country, particularly among blacks.
Infant mortality	The cause most associated with infant mortality is low birth weight; black American infants have the highest incidence (13% in 1988) of low birth weight among all ethnic groups—greater than twice the rate for whites (5.5%).

From: Livingston, I. L., ed. *Handbook of Black American Health.* (Westport, Conn.: Greenwood Publishing Group, 1994), pp. 3, 24, 33, 47, 60, 70, 78, 111, 117, 118, 125, 140, 160, 170, 179, 190, 205–206, and 219. Reprinted with permission.

den. As a result, blacks may stay away from clinics or outpatient departments or receive their care with passivity while appearing to the provider to be evasive. Some black patients believe that they are being talked down to by health-care providers and that the providers fail to listen to them. They choose, consequently, to "suffer in silence." Many of the problems that blacks relate in dealing with the health-care system can apply to anyone, but the inherent racism within the health system cannot be denied. Currently, efforts are being made to overcome these barriers.

Since the 1960s health-care services available to blacks and other people of color have improved. A growing number of community health centers have emphasized health maintenance and promotion. Community residents serve on the boards.

Table 10–4 | **Selected Black Culture–Bound Mental Illnesses**

Traditional Malady	Symptoms	Regions Encountered
Boufée delirante	Sudden outburst of agitated and aggressive behavior, marked confusion, and psychomotor excitement; occasional visual and auditory hallucinations or paranoid ideation	West Africa and Haiti
Falling-out or blacking-out	Sudden collapse without warning but preceded by a feeling of dizziness or "swimming" in the head	Southern United States and Caribbean groups
Rootwork	Illness is ascribed in the folk tradition to hexing, witchcraft, sorcery, or evil influence of another person. Generalized anxiety, gastrointestinal complaints (nausea, vomiting, diarrhea), weakness, dizziness, and the fear of being poisoned or killed	Southern United States, among both African American and European Americans and in Caribbean societies
Spell	A trance state; person communicates with deceased relatives or with spirits	Southern United States, among both African Americans and European Americans
Zar	Person is possessed by a spirit and experiences dissociative episodes that may include shouting, weeping, laughing, hitting the head against the wall, or singing	North African countries, Ethiopia, Egypt, Sudan, Iran and Middle Eastern societies

Adapted from: American Psychiatric Association. 1994. *Diagnostic and Statistical Manual of Mental Disorders,* 4th ed. Washington DC.

Among the services provided by community health centers is an effort to discover children with high blood levels of lead in order to provide early diagnosis of and treatment for lead poisoning. Once a child is found to have lead poisoning, the law requires that the source of the lead be found and eradicated. Today, only apartments free of lead paint can be rented to families with young children. Apartments that are found to have lead paint must be stripped and repainted with nonlead paint. Another ongoing effort by the community health centers is to inform blacks who are at risk of producing children with sickle-cell anemia that they are carriers of this genetic disease. This program is fraught with conflict because many people prefer not to be screened for the sickle-cell trait, fearing they may become labeled once the tendency is discovered.

Birth control is another problem that is recognized with mixed emotions. To some, especially women who want to space children or who do not want to have numerous children, birth control is a welcome development. People who believe in birth control prefer selecting the time when they will have children, how many children they will have, and when they will stop having children. To many other people, birth control is considered a form of "black genocide" and a way of limiting the growth of the community. Health workers in the black community must be aware of both sides of this issue and, if asked to make a decision, remain neutral. Such decisions must be made by the clients themselves.

SPECIAL CONSIDERATIONS FOR BLACK HEALTH CARE

White health-care providers know far too little about how to care for a black person's skin or hair, or how to understand both black nonverbal and verbal behavior.

Physiological Assessment. Examples of possible physiological problems include the following (in observing skin problems, it is important to note that skin assessment is best done in indirect sunlight) (Bloch and Hunter 1981).

1. *Pallor*—There is an absence of underlying red tones; the skin of a brown-skinned person appears yellow-brown, and that of a black-skinned person appears ashen gray. Mucous membranes appear ashen, and the lips and nailbeds are similar.

2. *Erythema*—Inflammation must be detected by palpation; the skin is warmer in the area, tight, and edematous, and the deeper tissues are hard. Fingertips must be used for this assessment, as with rashes, since they are sensitive to the feeling of different textures of skin.

3. *Cyanosis*—Cyanosis is difficult to observe in dark-colored skin, but it can be seen by close inspection of the lips, tongue, conjunctiva, palms of the hands, and the soles of the feet. One method of testing is pressing the palms. Slow blood return is an indication of cyanosis. Another sign is ashen gray lips and tongue.

4. *Ecchymosis*—History of trauma to a given area can be detected from a swelling of the skin surface.

5. *Jaundice*—The sclera are usually observed for yellow discoloration to reveal jaundice. This is not always a valid indication, however, since carotene deposits can also cause the sclera to appear yellow. The buccal mucosa and the palms of the hands and soles of the feet may appear yellow.

Skin Problems. Several skin conditions are of importance in black patients (Sykes and Kelly 1979).

1. *Keloids*—Keloids are scars that form at the site of a wound and grow beyond the normal boundaries of the wound. They are sharply elevated and irregular and continue to enlarge.

2. *Pigmentary disorders*—Pigmentary disorders, areas of either postinflammatory hypopigmentation or hyperpigmentation, appear as dark or light spots.

3. *Pseudofolliculitis*—"Razor bumps" and "ingrown hairs" are caused by shaving too closely with an electric razor or straight razor. The sharp point of the hair, if shaved too close, enters the skin and induces an immune response

as to a foreign body. The symptoms include papules, pustules, and sometimes even keloids.

4. *Melasma*—The "mask of pregnancy," melasma, is a patchy tan to dark brown discoloration of the face more prevalent in dark pregnant women.

Hair-Care Needs. The care of the hair of blacks is not complicated, but special consideration must be given to help maintain its healthy condition (Bloch and Hunter 1972).

1. The hair's dryness or oiliness must be assessed, as well as its texture (straight or extra curly) and the patient's hairstyle preference.
2. The hair must be shampooed as needed and groomed according to the person's preference.
3. Hair must be combed well, with the appropriate tools, such as a "pic" or comb with big teeth, before drying to prevent tangles.
4. If the hair is dry and needs oiling, the preparations that the person generally uses for this purpose ought to be on hand.
5. Once dry, the hair is ready to be styled (curled, braided, or rolled) as the person desires.

❧ *Considerations for Health-Care Providers*

When they enter the profession, the majority of the members of the health-care profession are steeped in a middle-class white value system. In clinical settings, these people are being helped to become familiar with and to understand the value systems of other ethnic socioeconomic groups. They are being taught to recognize the symptoms of illness in blacks and to provide proper skin and hair care. The following are guidelines that a health-care provider can follow in caring for members of the black community.

1. The education of an ever-increasing number of blacks in the health professions must continue to be encouraged.
2. The needs of the patient must be assessed realistically.
3. When a treatment or special diet is prescribed, every attempt must be made to ascertain whether it is consistent with the patient's physical needs, cultural background, income, and religious practices.
4. The patient's belief in and practice of folk medicine must be respected; the patient must not be criticized for these beliefs. Every effort should be made to assist the patient to combine folk treatment with standard Western treatment as long as the two are not antagonistic. Most people who have a strong belief in folk remedies continue to use them with or without medical sanction.
5. Providers should be familiar with formal and informal sources of help in the black community. The former sources consist of churches, social clubs, and community groups. The latter include those women who provide care for members of their community in an informal way.
6. The beliefs and values of the health-care provider should not be forced on the client.

7. The treatment plan and the reasons for a given treatment must be shared with the patient.

BLACK AMERICAN HEALTH-CARE MANPOWER

The number of black Americans both enrolled in health programs and in practice in selected health professions is low, as illustrated in Tables 10–5 and 10–6. Efforts must be made to recruit and maintain more blacks in the health professions.

Table 10–5 | **Black Non-Hispanic Enrollment in Selected Health Professions Schools, 1995–1996**

	Total Program Enrollment	Black Enrollment
Allopathic medicine	66,970	5,337
Osteopathic medicine	8,475	318
Podiatry	2,312	112
Dentistry	16,374	951
Optometry	5,178	120
Pharmacy	33,205	2,548
Registered nursing	261,219	24,621

From: National Center for Health Statistics. 1998. *Health United States 1998 with Socioeconomic Status and Health Chartbook.* (Hyattsville, Md., 1998), pp. 331–332.

Table 10–6 | **Percentage of Black Non-Hispanics Enrolled in Selected Health Professions Schools Compared with Non-Hispanic Whites, 1995–1996**

Profession	Non-Hispanic Whites (%)	Non-Hispanic Blacks (%)
Allopathic medicine	66.6	8.0
Osteopathic medicine	80.3	3.8
Podiatry	77.2	4.8
Dentistry	68.0	5.8
Optometry	75.4	2.3
Pharmacy	71.9	7.7
Registered nurses	82.4	9.4

From: National Center for Health Statistics. 1998. *Health United States 1998 with Socioeconomic Status and Health Chartbook.* (Hyattsville, Md., 1998), pp. 331–332.

❦ References

American Psychiatric Association. 1994. *Diagnostic and Statistical Manual of Mental Disorders,* 4th ed. Washington, D.C.

Bloch, B., and Hunter, M. L. 1981. Teaching Physiological Assessment of Black Persons. *Nurse Educator* (January–February): 26.

Bullock, W. H., and Jilly, P. N. 1975. Hematology. In *Textbook of Black-Related Diseases*, R. A. Williams. New York: McGraw-Hill.

Bullough, B., and Bullough, V. L. 1972. *Poverty, Ethnic Identity, and Health Care*. New York: Appleton-Century-Crofts.

Davis, R. 1998. *American Voudou—Journey into a Hidden World*. Denton: University of North Texas Press.

Dunstin, B. 1969. Pica during Pregnancy. Chap. 26 in *Current Concepts in Clinical Nursing*. St. Louis: Mosby.

Gutman, H. G. 1976. *The Black Family in Slavery and Freedom, 1750–1925*. New York: Pantheon.

Haley, A. 1976. *Roots*. New York: Doubleday.

Hughes, L., and Bontemps, A., eds. 1958. *The Book of Negro Folklore*. New York: Dodd, Mead.

Jacques, G. 1976. Cultural Health Traditions: A Black Perspective. In *Providing Safe Nursing Care for Ethnic People of Color*. Edited by M. Branch and P. P. Paxton. New York: Appleton-Century-Crofts.

Kain, J. F. ed. 1969. *Race and Poverty*. Englewood Cliffs, N.J.: Prentice-Hall.

Livingston, I. L., ed. 1994. *Handbook of Black American Health*. Westport, Conn.: Greenwood.

Manderschied, R. W., and Sonnenschein, M. A., eds. 1992. *Mental Health, United States,* Washington, DC: Center for Mental Health Services and National Institute of Mental Health. DHHS Pub. No. (SMA) 92-1942) Government Printing Office.

National Center for Health Statistics. 1998. *Health United States, 1998, with Socioeconomic Status and Health Chartbook*. Hyattsville, Md.

Roach, L. B. Color Changes in Dark Skin. *Nursing* 77 (January): 48–51.

Spector, R. Culture, Ethnicity, and Nursing. In *Fundamentals of Nursing*, 3d ed., edited by P. Potter and A. Perry. St. Louis: Mosby-Year Book.

Spurlock, J. 1988. Black Americans. In *Cross-Cultural Mental Health*, edited by L. Comas-Diaz and E. E. H. Griffith. New York: Wiley.

Sykes, J., and Kelly, A. P. 1979. Black Skin Problems. *American Journal of Nursing* (June): 1092–1094.

Tallant, R. 1946. *Voodoo in New Orleans*, 7th printing. New York: Collier.

U.S. Department of Health and Human Services. 1992. *Healthy People 2000 National Health Promotion and Disease Prevention Objectives—Full Report with Commentary*. Boston: Jones and Bartlett.

———. 1993. *Health, United States, 1992; and Healthy People 2000 Review*. DHHS Pub. No. (PHS) 93-1232. Washington, D.C.: United States Department of Health and Human Services, Public Health Service Centers for Disease Control and Prevention, 44.

Webb, J. Y. 1971. Letter. Dr. J. R. Krevans to Y. Webb, 15 February 1967. Reported in *Superstitious Influence—VooDoo in Particular—Affecting Health Practices in a Selected Population in Southern Louisiana*. Paper. New Orleans.

Wintrob, R. 1972. Hexes, Roots, Snake Eggs? M.D. vs. Occults. *Medical Opinion* 1(7):54–61.

INTERNET SOURCE

http://www.census.gov

❋ *Resources*

- National Black Nurses Association, Inc.
  P.O. Box 1823
  Washington, D.C. 20013
  (202) 393-6870
  Publish: *Journal of the National Black Nurses Association*

- University Microfilms International
  300 North Zeeb Road
  P.O. Box 1764
  Ann Arbor MI 48106
  Publish: *Black Studies: A Catalog of Selected Doctoral Dissertation Research*

- Letteria Dalton Sigma Omega Foundation, Inc.
  P.O. Box 6479
  Cincinnati OH 45206-0479
  This organization is a public foundation founded on the principle that the empowerment of the black family is necessary for a strong viable community.

- Black Caucus
  American Public Health Association
  1015 Fifteenth Street, N.W.
  Washington, D.C. 20005
  Additional resources are included in Appendix VIII.

*Figure 10–1 from page 215
The chapter opening quilt panel of HEALTH-related images depicts the following objects people of Black American heritage may use to protect, maintain, and/or restore their HEALTH. The **beaded gourd** from Africa may be used to store traditional healing herbs. The **egg with mating couple** from Ethiopia represents the art forms linked to symbolic beliefs. Here, the couple is mating within the egg, and the shell is decorated with a tree—a symbol of life. The **drum** from Africa represents the role music plays in HEALTH. The drum serves as a reminder that African people came across the waters with more than one instrument and that music celebrates the Spirit of the African Celebration of Life. Music is sacred and plays an integral part in the life of people and is used to restore and maintain HEALTH. **Silver bangle bracelets** from Saint Thomas, the Virgin Islands, are open to let out evil yet closed to prevent evil from entering the body. They are said to tarnish when the person wearing them is vulnerable to illness; this alerts the person to take better care of themselves. They are worn from birth, and many people believe that they will die if they remove them. Often, many bracelets are worn together, and the sound that they make when they touch is said to scare the evil spirits away. These are worn to protect HEALTH. The **beadedbreast plate** from Africa is arrow shaped and may be worn for protection, as it contains an evil-eye motif. It may also be worn by the traditional healer during healing rituals. **Talismans** are believed

to hold even greater protective powers than amulets. This marionette protects the owner from all sickness. The piece of hand-engraved parchment is worn on a string around the waist or carried in a pocket or purse. **Rectified turpentine with sugar** is used by many Black Americans to treat a cough. Nine drops of turpentine nine days after intercourse acts as a contraceptive. Sugar and turpentine may be used to get rid of worms. **Dried snake** from Africa is ground up and brewed as a tea, and the liquid is used to treat skin blemishes. The **hat** is symbolic of the special clothing and hats that are worn to church by many Black American people. The spiritual importance of worship forms a strong link for members of the Black community.

Chapter 11

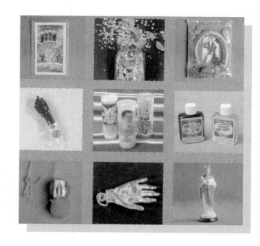

HEALTH and Illness in Hispanic American Communities

. . . AIDS haunts East Harlem. The neighborhood, north of 96th Street and east of Fifth Avenue is home to mostly poor Hispanics. On these streets, about 1 of every 35 adults has AIDS.

—Felicia R. Lee

The second largest emerging majority group, which is on the verge of being the largest, in the United States is composed of the Hispanic subgroups. In this chapter, the term *Hispanic Americans* refers to people who were born in or whose predecessors came from (even generations ago) Mexico, Puerto Rico, Cuba, Central and South America, Spain, and other Spanish-speaking communities and who now live in the United States. The term is then used to represent the diversity of the populations. The people constituted 9% of the population in the 1990 census and were estimated to make up 11.4% of the population in 1999 (www.census.gov). They are the fastest growing group. Over 70% of the people within this group were born in the United States (U.S. Department of Health and Human Services 1992, 34). Box 11–1 is an overview of Hispanic firsts from 1960 to 1997.

❀ *The Chicanos*

Who are the Chicanos? In answering this question, we hope to discover who the Mexican Americans are. What should the people be called? Depending on

---

Figure 11–1 (From left to right, top to bottom) Prayer card, herbal remedies, *rosa y cruz, mano negro,* candles, oils, deer's eye, *mano milagroso,* statue of Saint Barbara. *(For more information on each picture see explanation at the end of chapter.*)*

Box 11–1 ***Hispanic Firsts:***
1960–1998

1960	Mexican Americans become a sizable voting block and support the Kennedy–Johnson ticket
1965	Cesar Chavez forms the farmworkers union in Delano, California
1982	*Plyer* v. *Doe* case is won, giving children of undocumented workers in Texas the right to free public education
1984	Roberto Clemente, the baseball player, appears on a U.S. postage stamp
1986	Franklin Chang-Diaz is an astronaut on the space shuttle *Columbia*
1987	Geraldo M. Rivera hosts a nationally syndicated talk show
1989	Antonia Novella is appointed U.S. Surgeon General
1992	Voters Assistance Act passes making bilingual voter information available
1996	March for justice in Washington, DC, to protest attacks on affirmative action, immigration, welfare, and education
1997	Frederico Peña is appointed U.S. Secretary of Energy

From: Kanellos, N. (Detroit: Visible Ink Press, 1997). *Hispanic Firsts.* Reprinted with permission.

socioeconomic status, immigration or citizenship status, age, and the area in which the person lives, a member of this large emerging majority group refers to him- or herself as either Mexican American, Spanish American, Latin American, Latin, Latino or Mexican (Simmen 1972, 35). The term *Chicano* is used as an "identifying umbrella that identifies all Americans of Mexican descent" (p. 38). Hence the term is used here to refer to this particular cultural and ethnic group.

Americans of Hispanic origin, according to the 1990 census, numbered at least 13,600,190 people and of this number 7,225,591 were of Mexican origin. This figure is known to be an underenumeration and has increased since 1990. Figures will be available in early 2001 with the 2000 census data. This population is rapidly increasing because of a high birthrate and both legal and illegal immigration.

> We came to California long before the Pilgrims landed at Plymouth Rock. We settled California, and all the Southwestern part of the United States, including the States of Arizona, New Mexico, Colorado, and Texas. We built the missions and cultivated the ranches (Simmen 1970a, 38).

The Chicanos have been in the United States for a long time, moving from Mexico and later intermarrying with Indians and Spanish people in the southwestern parts of what is now the United States. Santa Fe, New Mexico, was settled in 1609. Most of the descendants of these early settlers now live in

Arizona, California, Colorado, New Mexico, and Texas. A large number of Chicanos also live in Illinois, Indiana, Kansas, Michigan, Missouri, Nebraska, New York, Ohio, Utah, Washington, and Wisconsin. Most Chicanos arrived in these latter states as migrant farm workers. While located there as temporary farm workers they found permanent jobs and stayed. Contrary to the popular views that Chicanos live in rural areas, most live in urban areas. Chicanos are employed in all types of jobs. Few, however, have high-paying or high-status jobs in labor or management. The majority work in factories, mines, and construction; others are employed in farm work and service areas. At present, only a small—though growing—number of the people are employed in clerical and professional areas. The number of unemployed in this group is high (estimated to be between 25 and 30%), and the earnings of those employed are well below the national average. The education of Chicanos, like that of most minorities in the United States, lags behind that of most of the population. Many Chicanos fail to complete high school. In the past few years, this situation has changed, and Chicano children are being encouraged to stay in school, go on to college, and enter the professions (Simmen 1970b, 45–52).

TRADITIONAL DEFINITIONS OF HEALTH AND ILLNESS

There are conflicting reports about the traditional meaning of health among Chicanos. Some sources maintain that health is considered to be purely the result of "good luck" and that a person loses his or her health if that luck changes (Welch, Comer, and Steinman 1973, 205). Some people describe health as a reward for good behavior. Seen in this context, health is a gift from God and should not be taken for granted. People are expected to maintain their own equilibrium in the universe by performing in the proper way, eating the proper foods, and working the proper amount of time. The protection of HEALTH is an accepted practice that is accomplished with prayer, the wearing of religious medals or amulets, and keeping relics in the home. Herbs and spices can be used to enhance this form of prevention, as can exemplary behavior (Lucero 1975). Illness is seen as an imbalance in an individual's body or as punishment meted out for some wrongdoing. The causes of illness can be grouped into five major categories.

1. The Body's Imbalance. Imbalance may exist between "hot" and "cold" or "wet" and "dry." The theory of hot and cold was brought to Mexico by Spanish priests and was fused with Aztec beliefs. The concept actually dates to the early Hippocratic theory of disease and four body humors. The disrupted relationship among these humors is often mentioned by Chicanos as the cause of disease (Lucero 1975).

There are four body fluids, or humors: (1) *blood,* hot and wet, (2) *yellow bile,* hot and dry, (3) *phlegm,* cold and wet, and (4) *black bile,* cold and dry. When all four humors are balanced, the body is healthy. When any imbalance occurs, an illness is manifested (Currier 1966). These concepts, of course, provide one way of determining the remedy for a particular illness. For example, if an illness is classified as hot, it is treated with a cold substance. A cold disease, in turn, must be treated with a hot substance. Food, beverages, animals, and people possess the characteristics of hot and cold to various degrees. Hot foods cannot be combined; they are to be eaten with cold foods. There is no general agreement as to what is a hot disease or food and what is a cold disease or food. The classification varies from person to person, and what is hot to one person may be cold to another (Saunders 1958, 13). Therefore, if a Chicano patient refuses to eat the meals offered to him in the hospital, it is wise to ask precisely what he can eat and what combinations of foods he thinks would be helpful for the existing condition. It is important to note that *hot* and *cold* do not refer to temperature but are descriptive of a particular substance itself.

For example, after a woman delivers a baby, a hot experience, she cannot eat pork, which is considered a hot food. She must eat something cold to restore her balance. Penicillin is a hot medication; therefore, it cannot be used to treat a hot disease. The major problem for the health-care provider is to *know* that the rules, so to speak, of hot and cold vary from person to person. If health-care providers understand the general nature of the hot and cold imbalance, they will be able to help the patient reveal the nature of the problem from the patient's perspective.

2. Dislocation of Parts of the Body. Two examples of "dislocation" are *empacho* and *caida de la mollera* (Nall and Spielberg 1967).

Empacho is believed to be caused by a ball of food clinging to the wall of the stomach. Common symptoms of this illness are stomach pains and cramps. This ailment is treated by rubbing and gently pinching the spine. Prayers are recited throughout the treatment. Another, more common, cause of such illness is thought to be lying about the amount of food consumed.

A 20-year-old Hispanic woman experienced the acute onset of sharp abdominal pain. She complained to her friend, and together they diagnosed the problem as *empacho* and treated it by massaging her stomach and waiting for the pain to dissipate. It did not, and they continued folk treatment for 48 hours. When the pain did not diminish, they sought help in a nearby hospital. The diagnosis was "acute appendicitis." The young woman nearly died and was quite embarrassed when she was scolded by the physician for not seeking help sooner.

Caida de la mollera is a more serious illness. It occurs in infants and young children aged under 1 year who are dehydrated for some reason (usually because of diarrhea or severe vomiting) and whose anterior fontanelle is depressed below the contour of the skull (Dorsey and Jackson 1976, 56). Much superstition and mystery surround this problem. Some of the poorly educated and rural people, in particular, believe that it is caused by a nurse's or physician's having touched the head of the baby. This can be understood if we take into account that (1) the fontanelle of an infant does become depressed if the infant is dehydrated, and (2) when physicians or nurses measure an infant's head they do touch this area. If a mother brings her baby to a physician for an examination and sees the physician touch the child's head, and if the baby gets sick thereafter with *caida de la mollera*, it might be very easy for this woman to believe it is the fault of the physician's or nurse's touch. Unfortunately, epidemics of diarrhea are common in the rural and urban areas of the Southwest, and a number of children tend to be affected. One case of severe dehydration that leads to *caida de la mollera* may create quite a stir among the people. The folk treatment of this illness has not been found to be effective. Unfortunately, babies are rarely brought to the hospital in time, and the mortality rate for this illness is high (Lucero 1975).

3. Magic or Supernatural Causes Outside the Body. Witchcraft or possession is considered to be culturally patterned role playing, a safe vehicle for restoring oneself. Witchcraft or possession legitimizes acting out bizarre behavior or engaging in incoherent speech.

A lesser disease that is caused from outside the body is *mal ojo*. *Mal ojo* means "bad eye," and it is believed to result from excessive admiration on the part of another. General malaise, sleepiness, fatigue, and severe headache are the symptoms of this condition. The folk treatment is to find the person who has caused the illness by casting the "bad eye" and have him care for the afflicted person (Nall and Spielberg 1967).

4. Strong Emotional States. *Susto* is described as an illness arising from fright. It afflicts many people—males and females, rich and poor, rural dwellers and urbanities. It involves *soul loss:* The soul is able to leave the body and wander freely. This can occur while a person is dreaming or when a person experiences a particularly traumatic event. The symptoms of the disease are (1) restlessness while sleeping, (2) listlessness, anorexia, and disinterest in personal appearance when awake, including disinterest in both clothing and personal hygiene, (3) loss of strength, depression, and introversion. The person is treated by a *curandero* (a folk healer, discussed in the section on *curanderismo*) who coaxes the soul back into the person's body. During the healing rites, the person is massaged and made to relax (Rubel 1964).

5. Envidia. *Envidia,* or envy, also is considered to be a cause of illness and bad luck. Many people believe that to succeed is to fail. That is, when one's success provokes the envy of friends and neighbors, misfortune can befall the person and his or her family. For example, a successful farmer, just when he is able to purchase extra clothing and equipment, is stricken with a fatal illness. He may well attribute the cause of this illness to the envy of his peers. A number of social scientists have, after much research, concluded that the "low" economic and success rates of the Chicano can ostensibly be attributed to belief in *envidia* (Lucero 1975).

RELIGIOUS RITUALS

Magicoreligious practices are quite common among the Chicano population. The more severe an illness, the more likely these practices are observed. There are four types of practices: (1) making promises, (2) visiting shrines, (3) offering medals and candles, and (4) offering prayers (Nall and Spielberg

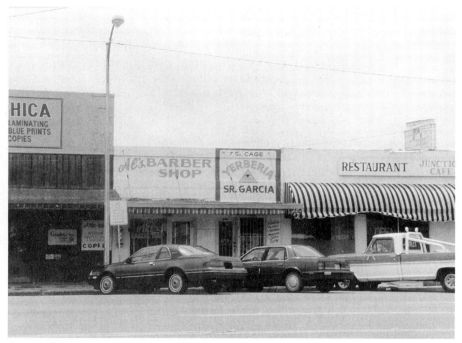

Figure 11–2 A traditional community resource (Yerberia) in Mission, Texas, where a person may purchase traditional remedies and amulets. (Photograph by the author.)

1967). It is not unusual for the people residing near the southern border of the continental United States to return home to Mexico on religious pilgrimages. The film mentioned in Chapter 6, *We Believe in Niño Fedencio,* demonstrates how these pilgrimages are conducted. The lighting of candles also is a frequently observed practice. These beautiful candles made of beeswax and tallow can be purchased in many stores, particularly grocery stores and pharmacies that are located in Chicano neighborhoods (Figs. 11–2 and 11–3). Many homes have shrines with statues and pictures of saints. The candles are lit here and prayers are recited. Some homes have altars with statues and pictures on them and are the focal point of the home. Some Chicanos are devoted to the Virgin de San Juan del Valle and make pilgrimages to the shrine in San Juan, Texas (Fig. 11–4).

When you visit a Catholic church in communities with Hispanic populations, such as San Antonio, Texas, or Chimayo, New Mexico (Fig. 11–5), it is not unusual to see statues covered with flowers and voltive figures such as those in Figure 11–6. These miniature articles are known in Spanish as *milagros,* meaning "miracles." *Milagros* are offered to a saint in thanks for answering a person's prayers. These are prayers for healing, success, a good marriage, and so forth. The *milagros* are made from wax, wood, bone, or a variety of metals and they are an integral part of an ancient folk tradition that is found in many cultures (Egan 1991, 1–2).

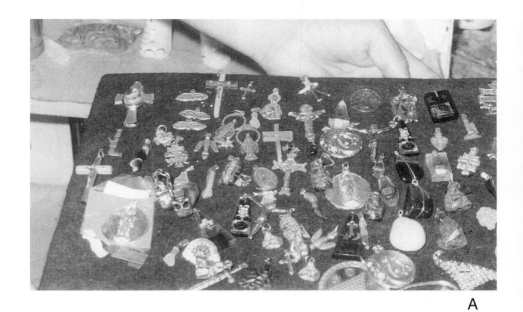

A

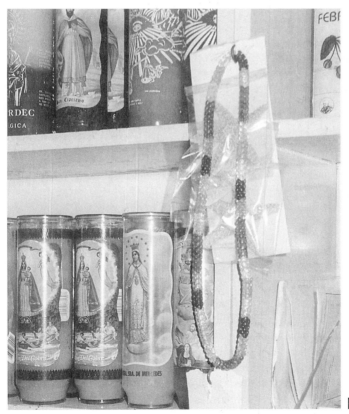

B

Figure 11–3 Samples of amulets (A) and candles (B) sold in Sr. Garcia's Yerberia. (Photographs by author.)

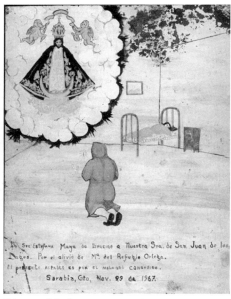

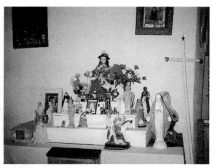

Figure 11–5   An altar in El Santuario de Chimayo, Chimayo, New Mexico. The figures are festooned with flowers and milagros. (Photograph by the author.)

Figure 11–4   A picture of a person giving thanks to the Virgin of San Juan de la Valle for the recovery of a loved one. (Spector Collection. Photograph by author.)

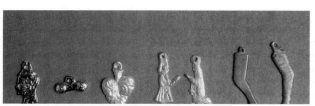

Figure 11–6   Milagros. (Spector Collection. Photograph by the author.)

CURANDERISMO

There are no specific rules for knowing who in the community uses the services of the folk healers. Not all Chicanos do, and not all Chicanos believe in their precepts. Initially, it was thought that only the poor used a folk healer, or *curandero*, because they were unable to get treatment from the larger, institutionalized health-care establishments. It now appears, however, that the use of healers occurs widely throughout the Chicano population. Some people try to use healers exclusively, whereas others use them along with institutionalized care. The healers do not advertise, but they are well known throughout the population because of informal community and kinship networks.

Curanderismo is defined as a medical system (Maduro 1976). It is a coherent view with historical roots that combine Aztec, Spanish, spiritualistic, homeopathic, and scientific elements.

The *curandero(a)* is a holistic healer. The people who seek help from him or her do so for social, physical, and psychological purposes. The *curandero(a)* can be either a "specialist" or a "generalist," a full-time or part-time practitioner. Chicanos who believe in *curanderos* consider them to be religious figures.

A *curandero(a)* may receive the "gift of healing" through three means. (1) He or she may be "born" to heal. In this case it is known from the moment of a *cuandero*'s birth that something unique about this person means that he is destined to be a healer. (2) He or she may learn by apprenticeship— that is, a person is taught the ways of healing, especially the use of herbs. (3) He or she may receive a "calling" through a dream, trance, or vision by which contact is made with the supernatural by means of a "patron" (or "caller"), who may be a saint. The "call" comes either during adolescence or during the midlife crises. This "call" is resisted at first. Later the person becomes resigned to his or her fate and gives in to the demands of the "calling."

Other folk healers include the *materia* or spirit channeler and the *partera* or lay midwife. Box 11–2 describes the scope of the *partera's* practice.

Box 11–2 *The Partera*

In Mexico and South Texas there is a long history of the use of midwives, or *parteras*. The practice of midwifery predates Cortes. The goddess Tlozoteotl was the goddess of childbirth, and the midwives were known as "Tlamatqui-Tuti." The *partera* is viewed as a healer by many members of the Mexican American and Mexican communities. She (most are women, although currently obstetricians from Mexico are providing this service in South Texas) is described as an individual who has the ability to heal and is outgoing, warm, gentle, caring, and cooperative. The *partera's* duties include (1) giving advice to the pregnant woman, (2) giving physical aid, such as treating any illness the woman may experience during pregnancy, (3) guiding the woman through her pregnancy in terms of nutrition or activities she can and cannot do, and (4) being in attendance during labor and delivery.

Patients are most often referred to the *parteras* by their friends or relatives. "A *partera* with a good reputation is always busy." Several *parteras* receive referrals from the health department with which they register, some advertise in the local newspaper, others in the telephone book, and several have signs on their homes or clinics (Fig. 11–7).

The *parteras* avoid delivering women with high blood pressure, anemia, a history of diabetes, multiple babies, and transverse presentations. Several *parteras* also prefer to send women with breech presentations to the hospital. If an unfamiliar woman in labor appears at their door "in the middle of the night" who is very poor with no place to go to deliver, most claim they will "take her in."

Most of the *parteras* keep records of their deliveries. Included in these records are such data as the name of the mother, date, time of admission, stage of labor, time in labor, contractions, time of delivery, presenting part, time of delivery and condition of placenta, and the physical condition of the mother and baby.

The amount of prenatal care the *parteras* deliver ranges from "a lot to a little." In general, the mothers seek assistance during their third or fourth month of pregnancy. When the *partera's* assistance is sought, the mother is sent either to the health department or to a doctor for routine blood work. The *partera*

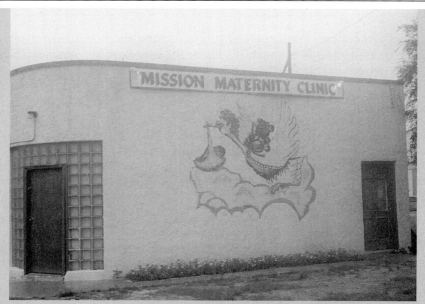

Figure 11–7 Sign for *partera* facilities. (Photograph by the author.)

is able to follow the mother's case and gives her advice and massages. One important service that the *partera* performs is the repositioning of the fetus in the womb through massage.

A *partera* may give several forms of advice to the pregnant woman. For example, she may advise the woman who is experiencing pica (the craving for and ingestion of nonfood substances, such as clay and laundry starch) to purchase solid milk of magnesia in Mexico. The milk of magnesia tastes like clay, thereby satisfying the pica, and is not considered harmful. The mother with food cravings is advised to satisfy them. The mothers also are instructed not to lift heavy objects, to take laxatives to prevent constipation, to exercise often by walking frequently, and to not cross their legs or bathe in hot water. The reason for the last two admonitions is the belief that crossing the legs and taking hot baths can cause the baby to assume the breech position.

If the *partera* knows the exact date of the mother's last period, she is able to accurately estimate when the woman is going to deliver by calculating eight lunar months and 27 days from the onset of the last period.

With the onset of labor, the mother contacts the *partera*. She goes to the birthing place—home or clinic of the *partera*—or the *partera* comes to her home. The mother is examined vaginally to determine how far along in labor she is and the position of the baby. She is instructed to shower and to empty her bowels, with an enema, if necessary; and she is encouraged to walk and move around until the delivery is imminent. Once the mother is ready to deliver, she is put to bed. Most of the mothers are delivered lying down in bed. If the mother chooses to do so, however, she is delivered in a squatting or sitting position. Several home remedies may be used during labor, including comino (cumin seed) tea or canela (cinnamon) tea to stimulate labor.

The baby is stimulated if needed, and the mucus is removed from the mouth and nose as needed with the use of a bulb syringe. The cord is clamped, tied with cord ties, and cut with scissors that have been boiled and soaked in alcohol. The stump is then treated with merbromin (Mercurochrome), alcohol, or a combination of the two. The baby is weighed, and some time after the delivery, it is bathed. Most of the *parteras* bind both the mother and the baby. The baby may be fed oregano or cumin tea right after birth or later to help it spit up the mucus. Eyedrops are instilled in the baby's eyes, in compliance with state laws (silver nitrate is used most frequently).

The *partera* stays at the mother's home for several hours after the delivery and then returns to check the mother and the baby the next day. If the mother delivers at the home of the *partera,* she generally stays 12 to 14 hours.

There are several ways of disposing of the placenta. It may just be placed in a plastic bag and thrown in the trash, or it may be buried in the yard. Some placentas are buried with a religious or folk ceremony. There are several folk reasons given for the burial of the placenta. The placenta must be buried so that the animals will not eat it. If it is eaten by a dog, the mother will not be able to bear any more children. If it is thrown in the trash, the mother's womb may become "cold." If the baby is a girl, the placenta is buried near the home so the daughter will not go far away. If it is a boy, it is buried far away.

The practice of the *partera* in the Rio Grande Valley is the life of the past, the present, and of the future: "a way of life de ayer, hoy y mañana" (Julian Castillo 1982).

Adapted from: Spector, R. *Cultural Diversity in Health and Illness,* 4th ed. (Stamford, Conn.: Appleton & Lang, 1996), pp. 305–325.

TREATMENT

The most popular form of treatment used by folk healers involves herbs, especially when used as teas. The *curandero* knows what specific herbs to use for a problem. This information is revealed in dreams in which the "patron" gives suggestions.

Because the *curandero* has a religious orientation, much of the treatment includes elements of both the Catholic and Pentecostal rituals and artifacts: offerings of money, penance, confession, lighting candles, wooden or metal offerings in the shape of the afflicted anatomical parts *(milagros)*, and laying on of hands. Massage is used in illnesses, such as *empacho* (discussed in the section on body imbalance).

Cleanings, or *limpias,* are done in two ways. The first is by passing an unbroken egg over the body of the ill person. The second method entails passing herbs tied in a bunch over the body. The back of the neck, which is considered a vulnerable spot, is given particular attention.

In contrast to the depersonalized care Chicanos expect to receive in medical institutions, their relationship with and care by the *curandero* are uniquely personal, as described in Table 11–1. This special relationship between the Chicano and the *curandero* may well account for this folk healer's popularity.

Table 11–1 | **Comparisons Between Curandero and Allopathic Health-Care Provider**

Curandero	Physician
1. Maintains informal, friendly, affective relationship with entire family	1. Businesslike, formal relationship; deals only with the patient
2. Comes to house day or night	2. Patient must go to physician's office or clinic, and only during the day; may have to wait for hours to be seen; home visits are rarely made
3. For diagnosis, consults with head of house, creates a mood of awe, talks to all family members, is not authoritarian, has social rapport, builds expectation of cure	3. Rest of family is usually ignored; deals solely with the ill person, and may deal only with the sick part of the patient; authoritarian manner creates fear
4. Is generally less expensive than physicians	4. More expensive than *curanderos*
5. Has ties to the "world of the sacred"; has rapport with the symbolic, spiritual, creative, or holy force	5. Secular; pays little attention to the religious beliefs or meaning of a given illness
6. Shares the world view of the patient—that is, speaks the same language, lives in the same neighborhood or in some similar socioeconomic conditions, may know the same people, understands the lifestyle of the patient	6. Generally does not share the world view of the patient—that is, may not speak the same language, does not live in the same neighborhood, does not understand the socioeconomic conditions or lifestyle of the patient

In addition to the close, personal relationship between patient and healer, other factors may explain the continuing belief in *curanderismo.*

1. The mind and body are inseparable.
2. The central problem of life is to maintain harmony, including social, physical, and psychological aspects of the person.
3. There must be harmony between the hot and cold, wet and dry. The treatment of illness should restore the body's harmony, which has been lost.
4. The patient is the passive recipient of disease when the disease is caused by an external force. This external force disrupts the natural order of the internal person, and the treatment must be designed to restore this order. The causes of disharmony are evil and witches.
5. A person is related to the spirit world. When the body and soul are separated, "soul loss can occur." This loss is sometimes caused by *susto,* a disease or illness resulting from fright, which may afflict individuals from all socioeconomic levels and lifestyles.
6. The responsibility for recovery is shared by the ill person, the family, and the *curandero.*

HEALTH and Illness in Hispanic American Communities ■ 249

Table 11–2 **Classification of Selected Emotional Illnesses in Segments of the Hispanic Population**

Disease Type	Common Cause	Specific Diseases
Mental illness	Heredity	Epilepsy *(epilepsia)*
	Hex	Evil eye *(mal ojo)*
		Witchcraft *(hechiceria)*
	Worry	Anxiety *(tirisia)*
	Fright *(susto)*	Hysteria *(histeria)*
		Nervous breakdown *(ataque de nervios)*
	Blow to the head	Craziness *(locura)*
Moral illness	Vice	User of—drugs *(drogadicto)*
		—marijuana *(marijuanero)*
	Character weakness	Alcoholism *(alcoholismo)*
	Emotions	Jealousy *(celos)*
		Rage *(coraje)*

From: Spencer, R. T., Nichols, L. W., Lipkin, G. B., et al. *Clinical Pharmacology and Nursing Management,* 4th ed. (Philadelphia: Lippincott, 1993), p. 133. Reprinted with permission.

7. The natural world is not clearly distinguished from the supernatural world. Thus, the *curandero* can coerce, curse, and appease the spirits. The *curandero* places more emphasis on his or her connections with the sacred and the gift of healing than on personal properties. (Such personal properties might include, for example, social status, a large home, and expensive material goods.)

Several examples of emotional illnesses (Table 11–2) are found in the Hispanic, and frequently in Chicano, populations. These are further divided into mental illness (in which the illness is not judged) and moral illness (in which others can judge the victim). Ethnopharmacologic teas may be used to treat these maladies (Table 11–3).

Table 11–3 **Ethnopharmacologic Teas Commonly Used to Treat Mental Ailments**

Spanish Name	English Name	Botanical Name	Ailment Treated
Manzanilla	Camomile	*Matricaria chamomilla*	Cure fright *(susto)*
Yerba buena	Spearmint	*Mentha spicata*	Nervousness
Te de narranjo	Orange leaves	*Citrus aurantium*	Sedative, nervousness
Albacar	Sweet basil	*Ocimum basilicum*	Treat *susto;* ward off evil spirits

From: Spencer, R. T., Nichols, L. W., Lipkin, G. B. et al. *Clinical Pharmacology and Nursing Management,* 4th ed. (Philadelphia: Lippincott, 1993), p. 133. Reprinted with permission.

❋ *Puerto Ricans*

Puerto Rican migrants to the United States mainland are American citizens, albeit with a different language and culture. They are neither immigrants nor aliens. According to the 1990 census, at least 1,895,981 Puerto Ricans live on the mainland. They live mostly on the East Coast, with the greatest number living in New York City and metropolitan New Jersey. Most Puerto Ricans migrate to search for a better life or because relatives, particularly spouses and parents, have migrated previously. Life on the island of Puerto Rico is difficult because there is a high level of unemployment. Puerto Ricans are not well known or understood by the majority of people in the continental United States. Little is known about their cultural identity. Mainlanders tend to forget that Puerto Rico is, for the most part, a poor island whose people have many problems. When many Puerto Ricans migrate to the mainland, they bring many of their problems—especially those with poor health and social circumstance (Cohen 1972).

Puerto Ricans, along with Cubans, constitute the most recent major immigration group to these shores. They cover the spectrum of racial differences and have practiced racial intermarriage. Many are Catholic, but some belong to Protestant sects.

Many people from Puerto Rico perceive health and illness and use folk healers and remedies in ways similar to those used by other Hispanics, whereas others practice santeria. Most studies on health and illness beliefs and healing have been conducted on Chicanos. It is not easy to find information about the beliefs of Puerto Ricans. Much of the information presented here was gleaned from students and patients. Both groups feel that their beliefs should be known by health-care deliverers. One student, whose mother is a healer and is teaching her daughter the art, corroborated much of the following material.

COMMON FOLK DISEASES AND THEIR TREATMENT

Table 11–4 lists a number of folk diseases and the usual source and type of treatment.* Many of these diseases or disharmonies have been mentioned in the section on Chicano approaches. Nonetheless, there are subtle differences in the ways folk diseases are perceived by Chicanos and Puerto Ricans. For example, although diseases are classified as hot and cold, treatments—that is, food and medications—are categorized as hot *(caliente)*, cold *(frio)*, and cool *(fresco)*. Cold illnesses are treated with hot remedies; hot diseases are treated with cold or *cool* remedies. Table 11–5 lists the major illnesses, foods, and medicines and herbs associated with the hot–cold system as it is applied among Puerto Ricans in New York City.

---

*The data contained in Table 11–4 were provided by Puerto Rican students and patients who were interviewed carefully several times.

Table 11–4 Folk Diseases

Name	Description	Treatment	Source of Treatment
Susto	Sudden fright, causing shock	Relaxation	Relative or friend
Fatigue	Asthmalike symptoms	Oxygen; medications	Western health-care system
Pasmo	Paralysis-like symptoms, face or limbs	Prevention; massage	Folk
Empacho	Food forms into a ball and clings to the stomach, causing pain and cramps	Strong massage over the stomach; medication; gently pinching and rubbing the spine	Folk
Mal ojo	Sudden, unexplained illness in a usually well child or person	Prevention; babies wear a special charm	Depends on the severity of the symptoms; usually home or folk
Ataque	Screaming, falling to ground, wildly moving arms and legs	None—ends spontaneously	

Table 11–5 The Hot–Cold Classification Among Puerto Ricans

	Frio (cold)	Fresco (cool)	Caliente (hot)
Illness or bodily conditions	Arthritis Menstrual period Joint pains	Colds	Constipation Diarrhea Pregnancy Rashes Ulcers
Medicine and herbs		Bicarbonate of soda Linden flowers Milk of magnesia Nightshade Orange flower water Sage Tobacco	Anise Aspirin Castor oil Cinnamon Cod-liver oil Iron tablets Penicillin Vitamins
Foods	Avocado Banana Coconut Lima beans Sugar cane White beans	Barley water Whole milk Chicken Fruits Honey Raisins Salt cod Watercress Onions Peas	Alcoholic beverages Chili peppers Chocolate Coffee Corn meal Evaporated milk Garlic Kidney beans

From: Schilling, B., and Brannon, E. "Health Related Dietary Practices," in *Cross-Cultural Counseling—A Guide for Nutrition and Health Counselors.* (Alexandria, Va.: U.S. Department of Agriculture, U.S. Department of Health and Human Services, Nutrition and Technical Services Division, September, 1986), p. 5. Reprinted with permission.

A number of activities are carried out to maintain the proper hot–cold balance in the body. The following list was prepared by a former patient.

1. *Pasmo,* a form of paralysis, usually is caused by an upset in the hot–cold balance. For example, if a woman is ironing (hot) and then steps out into the rain (cold), she may get facial or other paralysis.
2. A person who is hot cannot sit under a mango tree (cold) because he or she can get a kidney infection or "back problems."
3. A baby should not be fed a formula (hot), as it may cause rashes; whole milk (cold) is acceptable.
4. A man who has been working (hot) must not go into the coffee fields (cold), or he could contract a respiratory illness.
5. A hot person must not drink cold water, as it could cause colic.

There is often a considerable time lag between disregarding these precautions and the occurrence of illness. A patient who had injured himself while lifting heavy cartons in a factory revealed that the "true" reason he was now experiencing prolonged back problems was because as a child he often sat under a mango tree when he was "hot" after running. This childhood habit had significantly damaged his back so that, as an adult, he was unable to lift heavy objects without causing injury.

The following are examples of selected behaviors a patient may manifest with an illness thought to be caused by an imbalance of hot and cold:

- During pregnancy a woman may avoid hot-classified foods and medicines and take cool-classified medicines
- During the postpartum period or during menstruation a woman may avoid cool-classified foods and medicines
- Infant formulas containing evaporated milk, which are hot-classified, may be avoided as the baby is fed cold-classified whole milk
- Penicillin, a hot-classified prescription, may not be taken for diarrhea, constipation, or a rash as these are hot-classified symptoms
- When a diuretic is prescribed that needs to supplemented with cold-classified bananas or raisins, the bananas or raisins may not be eaten when the disease is a cold-classified condition.

These examples serve to illustrate the use of foods or medicines to restore the sense of balance. (Harwood, 1971)

Puerto Ricans also share with others of Hispanic origin a number of beliefs in spirits and spiritualism. They believe that mental illness is caused primarily by evil spirits and forces. People with such disorders are preferably treated by a "spiritualist medium" (Cohen 1972). The psychiatric clinic is known as the place where *locos* go. This attitude is exemplified in the Puerto Rican approach to visions and the like. The social and cultural environment encourages the acceptance of having visions and hearing voices. In the dominant culture of the continental United States, when one has visions or hears voices, one is encouraged to see a psychiatrist. When a Puerto Rican regards this experience as a problem, he or she may seek help through *santeria* (Mumford 1973).

Santeria is the form of Latin American magic that had its birth in Nigeria, the country of origin of the Yoruba people, who were brought to the New World as slaves over 400 years ago. The *santeria,* or *santero,* may use story telling as a way of helping people cope with day-to-day difficulties (Flores 1991). They brought with them their traditional religion, which was in time synthesized with Catholic images. The believers continue to worship in the traditional way, especially in Puerto Rico, Cuba, and Brazil. The Yorubas identified their gods—*orishas*—with the Christian saints and invested in these saints the same supernatural powers of gods. The *orishas*/saints related to health situations include the following (Gonzalez-Wippler 1987, 1–30; Riva 1990, 91–93):

Orisha	Saint	Health Problem
Chango	Saint Barbara	Violent death
Babalu-Aye	Saint Lazarus	Sickness
Bacoso	Saint Christopher	Infections
Ibeyi	Saints Cosmos and Damian	Infant illnesses
Ifa	Saint Anthony	Fertility
Yemaya	Our Lady of Regla	Maternity

Santeria is a structured system consisting of *espiritismo,* which is practiced by gypsies and mediums who claim to have *facultades.* These special *facultades* provide them with the "license" to practice. The positions of the practitioners form a hierarchy: the head is the *babalow,* a male; second is the *presidente,* the head medium; and third are the *santeros.* Novices are the "believers." The *facultades* are given to the healer from protective Catholic saints, who have African names and are known as *protecciones. Santeria* can be practiced in storefronts, basements, homes, and even college dormitories. *Santeros* dress in white robes for ceremonies and wear special beaded bracelets as a sign of their identity.

Puerto Ricans are able to accept much of what Anglos may judge to be idiosyncratic behavior. In fact, behavioral disturbances are seen as symptoms of illness that are to be treated, not judged. Puerto Ricans make a sharp distinction between "nervous" behavior and being *loco.* To be *loco* is to be bad, dangerous, evil. It also means losing all one's social status. Puerto Ricans who seek standard American treatment for mental illness are castigated by the community. They understandably prefer to get help for the symptoms of mental illness from the *santero,* who accepts the symptoms and attributes the cause of the illness to spirits outside the body. Puerto Ricans have great faith in this system of care and maintain a high level of hope for recovery.

The *santero* is an important person, respecting the patient and not gossiping about either the patient or his or her problems. Anyone can "pour his or her heart out" with no worry of being labeled or judged. The *santero* is able

Table 11–6	**Examples of Cultural Phenomena Affecting Health and Health Care Among Hispanic Americans**
Nations of origin:	Hispanic countries: Spain, Cuba, Mexico, Central and South America, Puerto Rico
Environmental control:	Traditional health and illness beliefs may continue to be observed by "traditional" people. Folk medicine tradition Traditional healers: *curandero, espiritista, partera, senoria*
Biological variations:	Diabetes mellitus Parasites Coccidioidomycosis Lactose intolerance
Social organization:	Nuclear families Large, extended family networks *Compadrazzo* (godparents) Strong church affiliations within community Community social organizations
Communication:	Spanish or Portuguese are the primary languages
Space:	Tactile relationships: touch, handshakes, embrace Value physical presence
Time orientation:	Present

Adapted from: Spector, R. "Culture, Ethnicity, and Nursing," in *Fundamentals of Nursing,* 3d. ed. eds. P. Potter and A. Perry. (St. Louis: Mosby-Yearbook, 1992), p. 101. Reprinted with permission.

to tell a person what the problem is, prescribe the proper treatment, and tell the person what to do, how to do it, and when to do it. A study in New York found that 73% of the Puerto Rican patients in an outpatient mental health clinic reported having visited a *santero.* Often a sick person is taken to a psychiatrist by his family to be "calmed down" and prepared for treatment by a *santero.* Families may become angry if the psychiatrist does not encourage belief in God and prayer during the psychiatrist's work with the patient. Because of cultural differences and beliefs, a psychiatrist often may diagnose as illness what Puerto Ricans may define as health. Frequently, a spiritualist treats the "mental illness" of a patient as *facultades,* which makes the patient a "special person." Thus, esteem is granted to the patient as a form of treatment. A number of cultural phenomena affect the health and health care of Hispanic Americans (Table 11–6) (Mumford 1973).

ENTRY INTO MAINLAND HEALTH SYSTEMS

Puerto Ricans living in New York City and other parts of the northern United States experience a high rate of illness and hospitalization during their first year on the mainland, as do other people of Hispanic origin. It is worthwhile considering the vast differences between living in New York and living in Puerto Rico. In Puerto Rico, winter weather is unheard of. The winters in the north can be bitter cold, and adjustment to climate change in itself is extremely difficult. Migrant people may be forced to live in crowded living quarters with poor sanitation.

Puerto Ricans seeking health care may go to a physician or to a folk practitioner or to both. The general progression of seeking care is as follows:

1. The person seeks advice from a daughter, mother, grandmother, or neighbor woman. These sources are consulted because the women of this culture are the primary healers and dispensers of medicine on the family level.
2. If the advice is not sufficient, the person may seek help from a *senoria* (a woman who is especially knowledgeable about the causes and treatment of illness).
3. If the *senoria* is unable to help, the person goes to a more sophisticated folk practitioner, an *espiritista* or a *curandera*. If the problem is "psychiatric," a *santero* may be consulted. These names describe similar people—those who obtain their knowledge from spirits and treat illness according to the instructions of the spirits. Herbs, lotions, creams, and massage often are used.
4. If the person is still not satisfied, he or she may go to a physician.
5. If the results are not satisfactory, the person may return to a folk practitioner. He or she may seek medical help sooner than step 4 or may go back and forth between the two systems.

Not all Puerto Ricans use the folk system. Health-care providers should remember that people who appear to have delayed seeking health care have most likely counted on curing their illness through the culturally known and well-understood folk process. Often when people disappear—or elope from the established health system—they may have elected to return to the folk system. Those who elope from the larger, institutionalized medical system may visit *botanica*. In these small *botanicas,* one can purchase herbs, potents, Florida water, ointments, and incense prescribed by the spiritualists. Some of these *botanicas* are so busy that each customer is given a number and is assisted only after the number is called (Mumford 1973). There are 24 *botanicas* located in one small area of New York City. A Spanish-speaking colleague and I visited a *botanica* in Boston that was similar to a pharmacy. The door was locked, but the proprietor admitted us when we revealed our identity. He explained the various remedies that were for sale. We were allowed to purchase only a few items because we did not have a spiritualist's prescription for herbs. The store also sold candles, religious statues, cards, medals, and relics.

A limited number of *santerias* place advertisements in local Spanish daily newspapers. Some of the more industrious ones distribute flyers in the New York City subways. Others maintain a low profile, and patients visit them because of their well-established reputations.

CURRENT HEALTH PROBLEMS

The Hispanic health profile is marked by diversity, and people of the Hispanic community experience perhaps the most varied set of health issues encountered by any of the emerging majority populations. The diversity in health problems is intertwined with the effects of socioeconomic status, and with geographic and cultural differences. The most important health issues for Hispanics are related to these demographic facts: the population is young and has a high birthrate (U.S. Department of Health and Human Services 1992, 30).

Mexican Americans have low rates of cerebrovascular disease, yet stroke rates among Puerto Ricans in New York are high. Infant mortality rates vary from group to group. The leading causes of death among Hispanic Americans illustrate differences between their health experiences and those of the total population, as can be seen in Table 11–7.

Hispanics experience a number of barriers when seeking health care. The most obvious one is language. In spite of the fact that Spanish-speaking people constitute one of the largest minority groups in this country, very few health-care deliverers speak Spanish. This is especially true in communities in which the number of Spanish-speaking people is relatively small. Hispanics who live in these areas experience tremendous frustration because of the language barrier. Even in large cities, there are far too many occasions when a sick person has to rely on a young child to act not only as a translator but also as interpreter. One way of sensitizing young nursing students to the pain of this situation is to ask them to present a health problem to a person who does not speak or understand a word of English. Needless to say, this is extremely difficult; it is also embarrassing. People who try this, rapidly comprehend and appreciate the feelings experienced by patients who are unable to speak or understand English. (After

Table 11–7	The 10 Leading Causes of Death for Hispanics and for All Persons, 1996
Hispanics	**All Persons**
1. Diseases of the heart	1. Diseases of the heart
2. Malignant neoplasms	2. Malignant neoplasms
3. Unintentional injuries	3. Cerebrovascular diseases
4. Cerebrovascular diseases	4. Chronic obstructive pulmonary diseases
5. Human immunodeficiency virus infection	5. Unintentional injuries
6. Diabetes mellitus	6. Pneumonia and influenza
7. Homicide and legal intervention	7. Diabetes mellitus
8. Pneumonia and influenza	8. Human immunodeficiency virus infection
9. Chronic liver disease and cirrhosis	9. Suicide
10. Chronic obstructive pulmonary diseases	10. Chronic liver disease and cirrhosis

From: National Center for Health Statistics. *Health United States 1998 with Socioeconomic Status and Health Chartbook.* (Hyattsville, Md.: Centers for Disease Control and Prevention), pp. 212–213.

this experience, two of my students decided to take a foreign-language elective.) Language will continue to be a problem until (1) there are more physicians, nurses, and social workers from the Spanish-speaking communities, and (2) more of the present deliverers of health care learn to speak Spanish.

A second crucial barrier that Hispanic people encounter is poverty. The diseases of the poor—for example, tuberculosis, malnutrition, and lead poisoning—all have high incidences among Spanish-speaking populations.

A final barrier to adequate health care is the time orientation of Hispanic Americans. To Hispanics, time is a relative phenomenon. Little attention is given to the *exact* time of day. The frame of reference is wider, and the issue is whether it is day or night. The American health-care system, on the other hand, places great emphasis on promptness. Health-care providers demand that clients arrive at the exact time of the appointment—despite the fact that clients are often kept waiting. Health-system workers stress the client's promptness rather than their own. In fact, they tend to deny responsibility for the waiting periods by blaming them on the "system." Many facilities commonly schedule all appointments for 9:00 A.M. when it is clearly known and understood by the staff members that the doctor will not even arrive until 11:00 A.M. or later. The Hispanic person frequently responds to this practice by coming late for appointments or failing to come at all. They prefer to attend walk-in clinics, where the waits are shorter. They also much prefer going to traditional healers.

HISPANIC AMERICAN HEALTH-CARE MANPOWER

The number of Americans of Hispanic origin who are enrolled in health programs or who in practice in selected health professions is low, as illustrated in Tables 11–8 and 11–9. Efforts must be made to recruit and maintain more Hispanics in the health professions.

Table 11–8 | **Hispanic Enrollment in Selected Health Professions Schools, 1995–1996**

	Total Program Enrollment	Hispanic Enrollment
Allopathic medicine	66,970	4,349
Osteopathic medicine	8,475	331
Podiatry	2,312	99
Dentistry	16,374	788
Optometry	5,178	196
Pharmacy	33,205	940
Registered nursing	261,219	9,039

From: National Center for Health Statistics. *Health, United States, 1998, with Socioeconomic Status and Health Chartbook.* (Hyattsville, Md., 1998), pp. 330–331.

Table 11–9 | **Percentage of Hispanics Enrolled in Selected Health Professions Schools Compared with Non-Hispanic Whites, 1995–1996**

Profession	Non-Hispanic White (%)	Hispanic (%)
Allopathic medicine	66.6	6.5
Osteopathic medicine	80.3	3.9
Podiatry	77.2	4.3
Dentistry	68.0	4.8
Optometry	75.4	3.8
Pharmacy	71.9	2.8
Registered nurses	82.4	3.5

From: National Center for Health Statistics. *Health, United States, 1998, with Socioeconomic Status and Health Chartbook.* (Hyattsville, Md., 1998), pp. 330–331.

❧ *References*

Castillo, J., director, Division of Health Related Professions. Personal letter of 6 April 1982.

Cohen, R. E. 1972. Principles of Preventive Mental Health Programs for Ethnic Minority Populations: The Acculturation of Puerto Ricans to the United States. *American Journal of Psychiatry* 128, no. 12 (June): 79.

Currier, R. L. 1966. The Hot-Cold Syndrome and Symbolic Balance in Mexican and Spanish-American Folk Medicine. *Ethnology* 5 (March): 251–263.

Dorsey, P. R., and Jackson, H. Q. 1976. Cultural Health Traditions: The Latino/Chicano Perspective. In *Providing Safe Nursing Care for Ethnic People of Color,* edited by M. F. Branch and P. P. Paxton. New York: Appleton-Century-Crofts.

Egan, M. 1991. *Milagros.* Santa Fe: Museum of New Mexico Press.

Flores, Y. Santero in Los Angeles, California. Personal interview, 10 June 1991.

Gonzalez-Wippler, M. 1987. *Santeria—African Magic in Latin America.* Bronx, N.Y.: Original Publications.

Harwood, A. 1971. The Hot–Cold Theory of Disease: Implications for Treatment of Puerto Rican Patients. *JAMA* 216:1154–1155.

Kanellos, N. 1997. *Hispanic Firsts.* Detroit: Visible Ink Press.

Lucero, G. 1975. Health and Illness in the Chicano Community. Lecture given at Boston College School of Nursing, March.

Maduro, R. J. 1976. *Curanderismo: Latin American Folk Healing.* Conference on Ways of Healing, Ancient and Modern. San Francisco, January.

Mumford, E. 1973. Puerto Rican Perspectives on Mental Illness. *Mount Sinai Journal of Medicine* 40, no. 6 (November–December): 771–773.

Nall, F. C. II, and Spielberg, J. 1967. Social and Cultural Factors in the Responses of Mexican-Americans to Medical Treatment. *Journal of Health and Social Behavior* 8: 302.

National Center for Health Statistics. 1998. Health United States 1998 with Socioeconomic Status and Health Chartbook. Hyattsville, Md.: Centers for Disease Control and Prevention.

Riva, A. 1990. *Devotions to the Saints.* Los Angeles: International Imports.

Rubel, A. J. 1964. The Epidemiology of a Folk Illness: Susto in Hispanic America. *Ethnology* 3, no. 3 (July): 270–271.

Saunders, L. 1958. Healing Ways in the Spanish Southwest. In *Patients, Physicians, and Illness,* edited by E. G. Jaco. Glencoe, Ill: Free Press.

Schilling, B., and Brannon, E. 1986. Health Related Dietary Practices. In *Cross-Cultural Counseling: A Guide for Nutrition and Health Counselors.* Alexandria, Va.: U.S. Department of Health and Human Services.

Simmen, E. 1970a. Anonymous, Who Am I? In *Educating the Mexican American,* edited by H. S. Johnson and W. J. Hernandez-M. Valley Forge, Penn.: Judson Press.

———. 1970b. We Mexican Americans. In *Educating the Mexican American,* edited by H. S. Johnson and W. J. Hernandez-M. Valley Forge, Penn.: Judson Press.

———. 1972. *Pain and Promise: The Chicano Today.* New York: New American Library.

Spector, R. 1996. *Cultural Diversity in Health and Illness,* 4th ed. Stamford, Conn.: Appleton & Lang.

Spencer, R. T., Nichols, L. W., Lipkin, G. B., et al. 1993. *Clinical Pharmacology and Nursing Management,* 4th ed. Philadelphia: Lipincott.

U.S. Bureau of the Census. 1992. *1990 Census of the Population, General Population Characteristics United States,* series 1990 CP-1-1. Washington, DC: Government Printing Office, 1992, p. 23.

U.S. Department of Health and Human Services. 1992. *Healthy People 2000, National Health Promotion and Disease Prevention Objectives—Full Report with Commentary.* Boston: Jones and Barlett.

Welch, S., Comer, J., and Steinman, M. 1973. Some Social and Attitudinal Correlates of Health Care among Mexican Americans. *Journal of Health and Social Behavior* 14 (September): 205.

INTERNET SOURCE

http://www.census.gov

❀ *Resources*

- National Coalition of Hispanic Health and Human Services (COSSMHO)
  1030 15th Street, N.W.
  Suite 1053
  Washington, DC 20005

- Latino Caucus
  American Public Health Association
  1015 15th Street, N.W.
  Washington, DC 20005

- National Association of Hispanic Nurses
  2300 West Commerce
  Suite 304
  San Antonio TX 78207
  (512) 226-9743

*Figure 11–1 from page 237
From left to right—top to bottom: The chapter opening quilt panel of HEALTH-related images depicts the following objects people of Hispanic heritage may use to protect, maintain, and/or restore their HEALTH. The **prayer card** depicts the miraculous hand; each finger has one of the Apostle's on it. It is carried for prayer. The Santeros in Puerto Rico carve them, and they are treasured objects. **Herbal remedies** purchased from an herbalist are brewed into a tea and used to treat hypertension. The **rosa y cruz,** from Mexico, is hung by the entrance to the home to protect it from the envy of others, for luck, health, happiness, love, and money. The **mano negro** is placed on babies to protect them from the evil eye and the envy of others. **Candles**—from left to right: The **Cross of Caravaca** is burned for health, courage, strength, fertility, and luck. This "wishing cross" is for good luck, health, and protection against evil. It is yellow to symbolize the power of the mind. The **Niño Fidencio candle** is burned for healing. Niño Fidencio was a famous healer in Mexico. This particular candle has a prayer for protection from suffering and is white, the color of purity. The third candle, **Vela Para Todo,** is an "all-purpose" candle and is burned for good luck, prosperity, luck in love, peace in the household, money, and success. It has many colors, including red for health and courage. **Oils,** from Puerto Rico—**Most Powerful Helping Hand oil** and **Keep Enemies Away oil**—are worn for protection from various feared evils. The **deer's eye** from Mexico is decorated with an image of the Virgin of Guadalupe and red string and a red pom-pom. This amulet is pinned on a baby to protect it from the evil eye and the envy of others. The **mano milagroso** from Mexico is a miraculous hand holding a cross and worn for protection from the evil eye and envy of others. **Saint Barbara statue,** from Cuba, represents the God Chango, and is believed to protect people from a violent death.

Chapter 12

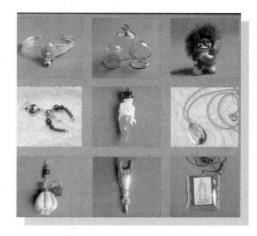

HEALTH and Illness in White European-American Communities

These are magic words. They'll make you feel better.
— *P. Malpezzi*

Members of white-European American communities have been immigrating to this country since the very first settlers came to the shores of New England. The white population has diverse and multiple origins. The recent literature in the area of ethnicity and health has focused on people of color, and little has been written about the white ethnic communities. In this chapter, an overview of the differences, by ethnicity, is presented. Earlier chapters have focused on religious differences with respect to HEALTH and healing. The focus on this chapter is on ethnic differences. Given that we are talking about 75% of the American population, the enormity of the task of attempting to describe each difference is readily apparent. Instead, this chapter highlights some of the basic beliefs of selected groups (those groups with which I have had the greatest exposure). The overview includes not only library research but also firsthand interviews and observations of people in their daily experiences with the health-care delivery system, both as inpatients and as community residents receiving home care.

❈ Background

The major groups migrating to this country between 1820 and 1990 included people from Germany—15%, Italy—11%, United Kingdom—11%,

Figure 12–1 (From left to right, top to bottom) Bracelet, bankes, troll, blue bead and horseshoe, *corno,* Saint Anthony medal, garlic with a blue bead, *figa,* green scapular. *(For more information on each picture see explanation at the end of chapter.*)*

261

$Table\ 12-1$	Examples of Cultural Phenomena Affecting Health Care Among European (White) Americans	
Nations of origin:	Germany, England, Italy, Ireland, former Soviet Union, and all other European countries
Environmental control:	Primary reliance on "modern, Western" health-care delivery system
	Remaining traditional health and illness beliefs and practices may be observed
	Some remaining traditional folk medicine
	Homeopathic medicine resurgent
Biological variations:	Breast cancer
	Heart disease
	Diabetes mellitus
	Thalassemia
Social organization:	Nuclear families
	Extended families
	Judeo-Christian religions
	Community and social organizations
Communication:	National languages
	Many learned English rapidly as immigrants
	Verbal, rather than nonverbal
Space:	Noncontact people—aloof, distant
	Southern countries—closer contact and touch
Time Orientation:	Future over present

Adapted from: Spector, R. "Culture, Ethnicity, and Nursing," in *Fundamentals of Nursing,* 3d ed., eds. P. Potter and A. Perry. (St. Louis: Mosby-Year Book, 1992), p. 101. Reprinted with permission.

Ireland—10%, Austro-Hungary—7%, Canada—8%, and Russia—7%: for a total of 69% of all the immigrants to arrive in this country (Lefcowitz 1996). In 1996, 16% of the total immigrants were from Europe (U.S. Immigration Service 1998). The most populous group—that is, people who are foreign-born Americans or native-born Americans with at least one foreign-born parent—includes people of Italian, German, Canadian, British, and Polish ancestry (Bernardo 1981, 474).

Ancestry refers to a person's nationality group, lineage, or the country in which the person or the person's parents or ancestors were born before they came to the United States. The 1980 census was the first to include a question about ancestry. The responses to the question were a reflection of the ethnic group(s) with which persons identified, and they were able to indicate their ethnic group regardless of how many generations they were removed from it (Bureau of the Census 1980). The following list shows the most common European ancestries in the U.S. population (Gaines 1993, 14).

Ancestry	Numbers Identifying Themselves as of This Ancestry (millions)
German	58
Irish	39
English	33
Italian	15
French	10
Polish	9
Dutch	6

The following discussion focuses on several white ethnic groups and attempts to describe some of the history of their migration to America, the areas where they now live, the common beliefs regarding health and illness, some kernels of information regarding family and social life, and problems that members from a given group may have in interacting with health-care providers. The intention is not to create a vehicle for stereotyping but to whet the reader's appetite to search out more information about the people in their care, given the vast differences among whites. There are countless cultural phenomena affecting health care; Table 12–1 suggests a few.

❋ *Italian Americans*

The Italian American community is made up of immigrants who came here from mainland Italy and from Sicily and Sardinia and other Mediterranean islands that are part of Italy. The number of Americans claiming Italian ancestry is 15 million.

Italian Americans indeed have a proud heritage in the United States, for America was "founded" by an Italian—Christopher Columbus, named for an Italian—Amerigo Vespucci, and explored by several Italian explorers, including Verrazano, Cabot, and Tonti (Bernardo 1981, 26).

HISTORY OF MIGRATION

Between 1820 and 1990, over 5 million people from Italy immigrated to the United States (Lefcowitz 1990, 6). The peak years were from 1901 to 1920, and only a small number of people continue to come today. Italians came to this country to escape poverty and to search for a better life in a country where they expected to reap rewards for their hard labor. The early years were not easy, but people chose to remain in this country and not return to Italy. Italians tended to live in neighborhood enclaves, and these neighborhoods, such as the North End in Boston and Little Italy in New York, still exist as Italian neighborhoods. Although the younger generation may have moved out, they still return home to maintain family, community, and ethnic ties (Nelli 1980, 545–560).

The family has served as the main tie keeping Italian Americans together because it provides the person with the strength to cope with the surrounding world and produces a sense of continuity in all situations. The family is the primary focus of the Italian's concern, and Italians take pride in the family and the home. Italians are resilient, yet fatalistic, and they take advantage of the present. Many upwardly mobile third- and fourth-generation Italian Americans often experience conflict between familial solidarity and society's emphasis on individualization and autonomy (Giordano and McGoldrick 1996, 571). As mentioned, the home is a source of great pride, and it is a symbol of the family, not a status symbol per se. The church also is an important focus for the life of the Italian. Many of the festivals and observances continue to exist today, and in the summer, the North End of Boston is alive each weekend with the celebration of a different saint (Fig. 12–2).

The father traditionally has been the head of the Italian household, and the mother is said to be the heart of the household.

Italian Americans have tended to attain low levels of education in the United States, but their incomes are comparable to or higher than those of other groups.

The Italian population falls into four generational groups: (1) the elderly, living in Italian enclaves, (2) a second generation, living both within the neigh-

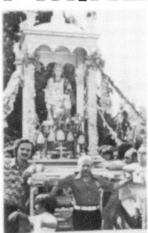

70th GRAND RELIGIOUS FEAST
IN HONOR OF THE PROTECTRESS
SAINT AGRIPPINA DI MINEO

THE THREE-DAY FEAST IS IN HONOR AND PRAISE OF SAINT AGRIPPINA, THE PROTECTRESS AND PATRON SAINT OF THE IMMIGRANTS FROM THE SMALL TOWN OF MINEO IN SICILY AND THEIR DESCENDANTS.

EACH YEAR FOR THE PAST 69 YEARS THIS GROUP OF DEVOTED 'PAESANI', NOW SCATTERED THROUGHOUT THE STATE, COME TOGETHER IN THE NORTH END SECTION TO PROCLAIM ANEW THEIR FAITH, AS WAS THE CUSTOM IN THEIR LAND OF ORIGIN. EACH YEAR EVERYONE IS INVITED TO PARTICIPATE AND WITNESS THE HONOR AND GLORY THAT IS BESTOWED TO THIS MARTYRED SAINT.

Advisory Consultant - Peter Tardo
Maestro di Banda - Gaetano Giaraffo
Capo di Banda - Stanley Pugliese

SANT'AGRIPPINA DI MINEO

A beautiful blonde maiden Saint'Agrippina was a princess by birth. This beautiful virgin martyr who was unmercifully scorged and tortured to death by the Emperor Valerion (256 AD). After her death, her relics were taken from Rome to Mineo by Saints Agatha Bassa and Paula.

The Greeks honor her in a lesser degree and claim to have relics of her. Also, in the city of Constantinople, they claim to have her body.

Saint Agrippina is the Patron Saint of thunderstorms, leprosy and evil spirits.

ST. AGRIPPINA PRAY FOR OUR DECEASED MEMBERS

A Tug of War will take place when the procession is over. The Saint is being carried by 20 men, namely Sicilians against the Romans.

Figure 12–2 Announcement of a North End (Boston) festival. (From the author's collection.)

borhoods and in the suburbs, (3) a younger, well-educated group, living mainly in the suburbs, and (4) new immigrants (Ragucci 1981, 216). More than 80% of Italian Americans marry people from a different ethnic group (Giordano and McGoldrick 1996).

HEALTH AND ILLNESS

Italians tend to present their symptoms to their fullest point and to expect immediate treatment for ailments. In terms of traditional beliefs, they may view the cause of illness to be one of the following: (1) winds and currents that bear diseases, (2) contagion or contamination, (3) heredity, (4) supernatural or human causes, and (5) psychosomatic interactions.

One such traditional Italian belief contends that moving air, in the form of drafts, causes irritation and then a cold that can lead to pneumonia. A belief an elderly person may express in terms of cancer surgery is that it is not a good idea to have surgery because surgery exposes the inner body to the air, and if the cancer is "exposed to the air the person is going to die quicker." Just as drafts are considered to be a cause of illness, fresh air is considered to be vital for the maintenance of health. Homes and the workplace must be well ventilated to prevent illness from occurring.

One sees the belief in contamination manifested in the reluctance of people to share food and objects with people who are considered unclean, and often in not entering the homes of those who are ill. Traditional Italian women have a strong sense of modesty and shame, resulting in an avoidance of discussions relating to sex and menstruation.

Blood is regarded by some, especially the elderly, to be a "plastic entity" that responds to fluids and food and is responsible for many variable conditions. Various adjectives, such as "high" and "low" and "good" and "bad," are used to describe blood. Some of the "old superstitions" include the beliefs that

1. Congenital abnormalities can be attributed to the unsatisfied desire for food during pregnancy.
2. If a woman is not given food that she smells, the fetus will move inside, and a miscarriage will result.
3. If a pregnant woman bends or turns or moves in a certain way, the fetus may not develop normally.
4. A woman must not reach during pregnancy because reaching can harm the fetus.

Italians may also attribute the cause of illness to the evil eye *(malocchio)* or to curses *(castiga)*. The difference between these two causes is that less serious illnesses, such as headaches, may be caused by *malocchio*, whereas more severe illness, which often can be fatal, may be attributed to more powerful *castiga*. Curses are sent either by God or by evil people. An example of a curse is the punishment from God for sins and bad behavior (Ragucci 1981, 216).

It is recognized by Italians that illness can be caused by the suppression of emotions, as well as stress from fear, grief, and anxiety. If one is unable to find an emotional outlet, one well may "burst." It is not considered healthy to bottle up emotions (Ragucci 1981, 232).

Often, the care of the ill is managed in the home, with all members of the family sharing in the responsibilities. The use of home remedies ostensibly is decreasing, although several students have reported the continued use of rituals for the removal of the evil eye and the practice of leeching. One practice described for the removal of the evil eye was to take an egg and olive oil and to drip them into a pan of water, make the sign of the cross, and recite prayers. If the oil spreads over the water, the cause of the problem is the evil eye, and the illness should get better. Mineral waters are also used, and tonics are used to cleanse the blood. There is a strong religious influence among Italians, who believe that faith in God and the saints will see them through the illness. One woman that I worked with had breast cancer. She had had surgery several years before and did not have a recurrence. She attributed her recovery to the fact that she attended mass every single morning and that she had total faith in Saint Peregrine, whose medal she wore pinned to her bra by the site of the mastectomy. Italian people tend to take a fatalistic stance regarding terminal illness and death believing that it is God's will. Death often is not discussed between the dying person and the family members. I recall when caring for an elderly Italian man at home that it was not possible to have the man and his wife discuss his impending death. Although both knew that he was dying and would talk with the nurse, to each other he "was going to recover," and everything possible was done to that end.

Italian families observe numerous religious traditions surrounding death, and funeral masses and anniversary masses are observed. It is the custom for the widow to wear black for some time after her husband's death (occasionally for the remainder of her life), although this is not as common with the younger generations.

HEALTH-RELATED PROBLEMS

Two genetic diseases commonly seen among Italians are (1) favism, a severe hemolytic anemia caused by deficiency of the X-linked enzyme glucose-6-phosphate dehydrogenase and triggered by the eating of fava beans, and (2) the thalassemia syndromes, also hemolytic anemias that include Cooley's anemia (or beta-thalassemia) and alpha-thalassemia (Ragucci 1981, 222).

Language problems frequently occur when elderly or new Italian immigrants are seeking care. Often, due to modesty, people are reluctant to answer the questions asked through interpreters, and gathering of pertinent data is most difficult.

Problems related to time also occur. Physicians tend to diagnose emotional problems more often for Italian patients than for other ethnic groups because of the Italian pattern of reporting more symptoms and reporting them more dramatically (Giordano and McGoldrick 1996, 576).

In general, Italian Americans are motivated to seek explanations with respect to their health status and the care they are to receive. If instructions and explanations are well given, Italians tend to cooperate with health-care providers. It is often necessary to provide directions in the greatest detail and then to provide written instructions to ensure compliance with necessary regimens.

❧ *German Americans*

(The following material, relating to both the German American and Polish American communities, was obtained from research conducted in southeastern Texas in May 1982. It is by no means indicative of the health and illness beliefs of the entire German American and Polish American communities. It is included here to demonstrate the type of data that can be gleaned using an "emic"* approach to collecting data. It cannot be generalized, but it allows the reader to grasp the diversity of beliefs that surround us!) (Lefcowitz 1990, 6).

Since 1830 more than 7 million Germans have immigrated to the United States. There are presently 58 million Americans who claim German ancestry. The Germans represented a cross section of German society and came from all social strata and walks of life. Some came to escape poverty, others came for religious or political reasons, and still others came to take advantage of the opportunity to open up the new lands. Many were recruited to come here, as were the Germans who settled in the German enclaves in Texas. The immigrants represented all religions, including primarily Lutherans, Catholics, and Jews. They represented the rich and the poor, the educated and the ignorant, and were of all ages. Present-day descendants are farmers, educators, artists. The Germans brought to the United States the cultural diversity and folkways they observed in Germany. The festivals of Corpus Christi, Kinderfeste (children's feast), and Sangerfeste (singing festival) all originated in Germany (Conzen 1980, 405–425).

The Germans began to migrate to the United States in the seventeenth century and have contributed 15% of the total immigration population. They are the least visible ethnic group in the United States, and people often are surprised to discover that there is such a large Germanic influence in this country. In some places, the German communities maintain strong identification with their German heritage. For example, the city of Fredericksberg, Texas, maintains an ambience of German culture and identity. Some people born there who are fourth generation and more continue to learn German as their first spoken language (Spector 1983).

The German ethnic community is the second largest in the state of Texas and is exceeded only by the Mexican community. Germans have been immigrating to Texas since 1840 and continue to arrive. They are predominantly Catholic, Lutheran, and Methodist. Many of these people have maintained their German identity. The major German communities in Texas are Victoria, Cuero, Gonzales, New Braunfels, and Fredericksberg.

Emic: description of behavior dependent on the person's categorization of the action. *Etic:* description of behavior based on categories created by the investigator and employed to compare phenomena cross-culturally. These are two forms of anthropological research described by Pelto, P. J., and Pelto, G. H. in *Anthropological Research: The Structure of Inquiry,* 2d ed. (Cambridge: Cambridge University Press, 1978).

During the European freedom revolutions of 1830 and 1848, Texas was quite popular, especially in Germany, and was seen as a "wild and fabulous land." For tradition-bound German families, however, the abandonment of the homeland was difficult. They were enticed, however, by the hopes of economic and social improvement and political idealism. An additional reason for the mass migration was the overpopulation of Germany and the immigrants' desire to escape an imminent European catastrophe. By the 1840s, several thousand northern Germans had come to Texas, and another large migration occurred in 1890. This second cluster of people came because there was a severe crop failure in Russian-occupied Germany, and the Russian language had become a required subject in German schools. Other German migrations occurred from 1903 to 1905.

The Germans found pleasure in the small things of everyday life. They were tied together by the German language because it bound them to the past, entertaining them with games, riddles, folk songs and literature, and folk wisdom. The greatest amusement was singing and dancing. Religion for the Lutherans, Catholics, and Methodists was a part of everyday life. The year was measured by the church calendar; observance of church ritual paced the milestones of the life cycle. The Germans believed that each individual was a "part of the fabric of humanity," that "history was a continued process," and "everything had a purpose as mankind strove to something better" (Lich 1982, 33–72).

The Germans had a penchant for forming societies and clubs, the longest lasting of which are the singing societies. The first was organized in 1850 and exists still today. The Germans brought with them their customs and traditions, their cures, curses, and recipes, and their tools and ways of building (Lich 1982).

HEALTH AND ILLNESS

Among the Germans, health is described as more than not being ill but as a state of well-being—physically and emotionally; the ability to do your duty, positive energy to do things, and the ability to do and think and act the way you would like, to go and congregate, to enjoy life. Illness may be described as the absence of well-being: pain, malfunction of body organs, not being able to do what you want, a blessing from God to suffer, and a disorder of body, imbalance.

CAUSES OF ILLNESS

Most German Americans believe in the germ theory of infection and in stress-related theories. Other causes of illness are identified, however, such as drafts, environmental changes, and belief in the evil eye and punishment from God.

The methods of maintaining health include the requirement of dressing properly for the season, proper nutrition, and the wearing of shawls to protect oneself from drafts—also, the taking of cod-liver oil, exercise, and hard work. Methods for preventing illness include wearing an asafetida bag around the neck in the winter to prevent colds, wearing scapulars, religious practices, sleeping with the windows open, and cleanliness.

The use of home remedies to treat illness continues to be practiced. Table 12–2 gives examples of commonly used home remedies.

CURRENT HEALTH PROBLEMS

There do not appear to be any unusual health problems particular to German Americans.

Table 12–2 **Illness Symptoms and Remedies Among German Americans**

Gastrointestinal Problems

Symptom	Remedy
Constipation	Castor oil
	Black draught
Diarrhea or vomiting	Do not eat for 24 hours
	Chicken soup
Stomachache	Peppermint tea
	Tea and toast
	Berries, elderberries

Respiratory Problems

Symptom	Remedy
Cold	Wet compress around throat—cover with wool
	Lemon juice and whiskey
	Apply chopped onions in a sack to the soles of the feet
	Olbas oil (made in Germany)
Cough	Goose fat—rub on chest
	Honey and milk
	Tausend Gülden Kraut (thousand golden cabbage)—rum
Earache	Put warm oil in ear
	Warm towels
	Bitter geranium leaves
Sore throat	Put camphor on a wet rag—wrap around the throat
	Gargle with salt water
	Onion compress
	Chicken soup
	Liniments

Physical Injuries

Symptom	Remedy
Bumps	Hard knife (cold metal), place on bump
Cuts	Iodine—clean well
Puncture wound (nail)	Soak in kerosene
Wounds	Clean well with water—apply iodine

(continued)

| Table 12-2 | —Continued |

Miscellaneous Problems

Symptom	Remedy
Aches and pains	Kytle's liniment
	Olbas oil
	Volcanic oil
	Salves and liniments
Arthritis	Warm water soaks
	Honey, vinegar, and water soaks
Boils	"Capital water"—sulfur water—drink this
	(this is available at the Texas capital)
Clean body after winter	Kur (similar to hot springs) drink
Fever	Cold compress on head—fluids
Headache	Iced cloth on head
Menstrual cramps	Cardui
Rheumatism	Aloe vera—rub on sore area
	Cod-liver oil—massage
	Apply fig juice
Ringworm	Camomile tea compress
Stye	One half of hard-boiled egg—apply warm white on eye
Toothache	Cloves
	Salbec tea
	Olbas oil
Warts	Apply fig juice and fig leaf milk

From: Spector, R. E. "A Description of the Impact of Medicare on Health-Illness Beliefs and Practices of White Ethnic Senior Citizens in Central Texas." Ph.D. diss. University of Texas at Austin School of Nursing, 1983; Ann Arbor, Mich.: University Microfilms International, 1983. Reprinted with permission.

❧ *Polish Americans*

The first people immigrating to this country from Poland came with Germans in 1608 to Jamestown, Virginia, to help develop the timber industry. Since that time, Poland, too, has given America one of its largest ethnic groups, with over 9 million people claiming Polish ancestry. The peak year for Polish immigration was 1921, and well over 578,875 people immigrated here. Many of the people arriving before 1890 came for economic reasons. Those coming here since that time have come for both economic and political reasons and for religious freedom. Polish heroes include Casimir Pulaski and Thaddeus Kosciuszko, who were heroes in the American Revolution. The major influx of Poles to the United States began in 1870 and ended in 1913. The people who arrived were mainly peasants seeking food and release from the political oppression of three foreign governments in Poland. The immigrants who came both before and after this mass migration were better educated and not as poor. In the United States, Polish immigrants lived in poor conditions either because they had no choice or because that was the way they were able to meet their own priorities. They were seen by other Americans to live as animals and were often mocked and called stupid. Quite often, the Polish people spoke and understood several European languages but had difficulty learning English and were therefore scorned. Polish people shared the problem as a community and banded together in tight enclaves called "Polonia." They attempted to be as self-sufficient as possible. They worked at preserving their native culture, and voluntary Polish ghettos grew up in close proximity to the parish church (Green 1982, 787–803).

An example of the Polish experience in the United States is that of the Polish immigrants in Texas. The first Poles came to Texas in the second half of the nineteenth century, and most of them settled in Victoria, San Antonio, Houston, and Bandera. The first Polish colonies in America were located in Texas, the oldest being Panna Maria (Virgin Mary) in Karnes County, 50 miles southeast of San Antonio. Unlike other Poles who wanted to return to Poland, the colonists who arrived in Texas after 1850 came to settle permanently and had no intention of returning to their homeland. Although these people came to Texas for economic, political, and religious reasons, severe poverty was their major reason for leaving Poland.

The first collective Polish immigration to America was in 1854, when 100 families came to Texas. They landed in Galveston, where a few in the party remained. The rest traveled in a procession northwestward, bringing with them a few belongings, such as featherbeds, crude farm implements, and a cross from their parish church. Their dream was to live in the fertile lands of Texas and raise crops, speak their own language, educate their children, and worship God as they pleased. This dream did not materialize, and members of the band grew discouraged. Some of the immigrants remained in Victoria and others went to San Antonio.

The people who went to San Antonio continued to travel, and on Christmas Eve, 1854, they stopped at the junction of the San Antonio and Cibolo Rivers. Here, under a live oak tree, they celebrated mass and founded Panna Maria. In 1855, 1856, and 1857, others followed this small group in moving to this part of Texas.

These settlers were exposed to many dangers from nature, such as heat, drought, snakes, and insects. The Polish settlers were not accepted by the other settlers in the area because their language, customs, and culture were different, but the immigrants survived, and many moved to settle other areas near Panna Maria. Today, the people of Panna Maria continue to live simple lives close to nature and God and speak mainly Polish.

Much of the history of the Polish people in Texas is written around the founding and the location of the various church parishes. For example, in 1873 the Parish of the Nativity of the Blessed Virgin Mary was begun in Cestohowa. Within this church above the main altar is a large picture of the Virgin Mary of Czestochowa. This picture was taken to the church from Panna Maria. It is a copy of the famous Black Madonna of Czestochowa, Poland, a city 65 miles east of where the immigrants to Texas originated. The Black Madonna is a beloved, miraculous image and a source of faith to the Polish people. The shrine of Our Lady in Czestochowa, Poland, is one of the largest shrines in the world. Since the fourteenth century, that picture had been the object of veneration and devotion of Polish Catholics. It is claimed to have been painted by Saint Luke the Evangelist. Its origin is traced to the fifth or sixth century and is the oldest picture of the Virgin in the world. The scars on the face date from 1430 when bandits struck it with a sword. The history, traditions, and miracles of Czestochowa are the heritage of the Polish people (Dworaczyk 1976). One woman I interviewed said she had been ill with a fatal disease. The entire time that she lay close to death she prayed to the Virgin. When she finally did recover, she made a pilgrimage back to her homeland in Poland and visited the shrine to give thanks to the Virgin. The woman was positive that this was the source of her recovery.

HEALTH AND ILLNESS

The definitions of health among the Polish people I interviewed included: feeling O.K.—as a whole—body, spirit, everything a person cannot separate; happy, until war, do not need doctor, do not need medicine; active, able to work, feel good, do what I want to do; and good spirit, good to everybody, never cross. The definitions for illness may include: something wrong with body, mind, or spirit; one wrong affects them all; not capable of working, see the doctor often; not right, something ailing you; not active; feeling bad; and opposite of health, not doing what I want to do. The methods for maintaining health include maintaining a happy home, being kind and loving, eating healthy food, remaining pure, walking, exercising, wearing proper clothing, (sweaters), eating a well-balanced diet, trying not to worry, having faith in God, being active, dressing warmly, going to bed early, and working hard. The methods for preventing illness include: cleanliness, the wearing of scapulars, avoiding drafts, following the proper diet, not gossiping, keeping away from people with colds, and wearing medals because "God is with you all the time to protect you and take care of you." Other ideas about illness include the beliefs that illnesses are caused by poor diets and that the evil eye may well exist as a causative factor (but not really sure). This belief was attributed to the older generations and is not regarded as prevalent among younger Polish Americans.

The home remedies listed in Table 12–3 were described by and were in common use among Polish Americans.

HEALTH-CARE PROBLEMS

The Polish community has not tended to have any major problems with the health-care deliverers. Language may be a barrier if members of the older generation do not speak English, and the taking of health histories is complicated when the providers cannot communicate directly with the informant. Again, problems may develop when there is difficulty finding someone who is conversant in Polish, whom the informant can trust to reveal personal matters to, and who can translate medical terms accurately.

In Poland, there is a shortage of medical supplies, so the people tend to use faith healers and believe in miracle workers. On the main street of Warsaw

Table 12–3 **Illness Symptoms and Remedies among Polish Americans**

Gastrointestinal Problems

Symptom	Remedy
Colic	Tea—peppermint or camomile
	Sugar, water, vinegar, and soda, makes soda water
	Bess-plant tea
	Homemade sauerkraut
Constipation	Epsom salts—teaspoon in water—cleans out stomach
	Cascara
	Castor oil
	Senna-leaf tea
Cramps	Camomile tea
Diarrhea	Paregoric
	Cinnamon tea
	Dried blueberries
	Chew coffee beans
Gas	Drink soda water
Indigestion	Aloes vulgaris—juniper and elderberries
	Peppermint and spearmint teas
	Blackberries

Respiratory Problems

Symptom	Remedy
Cold	Castor oil—mentholatum
	Flaxseed or mustard poultice on chest
	Dried raspberries and tea with wine
	Mustard plaster
	Oatmeal poultice—hot bricks to feet
	Cupping
	Camphor salve
	Oxidine
	Rub goose fat on chest
Cough	Honey and hot water; bedrest
	Hot lemonade with whiskey; honey
	Few drops of turpentine and sugar
	"Gugel Mugel"—warm milk with butter, whiskey, and honey
	Honey and warm milk
	Milk with butter and garlic
	Mustard plaster
	Linden tea
	Onion poultice
Croup	Few drops of kerosene and sugar
Sore throat	Honey
	Warm water, salt—gargle
	Goose grease around throat covered with dry rag
	Paint throat with kerosene
	Goose fat in milk

(continued)

| Table 12–3 | —Continued |

Physical Injury

Symptom	Remedy
Burns	Aloe vera
Cuts	Vinegar, water, flour paste
	Clean with urine
	Carbolic salve
Puncture wounds (nail)	Turpentine and liniment
	Put salt pork on wound and soak in hot water
	Hunt's lightning oil
Frostbite	Put snow on frozen place
Scratches, sores	Liniment
	Moss
	Spider webs
Sprains	Liniments—Sloan's Volcanic

Miscellaneous Problems

Symptom	Remedy
Earache	Hot-water bottle to ear
	Camphor on cotton—place in ear
Fever	Camomile tea
Flu	Novak oil—rub on head
	Knorr's Green Drops
Headache	Vinegar on a cloth applied to head
	Steam kettle—cover head and inhale
High blood pressure	Cooked garlic
	Garlic oil
Lice	Cover head with kerosene
Toothache	Hot salt compress
Neuralgia	Bedrest
Pyorrhea	Drink yarrow tea
Rheumatism	Lemon juice—rub on sore places
Trouble urinating	Juice of pumpkin seeds made into a tea
	Swamp root medicine

From: Spector, R. E. "A Description of the Impact of Medicare on Health-Illness Beliefs and Practices of White Ethnic Senior Citizens in Central Texas." Ph.D. diss. University of Texas at Austin School of Nursing, 1983; Ann Arbor, Mich.: University Microfilms International, 1983. Reprinted with permission.

all sorts of folk-medicine and miracle-worker paraphernalia are on sale: divining rods, cotton sacks filled with herbs to be worn over an ailing heart or liver, coils of copper wire to be placed under food to rid it of poisons, and pendulums (Letter from Poland 1983).

In this chapter I have attempted to open the door to the enormous diversity in health and illness beliefs that exists in European American (white) communities. I have only opened the door and peeked inside. There is a richness of knowledge to be gained. It is for you to acquire it as you care for all patients. Ask them what they believe about health and illness and what their practices and remedies may be. The students that I am working with find this to be a most enlightening experience.

❧ *References*

Bernardo, S. 1981. *The Ethnic Almanac.* New York: Doubleday.

Conzen, K. N. 1980. Germans. In *Harvard Encyclopedia of American Ethnic Groups,* edited by S. Thernstrom. (Cambridge: Harvard University Press, 1980), pp. 405–425.

Dworaczyk, E. J. 1979. The First Polish Colonies of America in Texas. San Antonio: Naylor.

Folwarski, J., and Marganoff, P. P. Polish Families. In *Ethnicity and Family Therapy,* 2d ed., edited by M. McGoldrick, J. Giordano, and J. K. Pearce. New York: Guilford.

Gaines, J. R. 1993. The New Face of America. *Time* 142 (21): 14.

Giordano, J., and McGoldrick, M. 1996. Italian Families. In *Ethnicity and Family Therapy,* 2d ed., edited by M. McGoldrick, J. Giordano, and J. K. Pearce. New York: Guilford.

Green, V. Poles. In *Harvard Encyclopedia of American Ethnic Groups,* edited by S. Thernstrom, Cambridge: Harvard University Press.

Grzelonski, B. 1976. *Poles in the United States: 1776–1865.* Warsaw: Interpeirs.

Lefcowitz, E. 1990. *The United States Immigration History Timeline.* New York: Terra Firma Press.

Letter from Poland—of Faith Healers and Miracle Workers. *Boston Globe,* 21 August.

Lich, G. E. 1982. *The German Texans.* San Antonio: University of Texas Institute of Texan Cultures.

McGoldrick, M., Giordano, J., and Pearce, J. K. 1996. *Ethnicity and Family Therapy,* 2d ed. New York: Guildford.

Nelli, H. S. 1980. Italians. In *Harvard Encyclopedia of American Ethnic Groups,* edited by S. Thernstrom. Cambridge: Harvard University Press.

Ragucci, A. T. 1981. Italian Americans. In *Ethnicity and Medical Care,* edited by A. Harwood. (Cambridge: Harvard University Press.

Rotunno, M., and McGoldrick, M. 1982. *Italian Families.* In *Ethnicity and Family Therapy.* Edited by M. McGoldrick, J. K. Pearce, and J. Giordano, New York: Guilford.

Spector, R. E. 1983. A Description of the Impact of Medicare on Health-Illness Beliefs and Practices of White Ethnic Senior Citizens in Central Texas. Ph.D. diss. University of Texas at Austin School of Nursing; Ann Arbor, Mich.: University Microfilms International.

Spector, R. 1992. Culture, Ethnicity, and Nursing. In *Fundamentals of Nursing,* 3d ed., edited by P. Potter and A. Perry. St. Louis: Mosby, 101.

U.S. Bureau of the Census. 1983. *1980 Census of Population—Ancestry of the Population by State.* Washington, D.C.: Government Printing Office, 1983, p. 6.

Winawer, H., and Wetzel, N. A. 1996. German Families. In *Ethnicity and Family Therapy,* 2d ed. edited by M. McGoldrick, J. Giordano, and J. K. Pearce. New York: Guilford.

INTERNET SOURCE

http://www.ins.usdoj.gov/index.html
http://www.ins.usdoj.gov:statistics and definitions/stats/annual/fy96/
statsfy96a.htmlimmfy1996

*Figure 12–1 from page 261
From left to right—top to bottom: The chapter opening quilt panel of *health*-related images depicts objects people of white-European heritage may use to protect, maintain, and/or restore their HEALTH. The **bracelet,** from Armenia, with a large blue center and eye on it may be worn by a child for protection from the evil eye. **Bankes,** from Russia and Switzerland, are small, bulb-shaped, thick-glass jars that may be used to create negative pressure to break the congestion that occurs with bronchitis or pneumonia. (Directions: Place cotton saturated with alcohol in the jar and light it. Place grease on the skin in the area where you will place the jar. Turn the jar upside down on the skin. The flame goes out. Leave it for 5 minutes and then gently remove the jar. Go to bed and keep warm for several hours.) The *troll,* from Finland, may be used to protect the home from evil spirits. The **blue bead and horseshoe,** from Armenia, may be pinned on a baby or child for protection from the evil eye. The **corno** with a Gobo from Italy may be worn for protection and luck. The **Saint Anthony medal** from Italy is representative of the many saints who are thought to help with the countless dilemmas of life. Saint Anthony is thought to aid in the finding of lost items and is often petitioned for this purpose. **Garlic with a blue bead,** from Greece, may be pinned on a baby or child for protection from the evil eye. The **figa** from Portugal may be worn for protection from the evil eye. The **green scapular,** from France, is believed to bring healing to the person who wears or carries it. It can also be left in a sick person's room.

Epilogue

Why must health-care deliverers—nurses, physicians, public health and social workers, and other health-care professionals—study ethnicity, culture, and cultural sensitivity? Why must they know the difference between "hot" and "cold" and *yin* and *yang*? Why must they be concerned with the patient's failure to practice what professionals believe to be good preventive medicine or with the patient's failure to comply with a given treatment regimen or with the patient's failure to seek medical care during the initial phase of an illness? Is there a difference between *curing* and *healing*?

There is little disagreement that health-care services in this country are unevenly distributed and that the poor and the emerging majority get the short end of the stick in terms of the care they receive (or do not receive). There is the need to understand new immigrants as more and more people come to this country. Yet it is often maintained that when such care *is* provided, these same people fail to use it or use it inappropriately. Why is this seeming paradox so?

The major focus of this book has been on the provider's and the patient's differing perceptions of health and illness. These differences may account for the health-care provider's misconception that services are used inappropriately and that people do not care about their health. What to the casual observer appears to be "misuse" may represent our failure to understand and to meet the needs and expectations of the patient. This possibility may well be difficult for health-care providers to face, but careful analysis of the available information seems to indicate that this may—at least in part—be the case. How, then, can health-care providers change their method of operations and provide both safe and effective care for the emerging majority and, at the same time, for the population at large? The answer to this question is not an easy one, and some researchers think we are not succeeding. A number of measures can and must be taken to ameliorate the current situation. Multicultural health care and the educational preparation leading to this is a process, one that becomes a way of life and must be recognized as such. The changing of one's personal and professional ideas and stereotypes does *not* occur overnight, and the process, quite often, is neither direct nor easy. It is a multistep process, in which one must:

- Explore his or her own cultural identity and heritage and confront biases and stereotypes.
- Develop an awareness and understanding of the complexities of the modern health-care delivery system—its philosophy and problems, biases, and stereotypes.
- Develop a keen awareness of the socialization process that brings the provider into this complex system.

- Develop the ability to "hear" things that transcend language, foster an understanding of the patient and his or her cultural heritage and the resilience found within the culture that supports family and community structures.

Given the processes of acculturation, assimilation, and modernism, this is often difficult and painful. Yet, once the journey of exploring one's own cultural heritage and prejudices is undertaken, the awareness of the cultural needs of others becomes more subtle and understandable. This is well accomplished by using the umbrella of HEALTH traditions as the point of entry.

A student I once taught described the journey this way:

I was born in 1973 to fourth-generation Japanese American parents. I understood Japanese culture and the way of thinking and did not question when my parents told me to eat noodles on New Year's Day to bring long life. Then I changed schools and went to the Caucasian school. I came to *hate* my heritage and wanted to scream that "I'm as white on the inside as you are." I was bitter and embarrassed by my heritage and blamed my family, who were proud of their ancestry. When my parents tried to teach me about Japanese American history, I was not interested. I came to know, understand, and hate racism. On the inside I felt as "white American" as everyone else but I soon realized what I felt inside was not what other people saw. I now acknowledge who I am and I accept myself.

The voice of this young student speaks for many. In the course of having to explore the family's traditional health beliefs and practices, the student began to see, think through, understand, and accept herself.

Although curricula in professional education are quite full, multicultural health studies must be taken by all people who wish to deliver health care. It is no longer sufficient to teach a student in the health professions to "accept patients for who they are." The question arises: Who is the patient? Introductory sociology and psychology courses fail to provide this information. It is learned best by meeting with the people themselves and letting them describe who they are from their own perspective. I have suggested two approaches to the problem. One is to have people who work as patient advocates or as nurses and physicians come to the class setting and explain how people of their ethnic group view health and illness and describe the given community's HEALTH traditions. Another approach is to send students out into communities where they will have the opportunity to meet with people in their own settings. It is not necessary to memorize all the available lists of herbs, hot–cold imbalances, folk diseases, and so forth. The objective is to become more sensitive to the crucial fact that multiple factors underly given patient behaviors. One, of course, is that the patient may well *perceive* and *understand* HEALTH and illness from quite a different perspective than that of the health-care provider. Each person comes from a unique culture and a unique socialization process.

The health-care provider must be sensitive to his or her own perceptions of health and illness and the practices he or she employs. Even though the perceptions of most health professionals are based on a middle-class and medical-model viewpoint, providers must realize that there are other ways of regarding health and illness. The early chapters of this book are devoted to consciousness raising about self-treatment. It is always an eye-opening experience to publicly scrutinize ourselves in this respect. Quite often we are amazed to see how far we stray from the system's prescribed methods of keeping healthy. The journals confirm that we, too, delay in seeking health care and fail to comply with treatment regimens. Often our ability to comply rests on quite pragmatic issues, such as What is it doing for me? and Can I afford to miss work and stay in bed for two days? As we gain insight into our own health-illness attitudes and behaviors, we tend to be much more sympathetic to and empathetic with the person who fails to come to the clinic or who hates to wait for the physician or who delays in seeking health care.

The health-care provider should be aware of the complex issues that surround the delivery of health care from the patient's viewpoint. Calling the medical society for the name of a physician (because a "family member has a health problem") and visiting and comparing the services rendered in an urban and a suburban emergency room are exercises that can enable us to better appreciate some of the difficulties that the poor, the emerging majority, and the population at large all too often experience when they attempt to obtain health care. Members of the health-care team have a number of advantages in gaining access to the health-care system. For example, they can choose a physician whom they know because they work with him or her or because someone they work with has recommended this physician. Health-care providers must never forget, however, that most people do not have these advantages. It is indeed an unsettling, anxiety-provoking, and frustrating experience to be forced to select a physician from a list. It is an even more frustrating experience to be a patient in an unfamiliar location—for example, an urban emergency room, where, quite literally, anything can happen.

Another barrier to adequate health care is the financial burden imposed by treatments and tests. There are other issues as well. For example, a Chinese patient—who traditionally does not believe that the body replaces the blood taken for testing purposes—should have as little blood work as necessary, and the reasons for the tests should be explained carefully. A Hispanic woman who believes that taking a Pap smear is an intrusive procedure that will bring shame to her should have the procedure performed by a female physician or nurse. When this is not possible, she should have a female chaperone with her for the entire time that the male physician or nurse is in the room.

More members of the emerging majority must be represented in the health-care professions. Multiple issues are related to the problem of under-representation. Many of the programs designed to increase the number of emerging majority students in the health-care team have failed. Difficulties surrounding successful entrance into and completion of professional education programs are complex and numerous, having their roots in impoverished community structures and early educational deprivation. Although society is in some ways dealing with such issues—for example, initiating improvements in early education—we are faced with an *immediate* need to bring more emerging majority people into health-care services.

One method would be the more extensive use of patient advocates and outreach workers from the given ethnic community who may be recognized there as healers. These people can provide an overwhelmingly positive service to both the provider and the patient in that they can serve as the bridge in bringing health-care services to the people. The patient advocate can speak to the patient in language that he or she understands and in a manner that is acceptable. Advocates also are able to coordinate medical, nursing, social, and even educational services to meet the patient's needs as the patient perceives them. In settings where advocates are employed, many problems are resolved to the convenience of both the health-care member and, more importantly, the patient!

The nettlesome issue of language bursts forth with regularity. There is always a problem when a non–English-speaking person tries to seek help from the English-speaking majority. The more common languages, French, Italian, and Spanish, ideally should be spoken by at least some of the professional people who staff hospitals, clinics, neighborhood health-care centers, and home health agencies. The use of an interpreter is always difficult because the interpreter generally "interprets" what he or she translates. To bring this thought home, the reader should recall the childhood game of "gossip": a message is passed around the room from person to person, and by the time it gets back to the sender, its content is usually substantially changed. This game is not unlike trying to communicate through an interpreter, and the situation is even more frustrating when—as can often be the case in urban emergency rooms—the interpreter is a six-year-old child. It is, obviously, far more satisfying and productive if the patient, nurse, and physician can all speak the same language.

Health services must be made far more accessible and available to members of the emerging majority. I believe that one of the most important events in this modern era of health-care delivery is the advent of neighborhood health centers. They are successful essentially because people who work in them know the people of the neighborhood. In addition, the people of the community can contribute to the decision making involved in governing and running the agency so that services are tailored to meet the needs of the patients. Concerned members of the health-care team have a moral obligation to support the increased use of health-care centers and *not* their decreased use, as currently tends to occur because of cutbacks in response to allegations (frequently politically motivated) of too-high costs or the misuse of funds. These neighborhood health-care centers provide greatly needed personal services in addition to relief from the widespread depersonalization that occurs in larger institutions. When health-care providers who are genuinely concerned face this reality, perhaps they will be more willing to fight for the survival of these centers and strongly urge their increased funding rather than acquiesce in their demise. In rural areas, the problem is even greater, and far more comprehensive health planning is needed to meet patient needs.

CulturalCare is the term I have coined to express all that is inherent in this text. Countless conflicts in the health-care delivery arenas are predicated on cultural misunderstandings. Although many of these misunderstandings are related to universal situations, such as verbal and nonverbal language misunderstandings, the conventions of courtesy, sequencing of interactions, phasing of interactions, objectivity, and so forth, many cultural misunderstandings are unique to the delivery of health care. The necessity to provide CulturalCare— professional health care that is culturally sensitive, culturally appropriate, and culturally competent—is essential as we enter the new millennium, and it demands that providers be able to assess and interpret a given patient's health beliefs and practices. CulturalCare alters the perspective of health-care delivery as it enables the provider to understand, from a cultural perspective, the manifestations of the patient's HEALTH-care beliefs and practices.

I should like to reiterate that this book was written with the hope that by sharing the material I have taught over the years, some small changes will be made in the thinking of all health-care providers who read it. There is nothing new in these pages. Perhaps it is simply a recombination of material with which the reader is familiar, but I hope it serves its purpose: the sharing of beliefs and attitudes, and the stimulation of lots of consciousness raising concerning issues of vital concern to health-care providers who must confront the needs of clients with diverse cultural backgrounds.

Appendix 1

Selected Key Terms Related to Cultural Diversity in Health and Illness

Acculturation—The process of adapting to another culture. To acquire the majority group's culture.

Acupuncture—The traditional Chinese medical way of restoring the balance of *yin* and *yang* that is based on the therapeutic value of cold. Cold is used in a disease where there is an excess of *yang*.

Alien—Every person applying for entry to the United States. Anyone who is not a U.S. citizen.

Allopathic—Health beliefs and practices that are derived from current scientific models and involve the use of technology and other modalities of present-day health care, such as immunization, proper nutrition, and resuscitation.

Alternative health system—A system of health care a person may use that is not predicated within their traditional culture, but is not allopathic.

Amulet—An object with magical powers, such as a charm, worn on a string or chain around the neck, wrist, or waist to protect the wearer from both physical and psychic illness, harm, and misfortune.

Anamnesis—The traditional Chinese medical way of diagnosing a health problem by asking questions.

Aromatherapy—Ancient science that uses essential plant oils to produce strong physical and emotional effects in the body.

Assimilation—To become absorbed into another culture and to adopt its characteristics. To develop a new cultural identity.

Ayurvedic—Four-thousand-year-old method of healing originating in India, the chief aim of which is longevity and quality of life. The most ancient existing medical system that uses diet, natural therapies, and herbs.

Biofeedback—The use of an electronic machine to measure skin temperatures. The patient controls responses that are usually involuntary.

Biological variations—Biological differences that exist among races and ethnic groups in body structure, skin color, biochemical differences, susceptibility to disease, and nutritional differences.

Caida de la mollera—(Fallen fontanel) Traditional Hispanic belief that the fontanel falls if the baby's head is touched.

Care—Factors that assist, enable, support, or facilitate a person's needs to maintain, improve, or ease a health problem.

Charm—Objects that combine the functions of both amulets and talismans but consist only of written words or symbols.

Chinese doctor—Physician educated in China who uses traditional herbs and other therapeutic modalities in the delivery of health care.

Conjure—To effect magic.

CulturalCare—A concept that describes health care that is culturally sensitive, culturally appropriate, and culturally competent. CulturalCare is critical to meeting the complex nursing care needs of a given person, family, and community. It is the provision of health care across cultural boundaries and takes into account the context in which the patient lives as well as the situations in which the patient's health problems arise.

Culturally appropriate—Implies that the health-care provider applies the underlying background knowledge that must be possessed to provide a given patient with the best possible health care.

Culturally competent—Implies that within the delivered care the health-care provider understands and attends to the total context of the patient's situation. Cultural competence is a complex combination of knowledge, attitudes, and skills.

Culturally sensitive—Implies that the health-care providers possess some basic knowledge of and constructive attitudes toward the health traditions observed among the diverse cultural groups found in the setting in which they are practicing.

Culture—Nonphysical traits, such as values, beliefs, attitudes, and customs, that are shared by a group of people and passed from one generation to the next. A meta-communication system.

Culture shock—Disorder that occurs in response to transition from one cultural setting to another. Former behavior patterns are ineffective in such a setting, and basic cues for social behavior are absent.

Curandero—Traditional Hispanic holistic healer.

Curing*—Two-dimensional phenomenon that results in ridding the body or mind (or both) of a given disease.

Decoction—A simmered tea made from the bark, root, seed, or berry, of a plant.

Demography—The statistical study of populations, including statistical counts of people of various ages, sexes, and population densities for specific locations.

Disadvantaged background—Both educational and economic factors that act as barriers to an individual's participation in a health professions program.

Discrimination—Denying people equal opportunity by acting on a prejudice.

Divination—Traditional American Indian practice of calling on spirits or other forces to determine a diagnosis of a health problem.

Dybbuk—Wandering, disembodied soul that enters another person's body and holds fast.

Emerging majority—People of color—blacks; Asians/Pacific Islanders; American Indians, Eskimos, or Aleuts; and Hispanics—who are expected to constitute a majority of the American population by the year 2020.

Emic—Person's way of describing an action or event, an inside view.

Empacho—Traditional Hispanic belief that a ball of food is stuck in the stomach.

Envidia—Traditional Hispanic belief that the envy of others can be the cause of illness and bad luck.

Environmental control—Ability of a person from a given cultural group to actively control nature and to direct factors in the environment.

Epidemiology—The study of the distribution of disease.

Ethnicity—Cultural group's sense of identification associated with the group's common social and cultural heritage.

Ethnocentrism—Tendency of members of one cultural group to view the members of other cultural groups in terms of the standards of behavior, attitudes, and values of their own group. The belief that one's own cultural, ethnic, professional, or social group is superior to that of others.

Ethnomedicine—Health beliefs and practices of indigenous cultural development. Not practiced in many of the tenets of modern medicine.

Etic—The interpretation of an event by someone who is not experiencing that event, an outside view.

Evil eye—Belief that someone can project harm by gazing or staring at another's property or person.

Exorcism—Ceremonious expulsion of an evil spirit from a person.

Faith—Strong beliefs in a religious or other spiritual philosophy.

Folklore—Body of preserved traditions, usually oral, consisting of beliefs, stories, and associated information of people.

Geophagy—Eating of nonfood substances, such as starch.

Glossoscopy—Traditional Chinese medical way of diagnosing a health problem by examining the tongue.

Gris-gris—Symbols of voodoo. They may take numerous forms and be used either to protect a person or harm that person.

Haragei—Japanese art or practice of using nonverbal communication.

Healing*—Holistic, or three-dimensional, phenomenon that results in the restoration of balance, or harmony, to the body, mind, and spirit; or between the person and the environment.

Health*—A state of balance between the body, mind, and spirit.

HEALTH—The balance of the person, both within one's being, physical, mental, and spiritual—and in the outside world—natural, communal, and metaphysical.

Heritage consistency—Observance of the beliefs and practices of one's traditional cultural belief system.

Heritage inconsistency—Observance of the beliefs and practices of one's acculturated belief system.

Hex—Evil spell, misfortune, or bad luck that one person can impose on another.

Homeopathic—Health beliefs and practices derived from traditional cultural knowledge to maintain health, prevent changes in health status, and restore health.

Homeopathy—System of medicine based on the belief that a disease can be cured by minute doses of a substance that if given to a healthy person in large doses would produce the same symptoms that the person being treated is experiencing.

Hoodoo—A form of conjuring and a term that refers to the magical practices of voodoo outside New Orleans.

Hypnotherapy—The use of hypnosis to stimulate emotions and control involuntary responses such as blood pressure.

Illness*—State of imbalance among the body, mind, and spirit; a sense of disharmony both within the person and with the environment.

Immigrant—Alien entering the United States for permanent (or temporary) residence.

Indigenous—People native to an area.

Lay midwife—A person who practices lay midwifery.

Lay midwifery—Assisting childbirth for compensation.

Limpia—Traditional Hispanic practice of cleansing a person.

Macrobiotics—Diet and lifestyle from the Far East adapted for the United States by Michio Kushif. The principles of this vegetarian diet consist of balancing *yin* and *yang* energies of food.

Magicoreligious folk medicine—Use of charms, holy words, and holy actions to prevent and cure illness.

Mal ojo—(Bad eye) Traditional Hispanic belief that excessive admiration by one person can bring harm to another person.

Massage therapy—Use of manipulative techniques to relieve pain and return energy to the body.

Medically underserved community—Urban or rural population group that lacked or lacks adequate health care services.

Melting pot—The social blending of cultures.

Meridians—Specific points of the body into which needles are inserted in the traditional Chinese medical practice of acupuncture.

Metacommunication system—Large system of communication that includes both verbal language and nonverbal signs and symbols.

Miracle—Supernatural, unexplained event.

Modern—Present-day health and illness beliefs and practices of the providers within the American, or Western, health-care delivery system.

Motion in the hand—An example of a traditional American Indian practice of moving the diagnostician's hands in a ritual of divination.

Moxibustion—Traditional Chinese medical way of restoring the balance of *yin* and *yang* that is based on the therapeutic value of heat. Heat is used in a disease where there is an excess of *yin*.

Multicultural nursing—Pluralistic approach to understanding relationships between two or more cultures to create a nursing practice framework for broadening nurses' understanding of health-related beliefs, practices, and issues that are part of the experiences of people from diverse cultural backgrounds.

Mysticism—Aspect of spiritual healing and beliefs.

Natural folk-medicine—Use of the natural environment and use of herbs, plants, minerals, and animal substances to prevent and treat illness.

Nonimmigrant—People who are allowed to enter the country temporarily under certain conditions, such as crewmen, students, and temporary workers.

Occult folk medicine—The use of charms, holy words, and holy actions to prevent and cure illness.

Osphretics—Traditional Chinese medical way of diagnosing a health problem by listening and smelling.

Overheating therapy—(Hyperthermia) Used since the time of the ancient Greeks; the natural immune system is stimulated with heat to kill pathogens.

Partera—A Mexican American or Mexican lay midwife.

Pasmo—Traditional Hispanic disease of paralysis.

Pluralistic society—A society comprising people of numerous ethnocultural backgrounds.

Poultice—A hot, soft, moist mass of herbs, flour, mustard, and other substances spread on muslin and placed on a sore body part.

Powwow—A form of traditional healing practiced by German Americans.

Prejudice—Negative beliefs or preferences that are generalized about a group and that leads to "prejudgment."

Racism—The belief that members of one race are superior to those of other races.

Rational folk medicine—Use of the natural environment and use of herbs, plants, minerals, and animal substances to prevent and treat illness.

Raza-Latina—A popular term used as a reference group name for people of Latin American descent.

Reflexology—Natural science that manipulates the reflex points in the hands and feet that correspond to every organ in the body in order to clear the energy pathways and the flow of energy through the body.

Religion—Belief in a divine or superhuman power or powers to be obeyed and worshipped as the creator(s) and ruler(s) of the universe.

Resident alien—A lawfully admitted alien.

Restoration—Process used by a given person to return health.

Santeria—A syncretic religion comprising both African and Catholic beliefs.

Santero—Traditional priest in the religion of *santeria*.

Sexism—Belief that members of one sex are superior to those of the other sex.

Singer—A type of traditional American Indian healer who is able to practice singing as a form of treating a health problem.

Social organization—Patterns of cultural behavior related to life events, such as birth, death, child rearing, and health and illness, that are followed within a given social group.

Socialization—Process of being raised within a culture and acquiring the characteristics of the given group.

Soul loss—Belief that a person's soul can leave the body, wander around, and then return.

Space—Area surrounding a person's body and the objects within that area.

Spell—A magical word or formula or a condition of evil or bad luck.

Sphygmopalpation—Traditional Chinese medical way of diagnosing a health problem by feeling pulses.

Spirit—The noncorporeal and nonmental dimension of a person that is the source of meaning and unity. The source of the experience of spirituality and every religion.

Spirit possession—Belief that a spirit can enter people, possess them, and control what they say and do.

Spiritual—Ideas, attitudes, concepts, beliefs, and behaviors that are the result of the person's experience of the spirit.

Spirituality—The experience of meaning and unity.

Stargazing—Example of a traditional American Indian practice of praying the star prayer to the star spirit as a method of divination.

Stereotype—Notion that all people from a given group are the same.

Superstition—Belief that performing an action, wearing a charm or amulet, or eating something, will have an influence on life events. These beliefs are upheld by magic and faith.

Susto—(Soul loss) Traditional Hispanic belief that the soul is able to leave a person's body.

Taboo—A culture-bound ban that excludes certain behaviors from common use.

Talisman—Consecrated religious object that confers power of various kinds and protects people who wear, carry, or own them from harm and evil.

Tao—Way, path, or discourse. On the spiritual level, the way to ultimate reality.

Time—Duration, interval of time; also, instances, points in time.

Traditional—Ancient, ethnocultural-religious beliefs and practices that have been handed down through the generations.

Traditional epidemiology—Belief in agents—other than those of a scientific nature, causing disease.

Undocumented alien—Person of foreign origin who has entered the country unlawfully by bypassing inspection or who has overstayed the original terms of admission.

Voodoo—A religion that is a combination of Christianity and African Yoruba religious beliefs.

Witched—Example of a traditional American Indian belief that a person is harmed by witches.

Xenophobia—Morbid fear of strangers.

Yang—Male, positive energy that produces light, warmth, and fullness.

Yin—Female, negative energy; the force of darkness, cold, and emptiness.

---

*These terms are defined with their traditional connotations, rather than with modern denotations. *Source:* Compiled over time by R. Spector.

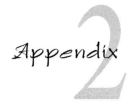

Appendix 2

Suggested Course Outline

❋ *NU301. Cultural Diversity in Health and Illness**

The purpose of this course is to bring the student into a direct relationship with health-care consumers from various cultural backgrounds—white, black, Asian, Hispanic, American Indian. The course content includes discussion of the following topics:

- The perception of health and illness among health-care providers and consumers
- The cultural and institutional factors that affect the consumers' access to and use of health-care resources
- Health-care providers' ways of coping with illness and related problems
- The manner in which people of different backgrounds and their problems have been depicted in the literature (e.g., the works of Lewis, Kiev, Clark) and the implications of historical treatment for health-care practice and health-care delivery.

GOAL

The goal of this course is to broaden the student's perception and understanding of health and illness and the variety of meanings these terms carry for members of differing groups.

OBJECTIVES

On completion of this course, the student should be able to

1. Understand more fully the perception and meaning of health and illness among various health-care consumers
2. Enter into dialogue with people who have experienced problems in dealing with the American health-care system

---

*From the Boston College School of Nursing, Chestnut Hill, Massachusetts 02167.

3. Understand the conflicts between the consumer and the American health-care system and the effect of those conflicts on health-care practice and action
4. Develop ideas about what health-care practice can do to intervene in this conflict and diminish it

TEXTS

The following texts should be read in their entirety: Spector, R. E. *Cultural Diversity in Health and Illness,* 5th ed. (Upper Saddle River, NJ: Prentice Hall Health, 2000). Starr, P. *The Social Transformation of American Medicine.* New York: Basic Books, 1982.

ASSIGNMENTS AND EVALUATION

1. Weekly readings, class attendance, preparedness, and participation   15%
2. Health interviews   5%
3. Health diaries   10%
4. Reaction papers   20%

The purpose of the reaction papers is to express the student's response to the assigned readings and to the classroom discussion.

5. Term paper (maximum 8 to 10 pages)   25%

The term paper must deal with the problems and issues presented in class and the student's interpretation of how professional nurses must cope with them in practice. All papers must be submitted in proper Turabian format, typed and double-spaced.

6. Term project   25%

The term project should be a small-group class presentation on perspectives of health and illness in one of the four communities studied. The class presentation must include the following data:

1. History of ethnic group in the United States
2. Traditional perceptions of HEALTH and illness
3. Traditional healing methods
4. Current health-care problems

Sources for the term project must include a bibliography, interviews with people within the given community, and personal observations.

❧ *Course Outline*

Week I   **Course Introduction: Discussion of General Concepts of Health**
Assignments for Class II:
1. Interview an older member of your family to determine
  (a) what practices were used to protect and maintain HEALTH

(b) what was done to restore HEALTH
2. Begin a daily diary of your HEALTH status for 1 month. (Both assignments must be handed in.)

Week II   **Discussion: Concepts of Illness and Practices for Maintaining Health and Preventing Illness**
Readings:[†]
- Spector, *Cultural Diversity*, Chapters 1 and 2
  Dubos, *Mirage of Health*
  Dubos, *Man Adapting*

Week III   **The Delivery of Health Care in the United States**
Readings:
- Spector, *Cultural Diversity*, Chapter 3
- Starr, *Social Transformation*, pp. 198–232, 379–419
- Califano, *Radical Surgery—What's Next for America's Health Care*

Week IV   **Culture: Its Effect on the Perception of Health and Illness**
Readings:
- Spector, *Cultural Diversity*, Chapter 4
- Zola, "Culture and Symptoms: An Analysis of Patients Presenting Complaints"

Week V   **Poverty and Its Effect on Health Care**
Readings:
- Spector, *Cultural Diversity*, Chapters 3 and 7
- Lavelle, *America's New War on Poverty—A Reader for Action*

Week VI   **Faith and Healing**
Readings:
- Spector, *Cultural Diversity*, Chapters 5 and 6
- Starr, *Social Transformation*, pp. 79–144, 198–234
  Kelsey, *Healing and Christianity*
  Film: *We Believe in Niño Fidencio*

Week VII   **Health and Illness in the Hispanic Communities**
Readings:
- Thomas, *Down These Mean Streets* or *Savior, Savior, Hold My Hand*
- Lewis, *La Vida*
  Clark, *Health in the Mexican-American Culture: A Community Study*
- Spector, *Cultural Diversity*, Chapter 11

[†]For complete bibliographic data on readings, see the Bibliography.
•The bullets indicate required reading.

Week VIII **Health and Illness in the American Indian Communities**
Readings:
- Spector, *Cultural Diversity,* Chapter 8
- Deloria, *Custer Died for Your Sins*
  Kluckhohn, *The Navaho*
  Brown, *Bury My Heart at Wounded Knee*

Week IX **Health and Illness in the Asian/Pacific Communities**
Readings:
- Spector, *Cultural Diversity,* Chapter 9

Week X **Health and Illness in the Black (African) Community**
Readings:
- Spector, *Cultural Diversity,* Chapter 10
  Haley, *Roots*
- Grier, *Black Rage*
  Wright, *Black Boy* or *Native Son*
  Gutman, *The Black Family in Slavery and Freedom*
  Angelou, *I Know Why the Caged Bird Sings*

Week XI **Health and Illness in the European (White) Communities**
Readings:
- Spector, *Cultural Diversity,* Chapter 12
  Background information about specific groups of instructor's or student's selection.

Week XII **Institutional Barriers and Advocacy**
Readings:
- Starr, *Social Transformation,* pp. 235–449
- Spector, *Cultural Diversity,* Epilogue

Week XIII **Implications for Health-Care Delivery**
Readings:
- Spector, *Cultural Diversity,* Epilogue

Week XIV **Evaluation and Interethnic Dinner**

Appendix 3

Suggested Course Activities

The study of cultural diversity comes alive the moment the student leaves the confines of the classroom and goes out into the community. One way to appreciate a given ethnoreligious community is to go into a particular community and observe firsthand what daily life is like for a member of that community. The following outline can serve as an assessment guide to the community and facilitate the student's understanding of CulturalCare.

Demographic data
  Total population size of entire city or town
  Breakdown by areas—residential concentrations
  Breakdown by ages
  Other breakdowns
    Education
    Occupations
    Income
  Nations of origin of residents of the location and the target neighborhood
Traditional health and illness beliefs
  Definition of health
  Definition of illness
  Overall health status
Causes of illness
  Poor eating habits
  Wrong food combinations
  Viruses, bacteria, other organisms
  Punishment from God
  The evil eye
  Hexes, spells, or envy
  Witchcraft
  Environmental changes
  Exposure to drafts
  Over- or underwork
  Grief and loss

Methods of protecting health
Methods of maintaining health
Methods of restoring health
Home remedies
Visits and use of M.D. or other health-care resources
Health-care resources, such as neighborhood health centers
Anyone else within community who looks after people, such as traditional healers
Childbearing beliefs and practices
Child-rearing beliefs and practices
Rituals and beliefs surrounding death and dying

A second phase of this activity is to go on a walk through the given community. Point out the various services that are available. If possible, visit a community health-care provider, visit a church or community center within the neighborhood, visit grocery stores and pharmacies and point out differences in foods and over-the-counter remedies, and eat a meal in a neighborhood restaurant.

I have shared this experience with many groups of students, and the experience has been well received.

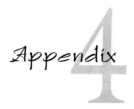

Appendix

Heritage Assessment Tool

This set of questions is to be used to describe a given client's—or your own—ethnic, cultural, and religious background. In performing a *heritage assessment* it is helpful to determine how deeply a given person identifies with his or her traditional heritage. This tool is most useful in setting the stage for assessing and understanding a person's traditional health and illness beliefs and practices and in helping to determine the community resources that will be appropriate to target for support when necessary. The greater the number of positive responses, the greater the degree to which the person may identify with his or her traditional heritage. The one exception to positive answers is the question about whether or not a person's name was changed. Background rationale for the development of this tool is found in Chapter 4.

1. Where was your mother born?_____

2. Where was your father born?_____

3. Where were your grandparents born?_____

    a. Your mother's mother?_____

    b. Your mother's father?_____

    c. Your father's mother?_____

    d. Your father's father?_____

4. How many brothers ____ and sisters ____ do you have?

5. What setting did you grow up in? Urban ____ Rural ____

6. What country did your parents grow up in?

    Father_____

    Mother_____

7. How old were you when you came to the United States? _____

8. How old were your parents when they came to the United States?

    Mother_____

    Father_____

9. When you were growing up, who lived with you?

_____

10. Have you maintained contact with
    a. Aunts, uncles, cousins? (1) Yes ___ (2) No ___
    b. Brothers and sisters? (1) Yes ___ (2) No ___
    c. Parents? (1) Yes ___ (2) No ___
    d. Your own children? (1) Yes ___ (2) No ___

11. Did most of your aunts, uncles, cousins live near your home?
    (1) Yes ___ (2) No ___

12. Approximately how often did you visit family members who lived outside of your home?
    (1) Daily ___ (2) Weekly ___ (3) Monthly ___
    (4) Once a year or less ___ (5) Never ___

13. Was your original family name changed?
    (1) Yes ___ (2) No ___

14. What is your religious preference?
    (1) Catholic ___ (2) Jewish ___
    (3) Protestant ___ Denomination ___
    (4) Other ___ (5) None ___

15. Is your spouse the same religion as you?
    (1) Yes ___ (2) No ___

16. Is your spouse the same ethnic background as you?
    (1) Yes ___ (2) No ___

17. What kind of school did you go to?
    (1) Public ___ (2) Private ___ (3) Parochial ___

18. As an adult, do you live in a neighborhood where the neighbors are the same religion and ethnic background as yourself?
    (1) Yes ___ (2) No ___

19. Do you belong to a religious institution?
    (1) Yes ___ (2) No ___

20. Would you describe yourself as an active member?
    (1) Yes ___ (2) No ___

21. How often do you attend your religious institution?

    (1) More than once a week ___ (2) Weekly ___ (3) Monthly ___

    (4) Special holidays only ___ (5) Never ___

22. Do you practice your religion in your home?

    (1) Yes ___ (2) No ___ (if yes, please specify)

    (3) Praying ___ (4) Bible reading ___ (5) Diet ___

    (6) Celebrating religious holidays ___

23. Do you prepare foods special to your ethnic background?

    (1) Yes ___ (2) No ___

24. Do you participate in ethnic activities?

    (1) Yes ___ (2) No ___ (if yes, please specify)

    (3) Singing ___ (4) Holiday celebrations ___

    (5) Dancing ___ (6) Festivals ___

    (7) Costumes ___ (8) Other ___

25. Are your friends from the same religious background as you?

    (1) Yes ___ (2) No ___

26. Are your friends from the same ethnic background as you?

    (1) Yes ___ (2) No ___

27. What is your native language? _____

28. Do you speak this language?

    (1) Prefer ___ (2) Occasionally ___ (3) Rarely ___

29. Do you read your native language?

    (1) Yes ___ (2) No ___

Quick Guide for CulturalCare

❄ *Preparing*

- Understand your own cultural values and biases.
- Acquire basic knowledge of cultural values and health beliefs and practices for client groups you serve.
- Be respectful of, interested in, and understanding of other cultures without being judgmental.

❄ *Enhancing Communication*

- Determine the level of fluency in English and arrange for an interpreter, if needed.
- Ask how the client prefers to be addressed.
- Allow the client to choose seating for comfortable personal space and eye contact.
- Avoid body language that may be offensive or misunderstood.
- Speak directly to the client, whether an interpreter is present or not.
- Choose a speech rate and style that promotes understanding and demonstrates respect for the client.
- Avoid slang, technical jargon, and complex sentences.
- Use open-ended questions or questions phrased in several ways to obtain information.
- Determine the client's reading ability before using written materials in the teaching process.

❄ *Promoting Positive Change*

- Build on cultural practices, reinforcing those that are positive, and promoting change only in those that are harmful.
- Check for client understanding and acceptance of recommendations.

- *Remember:* Not all seeds of knowledge fall into a fertile environment to produce change. Of those that do, some will take years to germinate. Be patient and provide nursing in a culturally appropriate environment to promote positive health behavior.

From: (Adapted for nursing) Schilling, B., and Brannon, E. 1986. *Cross-Cultural Counseling—A Guide for Nutrition and Health Counselors.* Alexandria, Va.: United States Department of Agriculture, United States Department of Health and Human Services, Nutrition and Technical Services Division, September, 19. Adapted with permission.

Appendix 6

Data Resources

Countless resources are available for information regarding the health-care delivery system. The following are a small sample:

Monthly Vital Statistics Report
U.S. Department of Health and
  Human Services
Public Health Service
Centers for Disease Control
National Center for Health
  Statistics
6525 Belcrest Road
Hyattsville MD 20782
(301) 436-8500

NCHS Advancedata
U.S. Department of Health and
  Human Services
Public Health Service
Centers for Disease Control
National Center for Health
  Statistics
3700 East-West Highway
Hyattsville MD 20782
(301) 436-8500

The Center for Public Policy and
  Contemporary Issues
2301 South Gaylord Street
University of Denver
Denver CO 80208

Committee for a National Health
  Program
15 Pearl Street
Cambridge MA 02139
(617) 868-3246

Health-Pac Bulletin Subscriptions
17 Murray Street
New York NY 10007

SCAPHA News
2516 N. Seminary
Chicago IL 60614

National AIDS Information
  Clearinghouse
P.O. Box 6003
Rockville MD 20850
1 (800) 458-5231

Appendix 7

NIH Office of Alternative Medicine

❋ *Directory of Alternative Health-Care Associations*

This list is not comprehensive but gives a range of professional associations grouped by type of alternative or complementary medical treatment. The categorization is not definitive; several therapies could be grouped differently. Generally, training institutions have not been included unless they provide a primary resource for information on a particular therapy.

Inclusion in this list does not constitute endorsement of any of the associations by the Office of Alternative Medicine, National Institutes of Health.

❋ *Holistic Health Care*

Association of Holistic Healing
Centers
109 Holly Crescent
Suite 201
Virginia Beach VA 23451
(804) 422-9033

Alliance/Foundation for
Alternative Medicine
160 NW Widmer Place
Albany OR 97321
(503) 926-4678

American College of Nurse-
Midwives
1522 K Street, NW
Washington DC 20005
(202) 289-0171

American Foundation for
Alternative Healthcare,
Research and Development
25 Landfield Avenue
Monticello NY 12701
(914) 794-8181

American Holistic Medical Association
4101 Lake Boone Trail
Suite 201
Raleigh NC 27607
(919) 787-5146

American Holistic Nurses Association
4101 Lake Boone Trail
Suite 201
Raleigh NC 27607
(919) 787-5181

American Holistic Veterinary
Medical Association
2214 Old Emmorton Road
Bel Air MD 21015
(410) 569-0795

American Medical Student
Association
1890 Preston White Drive
Reston VA 22091
(703) 620-6600

American Preventive Medical
Association
459 Walker Road
Great Falls VA 22066
(703) 759-0662

Canadian Holistic Medical
Association (CHMA/OMC)
491 Eglinton Avenue West, #407
Toronto, Ontario M5N 1A8
(416) 485-3071

Committee for Freedom of Choice
in Medicine
1180 Walnut Ave
Chula Vista CA 92011
(800) 227-4473

Holistic Dental Association
974 N. 21st Street
Newark OH 43055
(614) 366-3309

International Association of
Holistic Health Practitioners
3419 Thom Boulevard
Las Vegas NV 89130
(702) 873-4542

Mankind Research Foundation
1315 Apple Ave.
Silver Spring MD 20910
(301) 587-8686

❧ *Diet/Nutrition/Lifestyle Changes*

American College of Nutrition
722 Robert E. Lee Drive
Wilmington NC 28480
(919) 452-1222

American Natural Hygiene
Society
11816 Racetrack Road
Tampa FL 33626
(813) 855-6607

International Association of
Professional Natural Hygienists
204 Stambaugh Bldg.
Youngstown OH 44503
(216) 746-5000

ART, MUSIC, DANCE, HUMOR THERAPY

American Association for
Therapeutic Humor
12 S. Hanley St.
St. Louis MO 63105
(314) 863-6232

American Association of Music
Therapy
P.O. Box 80012
Valley Forge PA 19484
(215) 265-4006

American Art Therapy
Association, Inc.
1202 Allanson Rd.
Mundelein IL 60060
(708) 949-6064

American Dance Therapy
Association
2000 Century Plaza, Suite 108
Columbia MD 21044
(410) 997-4040

Dinshah Health Society
100 Dinshah Dr.
Malaga NJ 08328
(609) 392-4686

National Association for Music
Therapy
8455 Colesville Rd., Suite 930
Silver Spring MD 20910
(301) 589-3300

Radiance Technique Association
International
P.O. Box 40570
St. Petersberg FL 33743
(813) 347-3421

Trager Institute
33 Millwood
Mill Valley CA 94941-2091
(415) 388-2688

❧ *Traditional and Ethnomedicine*

ACUPUNCTURE AND TRADITIONAL CHINESE MEDICINE

Acupuncture Research Institute
313 W. Andrix St.
Monterey Park CA 91754
(213) 722-7353

American Association of
Acupuncture and Oriental
Medicine
4101 Lake Boone Trail, Suite 201
Raleigh NC 27607
(919) 787-5181

American Academy of Medical
Acupuncture
5820 Wilshire Blvd., Suite 500
Los Angeles CA 90036
(213) 937-5514

American Association of
Acupuncture and Oriental
Medicine
1400 16th St., N.W., Ste. 710
Washington DC 20036
(202) 265-2287

American Foundation of
Traditional Chinese Medicine
1280 Columbus Ave., Ste. 302
San Francisco CA 94133
(415) 776-0502

East–West Academy of Healing
Arts
450 Sutter, Ste. 916
San Francisco CA 94108
(415) 788-2227

International Foundation of
Oriental Medicine
42-62 Kissena Boulevard
Flushing NY 11355
(718) 321-8642

International Veterinary
Acupuncture Society
2140 Conestoga Rd.
Chester Springs PA 19425
(215) 827-7245

AYURVEDA

Ayurvedic Institute
11311 Menaul NE, Suite A
Albuquerque NM 87112
(505) 291-9698

Maharishi Ayurveda Assn. of
America
P.O. Box 282
Fairfield IA 52556
(515) 472-8477

KINESIOLOGY

International College of Applied
Kinesiology
P.O. Box 905
Lawrence KS 66044
(913) 542-1801

HERBALISM

American Botanical Council
P.O. Box 201660
Austin TX 78720
(512) 331-8868

American Herbalists Guild
P.O. Box 1683
Sequel CA 95073
(408) 438-1700

American Herb Assn.
P.O. Box 1673
Nevada City CA 95959
(916) 265-9552

Herb Research Foundation
1007 Pearl Street, Suite 200
Boulder CO 80302
(303) 449-2265

Herb Society of America
9019 Kirtland Chardon Road
Mentor OH 44060
(216) 256-0514

HOMEOPATHY

American Institute of Homeopathy
1585 Glencoe
Denver CO 80220
(303) 370-9164

Homeopathic Academy of
Naturopathic Physicians
14653 South Graves Road
Mulino OR 97042
(503) 829-7326

Homeopathic Medical
Association of America
18818 Teller Ave., Suite 230
Irvine CA 92715

International Foundation for
Homeopathy
2366 Eastlake Ave, E, #30
Seattle WA 98102
(206) 324-8230

National Center for Homeopathy
801 N. Fairfax St., Ste. 306
Alexandria VA 22314
(703) 548-7790

CRANIOSACRAL THERAPY

Cranial Academy
3500 Depaw Boulevard
Indianapolis IN 46268
(317) 879-0713

Upledger Institute
11211 Prosperity Farms Road
Palm Beach Gardens FL 33410
(407) 622-4706

❋ *Pharmacological and Biological Treatments*

CELL THERAPY

ICBR North American
Information Office
P.O. Box 509
Florissant MO 63032
(800) 826-5366

American Academy of Neural
Therapy
1468 South Saint Francis Drive
Santa Fe NM 87501
(505) 988-3086

DETOXIFICATION THERAPIES

American Colon Therapy
Association
11739 Washington Boulevard
Los Angeles CA 90066
(310) 390-5424

International Association of
Professional Natural Hygienists
Regency Health Resort and Spa
2000 South Ocean Drive
Hallandale FL 33009
(305) 454-2200

CHELATION

American Board of Chelation
Therapy
70 West Huron St.
Chicago IL 60610
(312) 787-ABCT

American College of Advancement
in Medicine
23121 Verdugo Dr.
Suite 204
Laguna Hills CA 92653
(714) 583-7666
(800) LEAD-OUT

Great Lakes Association of
Clinical Medicine, Inc.
70 West Huron Street
Chicago IL 60610
(312) 266-7246

Rheumatoid Disease Foundation
5106 Old Harding Road
Franklin TN 37064
(615) 646-1030

NATUROPATHY

American Association of
Naturopathic Physicians
2366 Eastlake Ave. E. Suite 322
Seattle WA 98102
(206) 323-7610

American Naturopathic
Association
1377 K Street NW, Suite 852
Washington DC 20005
(202) 682-7352

American Naturopathic Medical
Association
P.O. Box 96273
Las Vegas NV 89193
(702) 897-7053

OXYGEN THERAPY

International Association for
Oxygen Therapy
P.O. Box 1360
Priest River ID 83856
(208) 448-2504

International Bio-Oxidative
Medical Foundation
P.O. Box 61767
Dallas/Ft. Worth TX 75261
(817) 481-9772

International Ozone Association
31 Strawberry Hill Avenue
Stamford CT 06902
(203) 348-3542

✿ *Bioelectromagnetic Applications*

LIGHT THERAPY

American Optometric Association
(AOA)
243 N. Lindbergh Boulevard
St. Louis MO 63141
(314) 991-4100

College of Optometrists and
Vision Development
P.O. Box 285
Chula Vista CA 91912
(619) 425-6191

College of Syntonic
Optometry
1200 Robeson Street
Fall River MA 02720
(508) 673-1251

MAGNETIC FIELD THERAPY

Bio-Electro-Magnetics
Institute
2490 West Moana Lane
Reno NV 89509
(702) 827-9099

VISION THERAPY

Society for Light Treatment and
Biological Rhythms
P.O. Box 478
Wilsonville OR 97070
(503) 694-2404

Optometric Extension Program
Foundation, Inc. (OEP)
2912 Daimler St.
Santa Ana CA 92705
(714) 250-8070

American Optometric Association
243 N. Lindbergh Blvd.
St. Louis MO 63141
(314) 991-4100

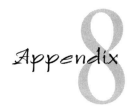

Appendix

Networks: Selected Health-Related Organizations

✺ African (Black) American

Association of Black Cardiologists
13404 S.W. 128th Street,
Suite A
Miami FL 33186
404/724-9199

Association of Black
Psychologists
P.O. Box 55999
Washington DC 20040-5999
202/722-0808

Association of Black Sociologists
Howard University
P.O. Box 302
Washington DC 20059
708/957-5025

Black Congress on Health, Law and
Economics
1025 Connecticut Ave., NW,
Suite 610
Washington DC 20036
202/659-4020

Black Psychiatrists of America
2730 Adelin St.
Oakland CA 94607
415/465-1800

Institute on Health Care for the
Poor and Underserved
Meharry Medical College
1005 D.B. Todd Boulevard
Nashville TN 37208
800/669-1269 or 615/327-6279

National Association for Sickle
Cell Disease
3345 Wilshire Blvd.
Suite 1106
Los Angeles CA 90010-1880
310/216-6363

National Association of Black Social
Workers
P.O. Box 92698
Atlanta GA 30314
313/862-6700

National Association of Blacks in
Criminal Justice
P.O. Box 66271
Washington DC 20035-6271
301/681-2365 or 713/484-4988

National Black Association for
Speech, Language and Hearing
P.O. Box 50605
Washington DC 20004-0605
202/727-2608

National Black Child Development
Institute
1023 Fifteenth Street, NW
Suite 600
Washington DC 20005
202/387-1281

National Black Nurses Association
1012 Tenth Street, NW
Washington DC 20001
202/393-6870

National Black Women's Health
Project
1237 R.D. Abernathy Boulevard,
SW
Atlanta GA 30310
800/275-2947

National Center for the
Advancement of Blacks in the
Health Professions (NCABHP)
P.O. Box 21121
Detroit MI 48221
(313) 345-4480

National Council of African
American Men
Academic and Professional
Programs
Department of Continuing
Education
University of Kansas
Lawrence KS 66045
913/864-3284

❧ *American Indian, Aleut, and Eskimo*

American Indian Health Care
Association
1550 Larimer Street
Suite 225
Denver CO 80202
303/607-1048

American Indian Institute
National American Indian
Conference on Child Abuse and
Neglect and Mental Health Issues
for the Emotionally Disturbed
North American Indian Child and
Adolescent
College of Continuing Education
University of Oklahoma
555 Constitution Street
Norman OK 73037-0005
405/842-6633

American Indian Rehabilitation
Research and Training Center
American Indians With Disabilities
Conference
P.O. Box 5630
Flagstaff AZ 86011-5630
602/523-4791 or 602/523-1695

Annual Wellness and Native Men
Conference
University of Oklahoma
Health Promotion Programs
555 E. Constitution Street
Norman OK 74037
405/325-1790

Association on American Indian
Affairs
245 Fifth Avenue
Suite 1801
New York NY 10016-8728
(212)689-8720

Association of American Indian
Physicians
1235 Sovereign Row, Suite C-7
Oklahoma City OK 73108
405/946-7072

U.S. Department of Health and
Human Services
Public Health Services
Health Administration
Indian Health Service
5600 Fishers Lane
Rockville MD 20857

National Congress of American
Indians
900 Pennsylvania Avenue, SE
Washington DC 20003
202/546-9404

Native Fitness Training and
Certification
University of Oklahoma
Health Promotion Programs
555 E. Constitution Street
Norman OK 74037
405/325-1790

National Indian Education
Association
1819 H Street, NW, Suite 800
Washington DC 20006
202/835-3001

National Indian Health Board
1385 South Colorado Blvd.
Suite A-708
Denver CO 80222
303/759-3075

National Native American AIDS
Prevention Center
6239 College Avenue, Suite 201
Oakland CA 94618
510/658-2051

Rural Alaskan Community Action
Program (RurAl CAP)
Alaskan Child Development and
Prevention Conference
P.O. Box 200908
Anchorage AK 99520
800/478-7227 or 907/279-2511

Society for the Advancement of
Chicanos and Native Americans in
Science (SACNAS)
University of California
Sinsheimer Lab
Santa Cruz CA 95064
408/459-4272

❀ *Asian/Pacific Islander*

Asian American Health Forum
116 New Montgomery Street
Suite 531
San Francisco CA 94105
415/541-0866

Asian Pacific Center
on Aging
1511 Third Avenue
Seattle WA 98101
206/624-1221

Association of Asian Pacific
Community Health Organizations
(AAPCHO)
1212 Broadway, Suite 730
Oakland CA 94612
510/272-9536

Association of Phillipine Physicians
of America
1129 20th Street, NW, Suite 400
Washington DC 20036
202/785-3336

Asian Pacific American Heritage
Council
1129 20th Street, NW
Suite 454
Washington DC 20036
703/356-2619

Cambodian Network Council
713 D Street, SE
Washington DC 20003
202/546-9144

Chinese American Medical Society
281 Edgewood Ave
Teaneck NJ 07666
201/833-1506

Filipino-American National Action
Foundation
5310 Macarthur Blvd., NW
Washington DC 20015
202/371-8933

Hawaiian Department of Health
Office of Refugee and Immigrant
Health
Pacific Islander Health Promotion
Office
1250 Punchbowl Street
Room 257
Honolulu HI 96813
808/586-4525

Hawaii University Program for
Development Disability
College of Education
SPED-UAP
1776 University Avenue:, UA4-6
Honolulu HI 96822
(808)956-5009

Korean Medical Association
162 Deer Run
Watchung NJ 07060-5938
908/755-5262

National Asian Pacific
American Families
Against Substance Abuse
(NAPAFASA)
420 E. Third Street, Suite 909
Los Angeles CA 90013-1647
213/617-8277

National Asian Pacific Center on
Aging
Melbourn Tower, Suite 914
1511 Third Avenue
Seattle WA 98101
206/624-1221

National Association for the
Education and Advancement of
Cambodian, Laotian, and
Vietnamese Americans Conference
(NAFEA)
2460 Cordova Lane
Rancho Cordova CA 95670
916/635-6815

National Research Center
on Asian American
Mental Health
405 Hilgard Avenue
Los Angeles CA 90024-1563
213/825-6251

Organization of Chinese Americans
1001 Connecticut Avenue, NW
Suite 707
Washington DC 20036
202/223-5500

Organization of Pan Asian
American Women
P.O. Box 39128
Washington DC 20016
202/659-9370

Philippine Medical Society
5220 N.W. 64th Street
Kansas City MO 64151
816/741-3969

Southeast Asian Refugee
Community Health (SEARCH)
4422 North Pershing Ave., Suite D-2
Stockton CA 95207
209/953-8843

Thailand Health Research Institute
1168 Phaholyothin 22,
Phalholyothin Road
Ladyao, Jatujak, Bangkok 10900,
Thailand
662/939-2239

❀ *Hispanic American*

ASPIRA
1112 16th Street, NW
Suite 2900
Washington DC 20036
202/835-3600

Hispanic Health Council
9648 Cedar Street
Hartford CT 06106
203/527-0856

Interamerican College of Physicians
and Surgeons
Hispanic National Medical
Association
1101 15th Street, NW, Suite 602
Washington DC 20005
202/467-4756

Midwest Hispanic AIDS Coalition
Conference
P.O. Box 470859
Chicago IL 60647
312/772-8195

National Coalition of Hispanic
Health and Human Services
Organizations (COSSMHO)
1501 16th Street, NW
Washington DC 20036
202/387-5100

National Coalition of Puerto Rican
Women
5 Thomas Circle, NW
Washington DC 20005
202/387-4716

National Council of La Raza
810 First Street, NE,
Suite 300
Washington DC 20002-4205
202/289-1380

National Hispanic Council on
Aging
2713 Ontario Road, NW
Washington DC 20009
202/265-1288

National Hispanic Nurses
Association
University of South Florida MDC
Box 2212901
Bruce B. Down Blvd.
Tampa FL 33162
813/974-2191

National Latina Health
Organization
P.O. Box 7567
Oakland CA 94601
510/534-1362

National Puerto Rican Coalition,
Inc.
1700 K Street, NW
Suite 500
Washington DC 20006
202/223-9315

National Puerto Rican Forum
National Association of Puerto
Rican Women
31 E. 32nd Street, 4th Floor
New York NY 10016
212/685-2311

Society for the Advancement of
Chicanos and Native Americans in
Science (SACNAS)
University of California,
Sinsheimer Lab
Santa Cruz CA 95064
408/459-4272

❀ *Multi Cultural*

American Public Health
Association
African American, Asian, Hispanic
and Native American Caucus
1015 Fifteenth Street, NW
Washington DC 20005
202/789-5600

Association of Minority Health
Professions Schools
Biomedical Symposium
720 Westview Drive, S.W.
Atlanta GA 30310
404/325-1790

Children's Defense Fund
25 E Street, NW
Washington, DC 20001
202/628-8787
3/9-11
Seattle WA

National Council for International
Health
1701 K Street, NW,
Suite 600
Washington DC 20006
202/833-5903

National Medical
Association
1012 Tenth Street, NW
Washington DC 20001
202/347-1895

National Migrant Resource
Program
1515 Capital of Texas Highway
South
Suite 220
Austin TX 78746
512/328-7682

National Minority AIDS Council
(NMAC) Public Policy Conference
300 Eye Street, NE, Suite 400
Washington DC 20002
202/544-1076

National Association of
Community Health Centers
1330 New Hampshire Avenue, NW
Suite 122
Washington DC 20036
202/659-8008

National Minority Health
Association
P.O. Box 11876
Harrisburg PA 17108-1876
717/763-1323

National Rural Health Association
301 E. Armour Boulevard, Suite 420
Kansas City MO 64111
816/756-3140

National Multicultural Institute
3000 Connecticut Avenue, NW
Suite 438
Washington DC 20008
202/483-0700

From: Jones, K. C. 1995. *Minority Health Calender*. Silver Spring, MD: International Minority Affairs Cooperative.
Reprinted with permission.
Calenders that list events sponsored by these organizations may be ordered by writing or calling:

- International Affairs Cooperative
- P.O. Box 10072
  Silver Spring MD 20914
  (301)890-0608

Bibliography

Abraham, L. K. *Mama Might Be Better Off Dead: The Failure of Health Care in Urban America*. Chicago: University of Chicago Press, 1993.

Abrahams, P. *Tell Freedom: Memories of Africa*. New York: Knopf, 1954.

Achebe, C. *Anthills of Savannah*. New York: Anchor Press/Doubleday, 1987.

———. *Things Fall Apart*. Greenwich, Conn.: Fawcett Crest, 1959.

Achterberg, J., Dossey, B., and Kolkmeier, L. *Rituals of Healing: Using Imagery for Health and Wellness*. New York: Bantam Books, 1994.

Aday, L. A. *At Risk in America—The Health and Health Care Needs of Vulnerable Populations in the United States*. San Francisco: Jossey-Bass, 1993.

Aiken, L. G. *Health Policy and Nursing Practice*. New York: McGraw-Hill, 1981.

Aiken, R. *Mexican Folk Tales from the Borderland*. Dallas: Southern Methodist University Press, 1980.

Albrecht, G. L., and Higgens, P. C., eds. *Health, Illness, and Medicine*. Chicago: Rand McNally, 1979.

Alcott, W. A. *The House I Live In; or the Human Body*. Boston: George W. Light, 1839.

Allende, I. *The House of the Spirits*. New York: Bantam Books, 1993.

Allison, D. *Bastard out of Carolina*. New York: Plume, 1992.

Allport, G. W. *The Nature of Prejudice* (abridged). Garden City, N.Y.: Doubleday, 1958.

Alvarez, H. R. *Health without Boundaries*. Mexico: United States–Mexico Border Public Health Association, 1975.

Alvarez, J. *How the Garcia Girls Lost Their Accents*. New York: Plume, 1992.

Ameer Ali, S. *The Spirit of Islam*. Delhi, India: IDARAH-I-ADABIYAT-I-DELLI, 1922, 1978.

American Nurses' Association. *A Strategy for Change*. Papers presented at the conference of the Commission on Human Rights, Albuquerque, N. Mex., 9–10 June 1979.

American Psychiatric Association: *Diagnostic and Statistical Manual of Mental Disorders*. 4th ed. Washington D.C. 1994.

Anderson, D. M. *Maasai People of Cattle*. San Francisco: Chronicle Books, 1995.

Anderson, E. T. and McFarlane, J. M. *Community as Client*. Philadelphia: J. B. Lippincott, 1988.

Anderson, J. Q. *Texas Folk Medicine*. Austin: Encino Press, 1970.

Andrade, S. J. *Chicano Mental Health: The Case of Cristal*. Austin: Hogg Foundation for Mental Health, 1978.

Andrews, E. D. *The People Called Shakers*. New York: Dover, 1953.

Andrews, M. M., and Boyle, J. S. *Transcultural Concepts in Nursing Care*. 2d ed. Philadelphia: J. B. Lippincott, 1995.

Angelou, M. *I Know Why the Caged Bird Sings*. New York: Random House, 1970.

Annas, G. J. *The Rights of Hospital Patients*. New York: Avon, 1975.

Appelfeld, A. *The Healer*. New York: Grove Weidenfeld, 1990.

Apple, D., ed. *Sociological Studies of Health and Sickness: A Source Book for the Health Professions*. New York: McGraw-Hill, Blakiston Division, 1960.

Archer, S. E., and Fleshman, R. P. *Community Health Nursing*. 3d ed. Monterey, Calif.: Wadsworth, 1985.

Armstrong, D., and Armstrong, E. M. *The Great American Medicine Show*. New York: Prentice Hall, 1991.

Arnold, M. G., and Rosenbaum, G. *The Crime of Poverty*. Skokie, Ill.: National Textbook Co., 1973.

Ashely, J. *Hospitals, Paternalism, and the Role of the Nurse*. New York: Teachers College Press, 1976.

Aurand, A. M. Jr. *The Realness of Witchcraft in America*. Lancaster, Pa.: Aurand Press, n.d.

Ausubel, N. *The Book of Jewish Knowledge*. New York: Crown, 1964.

Bahti, T. *Southwestern Indian Ceremonials*. Las Vegas: KC Publications, 1974.

———. *Southwestern Indian Tribes*. Las Vegas: KC Publications, 1975.

Bakan, D. *Disease, Pain, and Sacrifice: Toward a Psychology of Suffering*. Chicago: University of Chicago Press, 1968.

Baker, G. C. *Planning and Organizing for Multicultural Instruction*. 2d. ed. Menlo Park, Calif.: Addison-Wesley, 1994.

Balch, J. F., and Balch, P. A. *Prescription for Nutritional Healing*. Garden City Park, N.Y.: Avery, 1990.

Baldwin, R. *The Healers*. Huntington, Ind.: Our Sunday Visitor, 1986.

Banks, J. A., ed. *Teaching Ethnic Studies*. Washington, D.C.: National Council for Social Studies, 1973.

Bannerman, R. H., Burton, J., and Wen-Chieh, C. *Traditional Medicine and Health Care Coverage*. Geneva: World Health Organization, 1983.

Barden, T. E., ed. *Virginia Folk Legends*. Charlottesville: University Press of Virginia, 1991.

Bauwens, E. F. *The Anthropology of Health*. St. Louis: C. V. Mosby, 1979.

Beaudoin, T. *Virtual Faith: The Irreverent Spiritual Quest of Generation X*. San Francisco: Jossey Bass, 1998.

Becerra, R. M., and Shaw, D. *The Elderly Hispanic: A Research and Reference Guide*. Lanham, Md.: University Press of America, 1984.

Becker, M. H. *The Health Belief Model and Personal Health Behavior*. Thorofare, N.J.: Slack, 1974.

Beimler, R. R. *The Days of the Dead*. San Francisco: Collins Publishers, 1991.

Belgium, D., ed. *Religion and Medicine*. Ames: Iowa State University Press, 1967.

Ben-Amos, D., and Mintz, J. R. *In Praise of the Baal Shem Tov*. New York: Shocken Books, 1970.

Benedict, R. *Patterns of Culture*. New York: Penguin Books, 1946.

Benjamin, G. G. *The Germans in Texas*. 1910. Reprint, Austin: Jenkins, 1974.

Bennett, C. I. *Comprehensive Multicultural Education*. 2d ed. Boston: Allyn and Bacon, 1990.

Benson, H. *Timeless Healing*. New York: Scribner, 1996.

Berg, D. J., ed. *Homestead Hints*. Berkeley. Calif.: Ten Speed Press, 1986.

Berg, P. S., ed. *An Entrance to the Tree of Life*. Jerusalem, Israel: Research Center for Kabbalah, 1977.

Berman, E. *The Solid Gold Stethoscope*. New York: Macmillan Co., 1976.

Bermann, E. *Scapegoat*. Ann Arbor: University of Michigan Press, 1973.

Bernardo, A. *Lourdes: Then and Now*. Trans. Rand, P. T. Lourdes, France: Etablissements Estrade, n.d.

Bernardo, S. *The Ethnic Almanac*. Garden City, N.Y.: Doubleday, 1981.

Berwick, D. M., Godfrey, A. B., and Roessner, J. *Curing Health Care*. San Francisco: Josey-Bass, 1990.

Bienvenue, R. M., and Goldstein, J. E. *Ethnicity and Ethnic Relations in Canada*. 2d ed. Toronto: Butterworths, 1979.

Birnbaum, P. *Encyclopedia of Jewish Concepts*. New York: Hebrew, 1988.

Bishop, G. *Faith Healing: God or Fraud?* Los Angeles: Shervourne Press, 1967.

Bohannan P. *We, the Alien*. Prospect Heights Ill.: Waveland Press, Inc., 1992.

Boney, W. *The French Canadians Today*. London: J. M. Dent and Sons, 1939.

Bonfanti, L. *Biographies and Legends of the New England Indians*. Vol. 4. Wakefield, Mass.: Pride, 1974.

———. *Strange Beliefs, Customs, and Superstitions of New England*. Wakefield, Mass.: Pride, 1980.

Bottomore, T. B. *Classes in Modern Society*. New York: Vintage Books, 1968.

Bowen, E. S. *Return to Laughter*. Garden City, N.Y.: Doubleday, 1964.

Bowker, J. *The Meanings of Death*. Cambridge: Cambridge University Press, 1991.

Boyd, D. *Rolling Thunder*. New York: Random House, 1974.

Boyle, J. S., and Andrews, M. M. *Transcultural Concepts in Nursing Care*. 2d. ed. Philadelphia: J. B. Lippincott, 1995.

Bracq, J. C. *The Evolution of French Canada*. New York: Macmillan, 1924.

Bradley, C. J. "Characteristics of Women and Infants Attended by Lay Midwives in Texas, 1971: A Case Comparison Study." Master's thesis, University of Texas Health Science Center at Houston, School of Public Health, 1980.

Branch, M. F., and Paxton, P. P. *Providing Safe Nursing Care for Ethnic People of Color*. New York: Appleton-Century-Crofts, 1976.

Brand, J. *The Life and Death of Anna Mae Aquash*. Toronto: James Lorimer, 1978.

Brandon, G. *Santeria: From Africa to the New World*. Bloomington: University of Indiana Press, 1997.

Brink, J., and Keen, L. *Feverfew*. London: Century, 1979.

Brink, P. J., ed. *Transcultural Nursing: A Book of Readings*. Englewood Cliffs, N.J.: Prentice-Hall, 1976.

Brown, D. *Bury My Heart at Wounded Knee*. New York: Holt, Rinehart and Winston, 1970.

———. *Creek Mary's Blood*. New York: Holt, Rinehart and Winston, 1980.

Browne, G., Howard, J., and Pitts, M. *Culture and Children*. Austin: University of Texas Press, 1985.

Browne, K., and Freeling, P. *The Doctor–Patient Relationship*. Edinburgh: E & S Livingstone, 1967.

Brownlee, A. T. *Community, Culture, and Care: A Cross Cultural Guide for Healthworkers*. St. Louis: C. V. Mosby, 1979.

Bruchac, J. *Iroquois Stories Heroes and Heroines Monsters and Magic*. Freedom, Calif.: Crossing Press, 1985.

Bryant, C. A. *The Cultural Feast: An Introduction to Food and Society*. St. Paul, Minn.: West, 1985.

Buchman, D. D. *Herbal Medicine: The Natural Way to Get Well and Stay Well*. New York: Gramercy, 1979.

Budge, E. A. W. *Amulets and Superstitions*. New York: Dover, 1978.

Bullough, B. and Bullough, V. L. *Poverty, Ethnic Identity, and Health Care*. New York: Appleton-Century-Crofts, 1972.

Bullough, V. L., and Bullough, B. *Health Care for Other Americans*. New York: Appleton-Century-Crofts, 1982.

Butler, H. *Doctor Gringo*. New York: Rand McNally, 1967.

Buxton, J. *Religion and Healing in Mandari*. Oxford: Clarendon Press, 1973.

Cafferty, P. S. J., Chiswick, B. R., Greeley, A. M., et al. *The Dilemma of American Immigration: Beyond the Golden Door*. New Brunswick N.J.: Transaction Books, 1983.

Cahill, R. E. *Olde New England's Curious Customs and Cures*. Salem, Mass.: Old Saltbox Publishing House, 1990.

Cahill, R. E. *Strange Superstitions*. Salem, Mass.: Old Saltbox Publishing House, 1990.

Calhoun, M. *Medicine Show*. New York: Harper and Row, 1976.

Califano, J. *Radical Surgery*. New York: Random House, 1994.

Campos, E. *Medicina Popular: Supersticione Credios E Meizinhas*. 2d ed. Rio de Janeiro: Livraria-Editora da Casa. 1955.

Candill, H. M. *Night Comes to the Cumberlands*. Boston: Little, Brown, 1962.

Carnegie, M. E. *The Path We Tread: Blacks in Nursing 1854–1984*. Philadelphia: J. B. Lippincott, 1987.

Carson, V. B., ed. *Spiritual Dimensions of Nursing Practice*. Philadelphia: W. B. Saunders, 1989.

Catalog 70 and 75. *Immigration and Ethnic Studies*. Austin: The Austin Book Shop.

Catlin, G. *North American Indian Portfolios*. New York: Abbeville, 1993.

Chafets, Z. *Devil's Night and Other Tales of Detroit*. New York: Vintage Books, 1990.

Chan, L. S., McCandless, R., Portnoy, B., et al. *Maternal and Child Health on the U.S.–Mexico Border*. Austin: The University of Texas, 1987.

Chavira, L. Curanderismo: *An Optional Health-Care System*. Edinburg, Tex.: Pan American University, 1975.

Chenault, L. R. *The Puerto Rican Migrant in New York City*. New York: Columbia University Press, 1938.

Chiba, R. *The Seven Lucky Gods of Japan*. Rutland, Vt.: Charles E. Tuttle Co., 1966.

Choron, J. *Death and Modern Man*. New York: Collier Books, 1964.

Chun, M. N. *Hawaiian Medicine Book*. Honolulu: Bess Press, 1986.

Chute, C. *The Beans of Egypt, Maine*. New York: Ticknor & Fields, 1985.

Clark, A. *Culture, Childbearing Health Professionals*. Philadelphia: F. A. Davis, 1978.

Clark, A. L. *Culture and Child Rearing*. Philadelphia: F. A. Davis, 1981.

Clark, M. *Health in the Mexican-American Culture: A Community Study*. Berkeley: University of California Press, 1959.

Comas-Diaz, L., and Griffith, E. E. H. *Clinical Guidelines in Cross-Cultural Mental Health*. New York: Wiley, 1988.

Committee on Medical Care Teaching, eds. *Readings in Medical Care*. Chapel Hill: University of North Carolina Press, 1958.

Conde, M. I, *Tituba, Black Witch of Salem*. New York: Ballantine Books, 1992.

Conway, M. *Rise Gonna Rise*. New York: Anchor Books, 1974.

Corish, J. L. *Health Knowledge*. Vol. 1. New York: Domestic Health Society, 1923.

Cornacchia, H. J. *Consumer Health*. St. Louis: C. V. Mosby, 1976.

Corum, A. K. *Folk Remedies From Hawai'i*. Honolulu: Bess Press, 1985.

Council of Churches. *Knowing My Neighbor, Religious Beliefs and Traditions at Times of Illness and Death*. Springfield, Mass.: Visiting Nurse Hospice of Pioneer Valley, 1995.

Council on Cultural Diversity in Nursing Practice. *Proceedings of the Invitational Meeting on Multicultural Issues in the Nursing Workforce and Workplace.* Washington, D.C.: American Nurses' Association, 1994.

Cowan, N. M., and Cowan, R. S. *Our Parents' Lives.* New York: Basic Books, 1989.

Cramer, M. E. *Divine Science and Healing.* Denver: Colorado College of Divine Science, 1923.

Crichton, M. *Five Patients.* New York: Alfred A. Knopf, 1970.

Crispino, J. A. *Assimilation of Ethnic Groups: The Italian Case.* Newark, N.J.: New Jersey Center for Migration, 1980.

Cross T: "Understanding Family Resiliency from a Relational Worldview." In *Resiliency in Families: Racial and Ethnic Minority Families in America.* Madison: University of Wisconsin-Madison, 1994.

Crow Dog, L., and Erdoes, R. *Crow Dog.* San Francisco: Harper, 1996.

Culpeper, N. *Culpeper's Complete Herbal.* London: W. Foulsham, 1889.

Curry, M. A., project director. *Access to Prenatal Care: Key to Preventing Low Birth Weight.* Kansas City, Mo.: American Nurses' Association, 1987.

Curtis, E. *Native American Wisdom.* Philadelphia: Running Press, 1993.

Cutter, C. *First Book on Anatomy, Physiology, and Hygiene, for Grammar Schools and Families.* Boston: Benjamin B. Mussey, 1850.

Danforth, L. M. *The Death Rituals of Rural Greece.* Princeton: Princeton University Press, 1982.

Davis, F., ed. *The Nursing Profession: Five Sociological Essays.* New York: Wiley, 1966.

Davis, R. *American Voudou: Journey into a Hidden World.* Denton: University of North Texas Press, 1998.

DeBella, S., Martin, L., and Siddall, S. *Nurses' Role in Health Care Planning.* Norwalk, Conn.: Appleton-Century-Crofts, 1986.

De Castro, J. *The Black Book of Hunger.* Boston: Beacon Press, 1967.

Delaney, J., Lupton, M. J., and Toth, E. *The Curse: A Cultural History of Menstruation.* Chicago: University of Chicago Press, 1988.

Deller, B., Hicks, D., and MacDonald, G., coordinators. *Stone Boats and Lone Stars.* Hyde Park, Ontario: Middlesex County Board of Education, 1979.

Deloria, V. Jr. *Custer Died for Your Sins: An Indian Manifesto.* New York: Avon Books, 1969.

DeLys, C. *A Treasury of American Superstitions.* New York: Philosophical Library, 1948.

Densmore, F. *How Indians Use Wild Plants for Food, Medicine, and Crafts.* New York: Dover, 1974.

Deren, M. *Divine Horseman: The Living Gods of Haiti.* New York: McPherson, 1953.

Dey C. *The Magic Candle.* Bronx, N.Y.: Original Publications, 1982.

Dickerson, J. *Dixie's Dirty Secret.* Armonk, N.Y.: Sharpe, 1998.

Dickison, R., ed. *Causes, Cures, Sense, and Nonsense.* Sacramento, Calif.: Bishop Publishing Co., 1987.

Dinnerstein, L., and Reimers, D. M. *Ethnic Americans.* 3d ed. New York: Harper & Row, 1988.

Dioszegi, V. *Folk Beliefs and Shamanistic Practices in Siberia.* Budapest: Akademiai Kiado, 1996.

Doane, N. L. *Indian Doctor Book.* Charlotte, N.C.: Aerial, 1985.

Doka, K. J., and Morgan, J. D., eds. *Death and Spirituality.* Amityville, N.Y.: Baywood, 1993.

Donegan, J. B. *Women and Men Midwives: Medicine, Morality, and Misogyny in Early America*. Westport, Conn.: Greenwood Press, 1978.

Donin, H. H. *To Be a Jew*. New York: Basic Books, 1972.

Dorris, M. *The Broken Cord*. New York: Harper & Row, 1989.

Dorson, R. H. D., ed. *Folklore and Folklife*. Chicago: University of Chicago Press, 1972.

Dossey, L. *Healing Words*. San Francisco: Harper, 1993.

Dresser, N. Our Own Stories: *Cross-Cultural Communication Practice*. White Plains, N.Y.: Longman, 1993.

Dresser, N. *Multicultural Celebrations*. New York: Three Rivers Press, 1999.

———. *Multicultural Manners*. New York: Wiley, 1996.

Dubos, R. *Man, Medicine and Environment*. New York: Mentor, 1968.

———. *Mirage of Health*. Garden City, N.Y.: Anchor Books, Doubleday and Co., 1961.

Dubos, R. J. *Man Adapting*. New Haven: Yale University Press, 1965.

Dworaczyk, E. J. *The First Polish Colonies of America in Texas*. San Antonio: The Naylor Company, 1979.

Eck, D. L. *World Religions in Boston*. 2d. ed. Cambridge: Harvard University Press, 1998.

Egan, M. *Milagros*. Santa Fe: Museum of New Mexico Press, 1991.

Ehrenreich, B., and Ehrenreich, J. *The American Health Empire: Power, Profits, and Politics*. New York: Random House, Vintage Books, 1970.

Ehrenreich, B., and English, D. *Witches, Midwives, and Nurses: A History of Women Healers*. 2d ed. Old Westbury, N.Y.: Feminist Press, 1973.

Ehrlich, P. R. *The Golden Door: International Migration, Mexico and the United States*. New York: Wideview Books, 1979.

Eichler, L. *The Customs of Mankind*. Garden City, N.Y.: Doubleday, Page, 1923.

Eisenberg, D. *Encounters with Qi*. New York: W. W. Norton, 1985.

Eisinger, P. K. *Toward an End to Hunger in America*. Washington, D.C.: Brookings Institution, 1998.

Eliade, M., and Couliano, I. P. *The Eliade Guide to World Religions*. San Francisco: Harper, 1991.

Elling, R. H. *Socio-Cultural Influences on Health and Health Care*. New York: Springer, 1977.

Elworthy, R. T. *The Evil Eye: The Origins and Practices of Superstition*. New York: Julian Press, 1958. Originally published by John Murray, London, 1915.

Epstein, C. *Effective Interaction in Contemporary Nursing*. Englewood Cliffs, N.J.: Prentice-Hall, 1974.

Evans, E. F. *The Divine Law of Cure*. Boston: H. H. Carter, 1881.

Fadiman, A. *The Spirit Catches You and You Fall Down*. New York: Farrar, Straus and Giroux, 1997.

Farge, E. J. *La Vida Chicana: Health Care Attitudes and Behaviors of Houston Chicanos*. San Francisco: R and E Research Associates, 1975.

Feagin, J. R. *Subordinating the Poor: Welfare and American Beliefs*. Englewood Cliffs, N.J.: Prentice-Hall, 1975.

Feagin, J. R., and Feagin, C. B. *Discrimination American Style*. Englewood Cliffs, N.J.: Prentice-Hall, 1978.

Feldman, D. M. *Health and Medicine in the Jewish Tradition*. New York: Crossroads, 1986.

Finney, J. C., ed. *Culture Change, Mental Health, and Poverty*. New York: Simon and Schuster, 1969.

Fleming, A. S., chairman, U.S. Commission on Civil Rights. *The Tarnished Golden Door: Civil Rights Issues on Immigration.* Washington, D.C.: Government Printing Office, 1980.

Flores-Pena, Y., and Evanchuk, R. J. *Santeria Garments and Alters.* Jackson: University of Mississippi Press, 1994.

Fonseca, I. *Bury Me Standing: The Gypsies and Their Journey.* New York: Vintage, 1995.

Forbes, T. R. *The Midwife and the Witch.* New Haven: Yale University Press, 1966.

Ford, P. S. *The Healing Trinity: Prescriptions for Body Mind, and Spirit.* New York: Harper and Row, 1971.

Foy, F. A., ed. *Catholic Almanac.* Huntington, Ind.: Our Sunday Visitor, 1980.

Francis, P. Jr. *Beads of the World.* Atglen, Pa.: Schiffer, 1994.

Frankel, E., and Teutsch, B. P. *The Encyclopedia of Jewish Symbols.* Northvale, N.J.: Jason Aronson, Inc., 1992.

Frazer, J. G. *Folklore in the Old Testament.* New York: Tudor Publishing, 1923.

Freedman, L. *Public Housing: The Politics of Poverty.* New York: Holt, Rinehart and Winston, 1969.

Freeman, H., Levine, S., and Reeder, L. G., eds. *Handbook of Medical Sociology.* 2d ed. Englewood Cliffs, N.J.: Prentice-Hall, 1972.

Freidson, E. *Profession of Medicine.* New York: Dodd, Mead, 1971.

Freire, P. *Pedagogy of the Oppressed.* Trans. M. B. Ramos. New York: Seabury Press, 1970.

Friedman, M., and Friedland, G. W. *Medicine's Ten Greatest Discoveries.* New Haven: Yale University Press, 1998.

Frost, M. *The Shaker Story.* Canterbury, N.H.: Canterbury Shakers, n.d.

Fuentes, C. *The Old Gringo.* New York: Farrar, Straus and Giroux, 1985.

Fuller, J. G. Arigo: *Surgeon of the Rusty Knife.* New York: Pocket Books, 1974.

Galloway, M. R. U., ed. *Aunt Mary, Tell Me a Story.* Cherokee, N.C.: Cherokee Communications, 1990.

Gambino, R. *Blood of My Blood: The Dilemma of Italian-Americans.* Garden City, N.Y.: Doubleday, 1974.

Gans, H. J. *The Urban Villagers.* New York: Free Press, 1962.

Garcia, C. *Dreaming in Cuban.* New York: Ballantine Books, 1992.

Garner, J. *Healing Yourself.* 6th ed. Vashon, Wash.: Crossing Press, 1976.

Gaver, J. R. *Sickle Cell Disease.* New York: Lancer Books, 1972.

Gaw A, ed: *Cross-Cultural Psychiatry.* Boston: John Wright, 1982.

Geissler, E. M. *Pocket Guide Cultural Assessment.* 2d. ed. St. Louis: Mosby, 1998.

Gelfond, D. E., and Kutzik, A., eds. *Ethnicity and Aging: Theory, Research and Policy.* New York: Springer, 1979.

Genovese, E. D. *Roll, Jordan, Roll.* New York: Vintage Books, 1972.

Gibbs, J. T., Huang, L. N., Nagata, D. K., et al. *Children of Color.* San Francisco: Jossey-Bass, 1988.

Gibbs, T. *A Guide to Ethnic Health Collections in the United States.* Westport, Conn.: Greenwood, 1996.

Giger, J. N., and Davidhizar, R. E. *Transcultural Nursing Assessment and Intervention.* 2d ed. St. Louis: Mosby, 1995.

Giordano, J., and Giordano, G. P. *The Ethno-Cultural Factor in Mental Health.* New York: New York Institute of Pluralism and Group Identity, 1977.

Glazer, N., and Moynihan, D., eds. *Ethnicity: Theory and Experience.* Cambridge: Harvard University Press, 1975.

Goldberg B. *Alternative Medicine: The Definitive Guide.* Puyallup, Wash.: Future Medicine, 1993.

Gonzalez-Wippler, M. *Santeria: African Magic in Latin America.* Bronx, N.Y.: Original Publications, 1987.

———. *Tales of the Orishas.* New York: Original Publications, 1985.

———. *The Santeria Experience.* Bronx, N.Y.: Original Publications, 1982.

Gordon, A. F. and Kahan, L. *The Tribal Beads: A Handbook of African Trade Beads.* New York: Tribal Arts Gallery, 1976.

Gordon, D. M. *Theories of Poverty and Underemployment.* Lexington, Mass.: D. C. Heath, 1972.

Gordon, F. *Role Theory and Illness.* New Haven, Conn.: College and University Press, 1966.

Goswami, S. D. *Prabhupada: He Built a House in Which the Whole World Can Live.* Los Angeles: The Bhaktivedanta Book Trust, 1983.

Grant, G. *Obake: Ghost Stories in Hawaii.* Honolulu: Mutual, 1994.

Gray, K. *Passport to Understanding.* Denver: Center for Teaching International Relations, 1992.

Greeley, A. M. *The Irish Americans.* New York: Harper and Row, 1981.

———. *Why Can't They Be Like Us? America's White Ethnic Groups.* New York: E. P. Dutton, 1975.

Grier, W. H., and Cobbs, P. M. *Black Rage.* New York: Bantam Books, 1968.

Griffin, J. H. *Black Like Me.* New York: Signet, 1960.

Gruber R. *Rescue: The Exodus of the Ethiopian Jews.* New York: Atheneum, 1987.

Gutman, H. G. *The Black Family in Slavery and Freedom, 1750–1925.* New York: Pantheon Books, 1976.

Gutmanis, J. *Kahuna La'au Lapa'au.* Aiea, Hawaii: Island Heritage Press, 1994.

Hailey, A. *Strong Medicine.* Garden City, N.Y.: Doubleday, 1984.

———. *Roots.* Garden City, N.Y.: Doubleday, 1976.

Hallam, E. *Saints.* New York: Simon and Schuster, 1994.

Hammerschlag, C. A. *The Dancing Healers.* San Francisco: Harper & Row, 1988.

Hand, W. D. *American Folk Medicine: A Symposium.* Berkeley: University of California Press, 1973.

———. *Magical Medicine.* Berkeley: University of California Press, 1980.

Harney, R. F., and Troper, H. *Immigrants: A Portrait of Urban Experience 1890–1930.* Toronto: Van Nostrand Reinhold, 1975.

Harrington, C., and Estes, C. L. *Health Policy and Nursing.* Boston: Jones and Bartlett, 1994.

Harris, L. Holy Days: *The World of a Hasidic Family.* New York: Summit Books, 1985.

Harwood, A. 1971. "The Hot-Cold Theory of Disease: Implications for Treatment of Puerto Rican Patients," *Journal of the American Medical Asssociation* 216: 1154–1155.

———. ed. *Ethnicity and Medical Care.* Cambridge: Harvard University Press, 1981.

Haskins, J. *Voodoo and Hoodoo.* Bronx, N.Y.: Original Publications, 1978.

Hauptman, L. M., and Wherry, J. D. *The Pequots in Southern New England: The Fall and Rise of an American Indian Nation.* Norman: University of Oklahoma Press, 1990.

Hawkins, J. B. W., and Higgins, L. P. *Nursing and the Health Care Delivery System.* New York: Tiresias Press, 1983.

Hecker, M. *Ethnic American, 1970–1977.* Dobbs Ferry, N.Y.: Oceana, 1979.

Henderson, G., and Primeaux, M., eds. *Transcultural Health Care.* Menlo Park, Calif.: Addison-Wesley, 1981.

Hennessee, O. M. *Aloe: Myth-Magic Medicine.* Lawton, Okla.: Universal Graphics, 1989.

Hernandez, C. A., Haug, M. J., and Wagner, N. N. *Chicanos' Social and Psychological Perspectives.* St. Louis: C. V. Mosby, 1976.

Herzlich, C. *Health and Illness: A Social Psychological Analysis.* Trans. D. Graham. New York: Academic Press, 1973.

Hiatt, H. H. *America's Health in the Balance: Choice or Chance?* New York: Harper and Row, 1987.

Hickel, W. J. *Who Owns America?* New York: Paperback Library, 1972.

Himmelstein, D. U., and Woolhandler, S. *The National Health Program Book: A Source Guide for Advocates.* Monroe, Maine: Common Courage Press, 1994.

Hirsch, E. D. *Cultural Literacy: What Every American Needs to Know.* Boston: Houghton Mifflin, 1987.

Hongo, F. M., gen. ed. *Japanese American Journey: The Story of a People.* San Mateo, CA: JACP, 1985.

Honychurch P. N. *Caribbean Wild Plants and Their Uses.* London: Macmillan, 1980.

Howard M. *Candle Burning.* 2d ed. Weingborough, Northamptonshire, England: Aquarian Press, 1980.

Howe, I. *World of Our Fathers.* New York: Harcourt Brace Jovanovich, 1976.

Hufford, D. J. *American Healing Systems: An Introduction and Exploration.* Conference booklet. Philadelphia: University of Pennsylvania, 1984.

Hughes, H. S. *The United States and Italy.* Cambridge: Harvard University Press, 1953.

Hughes, L., and Bontemps, A., eds. *The Book of Negro Folklore.* New York: Dodd, Mead, 1958.

Hunter, J. D. *Before the Shooting Begins: Searching for Democracy in America's Culture War.* New York: Free Press, 1994.

Hunter, J. D. *Culture Wars: The Struggle to Define America.* New York: Basic Books, 1991.

Hurmence, B., ed. *My Folks Don't Want Me to Talk about Slavery.* Winston-Salem, N.C.: John F. Blair, 1984.

Hutchens, A. R. *Indian Herbalogy of North America.* Windsor, Ontario: Meico, 1973.

Hutton, J. B. *The Healing Power.* London: Leslie Frewin, 1975.

Illich, I. *Medical Nemesis: The Expropriation of Health.* London: Marion Bogars, 1975.

Illich, I., Zola, I. K., McKnight, J., et al. *Disabling Professions.* Salem, N.H.: Boyars,

Iorizzo, L. J. *Italian Immigration and the Impact of the Padrone System.* New York: Arno Press, 1980.

Jackson, J. S., Chatters, L. M., and Taylor, R. J. *Aging in Black America.* Newbury Park: Sage, 1993.

Jaco, E. G., ed. *Patients, Physicians, and Illness: Sourcebook in Behavioral Science and Medicine.* Glencoe, Ill.: Free Press, 1958.

Jacobs, H. A. *Incidents in the Life of a Slave Girl.* London: Oxford University Press, 1988.

Jacobs, L., ed. *The Jewish Mystics*. London: Kyle Cathie, 1990.

Jangl, A. M., and Jangl, J. F. *Ancient Legends of Healing Herbs*. Coeuor D'Alene, Idaho: Prisma Press, 1987.

Jarvis, D. C. *Folk Medicine: A Vermont Doctor's Guide to Good Health*. New York: Henry Holt, 1958.

Jennings, P., and Brewater, T. *The Twentieth Century*. New York: Doubleday, 1998.

Jilek W. G. *Indian Healing: Shamanic Ceremonialism in the Pacific Northwest Today*. Blaine, Wash.: Hancock House, 1992.

Johnson, C. J., and McGee, M. G., eds. *How Different Religions View Death and Afterlife*. Philadelphia: Charles Press, 1991.

Johnson, C. L. *Growing Up and Growing Old in Italian-American Families*. New Brunswick, N.J.: Rutgers University Press, 1985.

Johnson, E. A. *To the First Americans: The Sixth Report on the Indian Health Program of the U.S. Public Health Service*. Washington, D.C.: DHEW Publication (HSA) 77-1000, 1976.

Jonas, S., and Kovner, A. R., eds. *Health Care Delivery in the United States*. New York: Springer, 1998.

Jordan, B., and Heardon, S. *Barbara Jordan: A Self-Portrait*. Garden City, N.Y.: Doubleday, 1979.

Jung, C. G., ed. *Man and His Symbols*. Garden City, N.Y.: Doubleday, 1964.

Kain, J. F., ed. *Race and Poverty: The Economics of Discrimination*. Englewood Cliffs, N.J.: Prentice-Hall, 1969.

Kanellos, N. *Hispanic Firsts*. Detroit: Visible Ink, 1997.

Kaptchuk, T., and Croucher, M. *The Healing Arts*. New York: Summit Books, 1987.

Karolevitz, R. F. *Doctors of the Old West*. New York: Bonanza Books, 1967.

Katz, J. H. *White Awareness*. Norman: University of Oklahoma Press, 1978.

Kaufman, B. N., and Kaufman, S. L. *A Land beyond Tears*. Garden City, N.Y.: Doubleday, 1982.

Kavanagh, K. H., and Kennedy, P. H. *Promoting Cultural Diversity: Strategies for Health Care Professionals*. Newbury Park, Calif.: Sage, 1992.

Keith, J. *Old People as People: Social and Cultural Influences on Aging and Old Age*. Boston: Little, Brown, 1982.

———. *Old People New Lives*. Chicago: The University of Chicago Press, 1982.

Kekahbah, J., and Wood, R., eds. *Life Cycle of the American Indian Family*. Norman, Okla.: AIANA Publishing Co., 1980.

Kelly, I. *Folk Practice in North Mexico. Birth Customs, Folk Medicine, and Spiritualism in the Laguna Zone*. Austin: University of Texas Press, 1965.

Kelsey, M. T. *Healing and Christianity*. New York: Harper and Row, 1973.

Kennedy, E. M. *In Critical Condition: The Crises in America's Health Care*. New York: Simon and Schuster, 1972.

Kennett, F. *Folk Medicine, Fact and Fiction*. New York: Crescent Books, 1976.

Kiev, A. *Curanderismo: Mexican-American Folk Psychiatry*. New York: Free Press, 1968.

———. *Magic, Faith and Healing: Studies in Primitive Psychiatry Today*. New York: Free Press, 1964.

Killens, J. O. *The Cotillion*. New York: Ballantine, 1988.

Kilner, W. J. *The Human Aura*. Secaucus, N.J.: Citadel Press, 1965.

Kincaid, J. *A Small Place*. New York: Farrar, Straus and Giroux, 1988.

King, D. H. *Cherokee Heritage*. Cherokee, N.C.: Cherokee Communications, 1988.

Kingston, M. H. *Tripmaster Monkey: His Fake Book*. New York: Knopf, 1989.

Kirkland, J., Matthews, H. F. M., Sullivan, C. W. III, et al., eds. *Herbal and Magical Medicine: Traditional Healing Today*. Durham, N.C.: Duke University Press, 1992.

Klein, A. M. *Sugarball, The American Game, the Dominican Dream*. New Haven: Yale University Press, 1991.

Klein, J. W. *Jewish Identity and Self-Esteem: Healing Wounds through Ethnotherapy*. New York: Institute on Pluralism and Group Identity, 1980.

Klein: M. *A Time to Be Born: Customs and Folklore of Jewish Birth*. Philadelphia: Jewish Publication Society, 1998.

Kluckhohn, C. *Navaho Witchcraft*. Boston: Beacon Press, 1944.

Kluckhohn, C., and Leighton, D. *The Navaho*. Rev. ed. Garden City, N.Y.: Doubleday and Co., 1962.

Kmit, A., Luciow, L. L., Luciow, J., et al. *Ukrainian Easter Eggs and How We Make Them*. Minneapolis, Minn.: Ukrainian Gift Shop, 1979.

Knudtson, P., and Suzuki, D. *Wisdom of the Elders*. Toronto: Stoddart, 1992.

Knutson, A. L. *The Individual, Society, and Health Behavior*. New York: Russell Sage Foundation, 1965.

Komisar, L. *Down and Out in the USA: A History of Social Welfare*. New York: New Viewpoints, 1974.

Kordel, L. *Natural Folk Remedies*. New York: Putnam's, 1974.

Kosa, J., and Zola, I. K. *Poverty and Health: A Sociological Analysis*. 2d ed. Cambridge: Harvard University Press, 1976.

Kotelchuck, D., ed. *Prognosis Negative*. New York: Vintage Books, 1976.

Kotz, N. *Let Them Eat Promises*. Garden City, N.Y.: Doubleday, 1971.

Kovner, A., ed. *Health Care Delivery in the United States*. 4th ed. New York: Springer, 1990.

Kramer, R. M. *Participation of the Poor*. Englewood Cliffs, N.J.: Prentice-Hall, 1969.

Kraut, A. M. *Silent Travelers: Germs, Genes, and the Immigrant Menace*. New York: Basic Books, 1994.

Kraybeill, D. B. *The Riddle of Amish Culture*. Baltimore: Johns Hopkins, 1989.

Kreiger, D. *The Therapeutic Touch*. Englewood Cliffs, N.J.: Prentice-Hall, 1979.

Krippner, S., and Villaldo, A. *The Realms of Healing*. Millbrae, Calif.: Celestial Arts, 1976.

Kronenfeld, J. J. *Controversial Issues in Health Care Policy*. Newbury Park, Calif.: Sage, 1993.

Kunitz, S. J., and Levy, J. E. *Navajo Aging: The Transition from Family to Institutional Support*. Tucson: University of Arizona Press, 1991.

Lake, M. G. *Native Healer Initiation into an Art*. Wheaton, Ill.: Quest Books, 1991.

Landmann, R. S., ed. *The Problem of the Undocumented Worker*. Albuquerque: Latin American Institute, University of New Mexico, 1981.

Lasker, R. D. *Medicine and Public Health*. New York: New York Academy of Medicine, 1997.

Lassiter, S. *Multicultural Clients*. Westport, Conn.: Greenwood, 1995.

Last, J. M. *Public Health and Human Ecology*. Norwalk, Conn.: Appleton, 1987.

Lau, T. *The Handbook of Chinese Horoscopes*. Philadelphia: Harper and Row, 1979.

Laveau, M. *Black and White Magic: Burning of Candles, Use of Roots and Oils, Powders, and Incenses*. Purchased in New Orleans, La., in 1990.

Lavelle, R., ed. *America's New War on Poverty: A Reader for Action*. San Francisco: KQED Books, 1995.

Lawless, E. J. *God's Peculiar People*. Lexington: University of Kentucky Press, 1988.

Lee, P. R., and Estes, C. L., eds. *The Nation's Health*. 4th ed. Boston: Jones and Bartlett, 1994.

Leek, S. Herbs: *Medicine and Mysticism*. Chicago: Henry Regnery, 1975.

Leff, S., and Leff, V. *From Witchcraft to World Health*. New York: Macmillan, 1957.

Leininger, M. *Nursing and Anthropology: Two Worlds to Blend*. New York: Wiley, 1970.

———. *Transcultural Nursing: Concepts, Theories, and Practices*. New York: Wiley, 1978.

Leong, L. *Acupuncture: A Layman's View*. New York: Signet, 1974.

Lerner, M. *Choices in Healing*. Cambridge: MIT Press, 1994.

Leslau, C., and Leslau, W. *African Proverbs*. White Plains, N.Y.: Peter Pauper Press, 1985.

Lesnoff-Caravaglia, G., ed. *Realistic Expectations for Long Life*. New York: Human Sciences Press, 1987.

Lewis, O. *A Death in the Sanchez Family*. New York: Random House, 1966.

———. *Five Families: Mexican Case Studies in the Culture of Poverty*. New York: New American Library Basic Books, 1959.

———. *La Vida: A Puerto Rican Family in the Culture of Poverty—San Juan and New York*. New York: Random House, 1966.

———. *The Children of Sanchez: Autobiography of a Mexican Family*. New York: Random House, 1961.

Lewis, T. H. *The Medicine Men: Oglala Sioux Ceremony and Healing*. Lincoln: University of Nebraska Press, 1990.

Lich, G. E. *The German Texans*. San Antonio: The Institute of Texan Cultures, 1981.

Lieban, R. W. *Cebuano Sorcery*. Berkeley: University of California Press, 1967.

Linck, E. S., and Roach J. G. *Eats: A Folkhistory of Texas Foods*. Fort Worth: Texas Christian University Press, 1989.

Lipson, J. G., Dibble, S. L., and Minarik, P. A. *Culture and Nursing Care: A Pocket Guide*. San Francisco: UCSF Nursing Press, 1996.

Litoff, J. B. *American Midwives 1860 to the Present*. Westport, Conn.: Greenwood Press, 1978.

LittleDog, P. *Border Healing Woman: The Story of Jewel Babb*. 2d ed. Austin: University of Texas Press, 1994.

Livingston, I. L., ed. *Handbook of Black American Health*. Westport, Conn.: Greenwood Press, 1994.

Logan, P. *Irish Country Cures*. Dublin: Talbot Press, 1981.

Louv, R. *Southwind: The Mexican Migration*. San Diego: San Diego Union, 1980.

Lovering, A. T. 2 Vols. *The Household Physician*. Boston: Woodruff, 1923.

Lum, D. *Social Work Practice and People of Color: A Process-Stage Approach*. 2d ed. Pacific Grove, Calif.: Brooks/Cole, 1992.

Lynch, L. R., ed. *The Cross-Cultural Approach to Health Behavior*. Rutherford, N.J.: Fairleigh Dickenson University Press, 1969.

Mackintosh, J. *Principles of Pathology and Practice of Physic*. 3d ed. Vol. 1. Philadelphia: Key & Biddle, 1836.

MacNutt, F. *Healing*. Notre Dame, Ind.: Ave Maria Press, 1974.

———. *The Power to Heal*. Notre Dame, Ind.: Ave Maria Press, 1977.

Magida, A. J., ed. *How to Be a Perfect Stranger*. Vol. 1. Woodstock, Vt.: Jewish Lights Publishing, 1996.

Malinowski, B. *Magic, Science, and Religion*. Garden City, N.Y.: Doubleday, 1954.

Maloney, C., ed. *The Evil Eye*. New York: Columbia University Press, 1976.

Malpezzi, F. M., and Clement, W. M. *Italian American Folklore*. Little Rock, Ark.: August House Publishers, 1992.

Mandell, B. R., ed. *Welfare in America: Controlling the "Dangerous Classes."* Englewood Cliffs, N.J.: Prentice-Hall, 1975.

Manderschied, R. W., and Sonnenschein, M. A., eds. *Mental Health, United States, 1992*. Washington, D.C.: Center for Mental Health Services and National Institute of Mental Health. Government Printing Office, DHHS Pub. No. (SMA)92-1942, 1992.

Mann, F. Acupuncture: *The Ancient Chinese Art of Healing and How It Works Scientifically*. New York: Vintage Books, 1972.

Marquez, G. G. *Love in the Time of Cholera*. New York: Alfred A. Knopf, 1998.

Marsella, A. B., and Pedersens, P. B., eds. *Cross Cultural Counseling and Psychotherapy*. New York: Pergamon, 1981.

Marsella, A. J., and White G. M., eds. *Cultural Conceptions of Mental Health Therapy*. London: D. Reidel, 1982.

Martin, J., and Todnem, A. *Cream and Bread*. Hastings, Minn.: Redbird Productions, 1984.

Martin, J. L., and Nelson, S. J. *They Glorified Mary, We Glorified Rice*. Hastings, Minn.: Caragana Press, 1994.

———. *They Had Stories, We Had Chores*. Hastings, Minn.: Caragana Press, 1995.

Martin, L. C. *Wildflower Folklore*. Charlotte, N.C.: East Woods Press, 1984.

Martinez, R. A., ed. *Hispanic Culture and Health Care*. St. Louis: C. V. Mosby, 1978.

Matlins, S. M., and Magida, A. J., eds. *How to Be a Perfect Stranger*. Vol. 2. Woodstock, Vt.: Jewish Lights Publishing, 1997.

Matsumoto M. *The Unspoken Way*. Tokyo: Kodansha International, 1988.

Matthiessen, P. *In the Spirit of Crazy Horse*. New York: Viking Press, 1980.

McBrid, I. R. *Practical Folk Medicine of Hawaii*. Hilo: Petroglyph Press, 1975.

McBride, J. *The Color of Water*. New York: Riverhead Books.

McCall, N. *Makes Me Wanna Holler*. New York: Vintage Books, 1995.

McClain, M. *A Feeling for Life: Cultural Identity, Community, and the Arts*. Chicago: Urban Traditions, 1988.

McCubbin, H. I., Thompson, E. A., Thompson, A. I., et al. *Resiliency in Ethnic Minority Families*. Vol. 1, *Native and Immigrant American Families*. Madison: WI: University of Wisconsin, 1994.

McCubbin, H., Thompson, E. A., Thompson, A. I., et al. *Resiliency in Ethnic Minority Families*. Vol. 2, *African-American Families*. Madison: University of Wisconsin Center, 1995.

McCubbin, H. I., Thompson, E. A., Thompson, A. I., et al. *Sense of Coherence and Resiliency*. Madison: University of Wisconsin, 1994.

McGill, O. *The Mysticism and Magic of India*. South Brunswick, N.J., and New York: A. S. Baines, 1977.

McGoldrick, M., Giordano, J., and Pearce, J. K. *Ethnicity and Family Therapy*. 2d ed. New York: Guilford Press, 1996.

McGregor, J. H. *The Wounded Knee Massacre from the Viewpoint of the Sioux*. Rapid City, S.D.: Fenwyn Press, 1940.

McLary, K. *Amish Style*. Bloomington: Indiana Press, 1993.

McLemore, S. D. *Racial and Ethnic Relations in America*. Boston: Allyn and Bacon, 1980.

Means, R. *Where White Men Fear to Tread*. New York: St. Martin's Press, 1995.

Mechanic, D. *Medical Sociology: A Selective View.* New York: Free Press, 1968.

Menchu, R. *I, Rigoberta Menchu.* Trans. A. Wright. London: Verso, 1983.

Merrill, F. E. *Society and Culture.* Englewood Cliffs, N.J.: Prentice-Hall, 1962.

Metraux, A. *Voodoo in Haiti.* New York: Schocken Books, 1972.

Meyer, C. E. *American Folk Medicine.* Glenwood, Ill.: Meyerbooks, 1985.

Micozzi, M. S. *Fundamentals of Complementary and Alternative Medicine.* New York: Churchill, 1996.

Milio, N. *The Care of Health in Communities: Access for Outcasts.* New York: Macmillan, 1975.

Millman, M. *The Unkindest Cut.* New York: William Morrow, 1977.

Mindel, C. H., and Habenstein, R. W., eds. *Ethnic Families in America.* New York: Elsevier, 1976.

Miner, H. *St. Denis, A French Canadian Parish.* Chicago: University of Chicago Press, 1939.

Moldenke, H. N., and Moldenke, A. L. *Plants of the Bible.* New York: Dover Publications, 1952.

Montagu, A. *Touching.* New York: Harper & Row, 1971.

Montgomery, R. *Born to Heal.* New York: Coward, McCann, and Geoghegan, 1973.

Moody, R. A. *Life after Life.* New York: Bantam, 1976.

Mooney, J. *Myths of the Cherokee and Sacred Formulas of the Cherokees.* Nashville, Tenn.: Charles and Randy Elder—Booksellers, and Cherokee, N.C.: Museum of the Cherokee Indian, 1982.

Morgan, M. *Mutant Message Downunder.* Lees Summit, Mo.: MM CO, 1991.

Morgenstern, J. *Rites of Birth, Marriage, Death, and Kindred Occasions among the Semites.* Chicago: Quadrangle Books, 1966.

Morley, P., and Wallis, R., eds. *Culture and Curing.* Pittsburgh: University of Pittsburgh Press, 1978.

Morrison, T. *Beloved.* New York: Knopf/Random House, 1987.

———. *Tar Baby.* New York: Alfred A. Knopf, 1981.

Morton, L. T., and Moore, R. J. *A Chronology of Medicine and Related Sciences.* Cambridge: University Press, 1998.

Murray, P. *Song in a Weary Throat: An American Pilgrimage.* New York: Harper & Row, 1987.

Mushkin, S. V. *Consumer Incentives for Health Care.* New York: Prodist, 1974.

National Center for Health Statistics. *Health United States 1998 with Socioeconomic Status and Health Chartbook.* Hyattsville, Md., 1998.

Nelli, H. S. *From Immigrants to Ethnics: The Italian Americans.* Oxford: Oxford University Press, 1983.

Nelson, D. *Food Combining Simplified.* Santa Cruz, Calif.: The Plan, 1985.

Nemetz-Robinson, G. L. *Crosscultural Understanding.* New York: Prentice Hall, 1988.

Nerburn, K., and Mengelkoch, L., eds. *Native American Wisdom.* San Rafael, Calif.: New World Library, 1991.

Neugrossschel, J. *Great Tales of Jewish Occult and Fantasy.* New York: Wings Books, 1991.

Newman, K. D. *Ethnic American Short Stories.* New York: Pocket Books, 1975.

Norman, J. C., ed. *Medicine in the Ghetto.* New York: Appleton-Century-Crofts, 1969.

North, J. H., and Grodsky, S. J., comp. *Immigration Literature: Abstracts of Demographic, Economic, and Policy Studies.* Washington, D.C.: U.S. Department of Justice, Immigration & Naturalization Service, 1979.

Novak, M. *The Rise of the Unmeltable Ethnics.* New York: Macmillan, 1972.

Null, G. and Stone, C. *The Italian-Americans.* Harrisburg, Pa.: Stackpole Books, 1976.

O'Berennan, J., and Smith, N. *The Crystal Icon.* Austin, Tex.: Galahad Press, 1981.

Oduyoye, M. *Words and Meaning in Yoruba Religion.* London: Karnak House, 1996.

Opler, M. K., ed. *Culture and Mental Health.* New York: Macmillan, 1959.

Orlando, L. *The Multicultural Game Book.* New York: Scholastic Professional Books, 1993.

Orque, M. S., Block, B., and Monrray, L. S. A. *Ethnic Nursing Care: A Multi-Cultural Approach.* St. Louis: C. V. Mosby, 1983.

Osofsky, G. Harlem: *The Making of a Ghetto.* New York: Harper and Row, 1963.

Overfield, T. *Biologic Variation in Health and Illness.* Menlo Park, Calif.: Addison-Wesley, 1985.

Ozaniec, N. *Little Book of Egyptian Wisdom.* Rockport, Mass.: Element, 1997.

Padilla, E. *Up From Puerto Rico.* New York: Columbia University Press, 1958.

Paley, V. G. *White Teacher.* Cambridge: Harvard University Press, 1979.

Palos, S. *The Chinese Art of Healing.* New York: Herter and Herter, 1971.

Pappworth, M. H. *Human Guinea Pigs: Experimentation on Man.* Boston: Beacon Press, 1967.

Parsons, T., and Clark, K. B. *The Negro American.* Boston: Beacon Press, 1965.

Paul, B., ed. *Health, Culture, and Community: Case Studies of Public Reactions to Health Programs.* New York: Russell Sage Foundation, 1955.

Payer, L. *Medicine and Culture.* New York: Penguin Books, 1988.

Pearsall, M. *Medical Behavior Science: A Selected Bibliography of Cultural Anthropology, Social Psychology, and Sociology in Medicine.* Louisville: University of Kentucky Press, 1963.

Pelto, P. J., and Pelto, G. H. *Anthropological Research: The Structure of Inquiry.* 2d ed. Cambridge: Cambridge University Press, 1978.

Pelton, R. W. *Voodoo Charms and Talismans.* New York: Popular Library, 1973.

Perera, V. *The Cross and the Pear Tree.* Berkeley: University of California Press, 1995.

Petry, A. *The Street.* Boston: Beacon Press, 1985.

Philpott, L. L. "A Descriptive Study of Birth Practices and Midwifery in the Lower Rio Grande Valley of Texas." Ph.D. diss., University of Texas Health Science Center at Houston School of Public Health, 1979.

Pierce, R. V. *The People's Common Sense Medical Advisor in Plain English, or Medicine Simplified.* 12th ed. Buffalo, N.Y.: World's Dispensary, 1983.

Piven, F. F., and Cloward, R. A. *Regulating the Poor: The Functions of Public Welfare.* New York: Vintage Books, 1971.

Plotkin, M. J. *Tales of a Shaman's Apprentice.* New York: Viking, 1993.

Popenoe, C. *Wellness.* Washington, D.C.: YES!, 1977.

Powell, C. A. *Bound Feet.* Boston: Warren Press, 1938.

Power, S. *The Grass Dancer.* New York: Putnam, 1994.

Prabhupada, A. C. *Bhaktivedanta Swami. KRSNA: The Supreme Personality of Godhead.* Vol. 1. Los Angeles: The Bhaktivedanta Book Trust, 1970.

Prose, F. *Marie Laveau.* New York: Berkeley, 1977.

Proulx, E. A. *Accordion Crimes.* New York: Scribner, 1996.

Purnell, L. D., and Paulanka, B. J. *Transcultural Health Care.* Philadelphia: F. A. Davis, 1998.

Rand, C. *The Puerto Ricans.* New York: Oxford University Press, 1958.

Read, M. *Culture, Health, and Disease.* London: Javistock Publications, 1966.

Rector-Page, L. G. *Healthy Healing: An Alternative Healing Reference.* 9th ed. Calif.: Healthy Healing Publications, 1992.

Redman, E. *The Dance of Legislation.* New York: Simon and Schuster, 1973.

Reichard, G. A. *Navajo Medicine-Man Sandpaintings.* New York: Dover, 1977.

Reneaux, J. J. *Cajun Folktales.* Little Rock: August House Publishers, 1992.

Rist, R. C. *Desegregated Schools: Appraisals of an American Experiment.* New York: Academic Press, 1979.

Riva, A. *Devotions to the Saints.* Los Angeles: International Imports, 1990.

———. *Magic with Incense and Powders.* N. Hollywood, Calif.: International Imports, 1985.

———. *The Modern Herbal Spellbook.* N. Hollywood, Calif.: International Imports, 1974.

Rivera, J. R. *Puerto Rican Tales.* Mayaquez, Puerto Rico: Ediciones Libero, 1977.

Roby, P., ed. *The Poverty Establishment.* Englewood Cliffs, N.J.: Prentice-Hall, 1974.

Rodriquez, C. E. *Puerto Ricans Born in the U.S.A.* Boulder: Westview Press, 1991.

Roemer, M. I. *An Introduction to the U.S. Health Care System.* 2d ed. New York: Springer, 1990.

Rogler, L. H. *Migrant in the City.* New York: Basic Books, 1972.

Rohde, E. S. *The Old English Herbs.* New York: Dover, 1922, 1971.

Rose, P. I. *They and We: Racial and Ethnic Relations in the United States.* 3d ed. New York: Random House, 1981.

Rosen, P. *The Neglected Dimension: Ethnicity in American Life.* Notre Dame, London: University of Notre Dame Press, 1980.

Rosenbaum, B. Z. *How to Avoid the Evil Eye.* New York: St. Martin's Press, 1985.

Ross, N. W. *The World of Zen.* New York: Vintage Books, 1960.

Rossbach, S. *Interior Design with Feng Shui.* New York: Arkana, 1987.

Roter, D. L., and Hall, J. A. *Doctors Talking with Patients.* Westport, Conn.: Auburn House, 1993.

Rude, D., ed. *Alienation: Minority Groups.* New York: Wiley, 1972.

Russell, A. J. *Health in His Wings.* London: Metheun, 1937.

Ryan, W. *Blaming the Victim.* New York: Vintage Books, 1971.

S., E. M. *The House of Wonder: A Romance of Psychic Healing.* London: Rider, 1927.

Santillo, H. *Herbal Combinations from Authoritative Sources.* Provo, Utah: NuLife, 1983.

Santino, J. *All Around the Year.* Chicago, University of Illinois Press, 1994.

Santoli A. *New Americans.* New York: Ballantine, 1988.

Sargent, D. A. *Health, Strength, and Power.* New York: HM Caldwell, 1904.

Saunders, L. *Cultural Difference and Medical Care: The Case of the Spanish-Speaking People of the Southwest.* New York: Russell Sage Foundation, 1954.

Saunders, R. *Healing through the Spirit Agency.* London: Hutchinson, 1927.

Schneider, M. *Self Healing: My Life and Vision.* New York: Routledge & Kegan Paul, 1987.

Scholem, G. G. *Major Trends in Jewish Mysticism.* New York: Schocken Books, 1941.

School, B. F. *Library of Health Complete Guide to Prevention and Cure of Disease.* Philadelphia: Historical, 1924.

Schrefer, S., ed. *Quick Reference to Cultural Assessment.* St. Louis: Mosby, 1994.

Scott, W. R., and Volkart, E. H. *Medical Care.* New York: Wiley, 1966.

Senior, C. *The Puerto Ricans, Strangers—Then Neighbors.* Chicago: Quadrangle Books, 1961.

Serinus, J., ed. *Psychoimmunity and the Healing Process.* Berkeley, Calif.: Celestial Arts, 1986.

Sexton, P. C. *Spanish Harlem.* New York: Harper and Row, 1965.

Shaw, W. *Aspects of Malaysian Magic.* Kuala Lumpur, Malaysia: Naziabum. Nigara, 1975.

Sheinkin, D. *Path of the Kabbalah.* New York: Paragon House, 1986.

Shelton, F. *Pioneer Comforts and Kitchen Remedies: Oldtime Highland Secrets from the Blue Ridge and Great Smoky Mountains.* High Point, N.C.: Hutcraft, 1965.

———. ed. *Pioneer Superstitions.* High Point, N.C.: Hutcraft, 1969.

Shenkin, B. N. *Health Care for Migrant Workers: Policies and Politics.* Cambridge, Mass.: Ballinger, 1974.

Shepard, R. F., and Levi, V. G. *Live and Be Well.* New York: Ballantine Books, 1982.

Shih-Chen, L. *Chinese Medicinal Herbs.* Trans. F. P. Smith and G. A. Stuart. San Francisco: Georgetown Press, 1973.

Shor, I. *Culture Wars: School and Society in the Conservative Restoration 1969–1984.* Boston: Routledge & Kegan Paul, 1986.

Shorter, E. *The Health Century.* New York: Doubleday, 1987.

Shostak, A. B., Van Til, J., and Van Til, S. B. *Privilege in America: An End to Inequality?* Englewood Cliffs, N.J.: Prentice-Hall, 1973.

Silver, G. *A Spy in the House of Medicine.* Germantown, Md.: Aspen Systems Corp., 1976.

Silverman, D. *Legends of Safed.* Jerusalem: Gefen, 1989.

Silverstein, M. E., Chang, I-L., and Macon, N., trans. *Acupuncture and Moxibustion.* New York: Schocken Books, 1975.

Simmen, E., ed. *Pain and Promise: The Chicano Today.* New York: New American Library, 1972.

Simmons, A. G. *A Witch's Brew.* Coventry, Conn.: Caprilands Herb Farm, n.d.

Skelton, R. *Talismanic Magic.* York Beach, Maine: Samuel Weiser, 1985.

Slater, P. *The Pursuit of Loneliness.* Boston: Beacon Press, 1970.

Smith, H. *The Religions of Man.* New York: Harper and Row, 1958.

Smith, L. *Killers of the Dream.* Garden City, N.Y.: Doubleday, 1963.

Smith, P. *The Origins of Modern Culture, 1543–1687.* New York: Collier Books, 1962.

Sowell, T. *Ethnic America.* New York: Basic Books, 1981.

———. *Migrations and Cultures.* New York: Basic Books, 1996.

Spann, M. B. *Literature-Based Multicultural Activities.* New York: Scholastic Professional Books, 1992.

Spector, R. E. "A Description of the Impact of Medicare on Health-Illness Beliefs and Practices of White Ethnic Senior Citizens in Central Texas." Ph.D. diss., University of Texas at Austin School of Nursing, 1983; Ann Arbor, Mich.: University Microfilms International, 1983.

———. *CulturalCare: Maternal Infant Issues.* Baltimore: Williams and Wilkins, 1998 (video).

Spicer, E., ed. *Ethnic Medicine in the Southwest.* New York: Russell Sage Foundation, 1977.

Stack, C. B. *All Our Kin*. New York: Harper and Row, 1974.

Starr, P. *The Social Transformation of American Medicine*. New York: Basic Books, 1982.

Steele, J. D. *Hygienic Physiology*. New York: A. S. Barnes, 1884.

Steinberg, M. *Basic Judaism*. New York: Harcourt, Brace and World, 1947.

Steinberg, S. *The Ethnic Myth: Race, Ethnicity, and Class in America*. Boston: Beacon Press, 1989.

Steiner, S. *La Raza: The Mexican Americans*. New York: Harper and Row, 1969.

Steinsaltz, A. *The Thirteen Petalled Rose*. New York: Basic Books, 1980.

Stephan, W. G. and Feagin, J. R. *School Desegregation Past, Present, Future*. New York: Plenum, 1980.

Stevens, A. *Vitamins and Remedies*. High Point, N.C.: Hutcraft, 1974.

Stewart, J., ed. *Bridges Not Walls*. Reading, Mass.: Addison-Wesley, 1973.

Still, C. E., Jr. *Frontier Doctor Medical Pioneer*. Kirksville, Mo.: Thomas Jefferson University Press, 1991.

Stoll, R. I. *Concepts in Nursing: A Christian Perspective*. Madison, Wisc.: Intervarsity Christian Fellowship, 1990.

Stone, E. *Medicine among the American Indians*. New York: Hafner, 1962.

Storlie, F. *Nursing and the Social Conscience*. New York: Appleton-Century-Crofts, 1970.

Storm, H. *Seven Arrows*. New York: Ballantine Books, 1972.

Strauss, A. and Corbin, J. M. *Shaping a New Health Care System*. San Francisco: Josey-Bass, 1988.

Styron, W. *The Confessions of Nat Turner*. New York: Random House, 1966.

Swazey, J. P., and Reeds, K. *Today's Medicine, Tomorrow's Science*. Washington, D.C.: U.S. Government Department of Health, Education, and Welfare, 1978.

Sweet, M. *Common Edible Plants of the West*. Happy Camp, Calif.: Naturegraph, 1976.

Szasz, T. S. *The Myth of Mental Illness*. New York: Dell, 1961.

Takaki, R. *A Different Mirror: A History of Multicultural America*. Boston: Little, Brown, 1993.

Tallant, R. *Voodoo in New Orleans*. New York: Collier Books, 1946.

Tan, A. *The Joy Luck Club*. New York: Ivy Books, 1989.

Te Selle, S., ed. *The Rediscovery of Ethnicity: Its Implications for Culture and Politics in America*. New York: Harper and Row, 1973.

ten Boom, C. *The Hiding Place*. Washington Depot, Conn.: Chosen Books, 1971.

Thernstrom, S., ed. *Harvard Encyclopedia of American Ethnic Groups*. Cambridge: Harvard University Press, 1980.

Thomas, C. *They Came to Pittsburgh*. Pittsburgh: Post-Gazette, 1983.

Thomas, P. *Down These Mean Streets*. New York: Signet Books, 1958.

Thomas, P. *Savior, Savior, Hold My Hand*. Garden City, N.Y.: Doubleday, 1972.

Tierra, M. *The Way of Herbs*. New York: Pocket Books, 1990.

Titmuss, R. M. *The Gift Relationship*. New York: Vintage, 1971.

Tomasi, S. M., ed. *National Directory of Research Centers, Repositories, and Organizations of Italian Culture in the United States*. Torino: Fondazione Giovanni Agnelli, 1980.

Tompkins, P., and Bird C. *The Secret Life of Plants*. New York: Avon, 1973.

Tooker, E., ed. *Native American Spirituality of the Eastern Woodlands*. New York: Paulist Press, 1979.

Torres, E. *Green Medicine: Traditional Mexican-American Herbal Remedies.* Kingsville, Tex.: Nieves Press, 1982.

Torres-Gill, F. M. *Politics of Aging among Elder Hispanics.* Washington, D.C.: University Press of America, 1982.

Touchstone, S. J. *Herbal and Folk Medicine of Louisiana and Adjacent States.* Princeton, La.: Folk-Life Books, 1983.

Trachtenberg, J. *Jewish Magic and Superstition.* New York: Behrman House, 1939.

Trachtenberg, J. *The Devil and the Jews.* Philadelphia: The Jewish Publication Society of America, 1983. (Original publication, New Haven: Yale University Press, 1945).

Trattner, W. I. *From Poor Law to Welfare State: A History of Social Welfare in America.* New York: Free Press, 1974.

Trotter, R. II, and Chavira, J. A. *Curanderismo: Mexican American Folk Healing.* Athens, Ga.: University of Georgia Press, 1981.

Tucker, G. H. *Virginia Supernatural Tales.* Norfolk, Va.: Donning, 1977.

Tula, M. T. *Hear My Testimony.* Boston: South End Press, 1994.

Twining, M. A., and Baird, K. E., eds. *Sea Island Roots: African Presence in the Carolinas and Georgia.* Trenton, N.J.: Africa World Press, 1991.

Unger, S., ed. *The Destruction of American Indian Families.* New York: Association on American Indian Affairs, 1977.

U.S. Commission on Civil Rights. *Fulfilling the Letter and Spirit of the Law.* Washington, D.C.: Government Printing Office, 1976.

———. *Mexican Americans and the Administration of Justice in the Southwest.* Washington, D.C.: Government Printing Office, 1970.

U.S. Department of Commerce, Bureau of the Census. *Ancestry of the Population by State: 1980.* Washington, D.C.: Government Printing Office, 1980.

———. *Population Profile of the United States: 1981.* "Population Characteristics," ser. 20, no. 374, September 1982.

U.S. Department of Health and Human Services. *Comprehensive Health Care Program for American Indians and Alaska Natives.* Rockville, Md.: Public Health Service, Indian Health Service, 1997.

———. *Regional Differences in Indian Health.* Rockville, Md.: Public Health Service, Indian Health Service, 1997.

———. *Trends in Indian Health.* Rockville, Md.: Public Health Service, Indian Health Service, 1997.

———. *Health United States 1992 and Healthy People 2000 Review.* Washington, D.C.: United States Department of Health and Human Services, Public Health Service Centers for Disease Control and Prevention. DHHS Pub. No. (PHS) 93-1232, 1993.

———. *Healthy People 2000 National Health Promotion and Disease Prevention Objectives: Full Report with Commentary.* Boston: Jones and Bartlett, 1992.

U.S. Department of Health, Education, and Welfare. *Health in America: 1776–1976.* Washington, D.C.: DHEW pub. (HRA) 76-616, 1976.

U.S. Department of Justice, Immigration and Naturalization Service. *Immigration Literature: Abstracts of Demographic Economic and Policy Studies.* Washington, D.C.: Government Printing Office, 1979.

Valentine, C. A. *Culture and Poverty.* Chicago: University of Chicago Press, 1968.

Wade, M. *The French-Canadian Outlook.* New York: Viking Press, 1946.

———. *The French-Canadians, 1876–1945.* New York: Macmillan, 1955.

Walker, A. *The Temple of My Familiar.* New York: Harcourt, Brace, Jovanovich, 1989.

Wall, S. *Shadowcatchers.* New York: HarperCollins, 1994.

Wall, S., and Arden, H. *Wisdomkeepers Meetings with Native American Spiritual Elders.* Hillsboro, Ore.: Beyond Words Publishing Co., 1990.

Wallace, R. B., ed. *Public Health and Preventive Medicine.* 14th ed. Stamford, Conn.: Appleton & Lange, 1998.

Wallnöfer, H., and von Rottauscher, A. *Chinese Folk Medicine.* Trans. M. Palmedo. New York: New American Library, 1972.

Warner, D. *The Health of Mexican Americans in South Texas.* Austin, Tex.: Lyndon Baines Johnson School of Public Affairs, University of Texas at Austin, 1979.

Warner, D., and Red, K. *Health Care across the Border.* Austin, Tex.: LBJ School, 1993.

Warren, N., ed. *Studies in Cross-Cultural Psychology.* New York: Academic Press, 1980.

Weible, W. *Medjugore: The Message.* Orleans, Mass.: Paraclete Press, 1983.

Wei-kang, F. *The Story of Chinese Acupuncture and Moxibustion.* Peking: Foreign Languages Press, 1975.

Weil, A. *Health and Healing.* Boston: Houghton Mifflin, 1983.

Weinbach, S. *Rabbenu Yisrael Abuchatzira: The Story of His Life and Wonders.* Brooklyn, N.Y.: ASABA-FUJIE publication, 1991.

Weinberg, R. D. *Eligibility for Entry to the United States of America.* Dobbs Ferry, N.Y.: Oceana, 1967.

Weiss, G., and Weiss, S. *Growing and Using the Healing Herbs.* New York: Wings Books, 1985.

Wheelwright, E. G. *Medicinal Plants and Their History.* New York: Dover, 1974.

Wilen, J., and Wilen, L. *Chicken Soup and Other Folk Remedies.* New York: Fawcett Columbine, 1984.

Williams, R. A., ed. *Textbook of Black-Related Diseases.* New York: McGraw-Hill, 1975.

Williams, S. J., and Torrens, P. R. *Introduction to Health Services.* 3d ed. New York: Wiley, 1990.

Wilson, F. A., and Neuhauser, D. *Health Services in the United States.* 2d ed. Cambridge, Mass.: Ballinger, 1982.

Wilson, S. G. *The Drummer's Path: Moving the Spirit with Ritual and Traditional Drumming.* Rochester, Vt.: Destiny Books, 1992.

Winkler, G. *Dybbuk.* New York: Judaica Press, 1981.

Wright, E. *The Book of Magical Talismans.* Minneapolis, Minn.: Marlar Publishing, Co., 1984.

Wright, R. *Black Boy.* New York: Harper and Brothers, 1937.

———. *Native Son.* New York: Grosset and Dunlop, 1940.

Wright-Hybbard, E. *A Brief Study Course in Homeopathy.* Philadelphia: Formur, 1977–1992.

Yambura, B. S. *A Change and A Parting.* Ames: University of Iowa Press, 1960.

Young, J. H. *The Medical Messiahs.* Princeton: Princeton University Press, 1967.

Zambrana, R. E., ed. *Work, Family, and Health: Latina Women in Transition.* New York: Fordham University, 1982.

Zborowski, M. *People in Pain.* San Francisco: Jossey-Bass, 1969.

Zeitlin, S. J., Kotkin, A. J., and Baker, H. C. *A Celebration of American Family Folklore: Tales and Traditions from the Smithsonian Collection.* New York: Pantheon Books, 1977.

Zolla, E. *The Writer and the Shaman*. New York: Harcourt Brace Jovanovich, 1969.

Zook, J. *Exploring the Secrets of Treating Deaf-Mutes*. Peking: Foreign Languages Press, 1972.

———. *Oneida, The People of the Stone*. The Church's Mission to the Oneidas. Oneida Indian Reservation, Wisconsin, 1899.

———. *Your New Life in the United States*. Washington, D.C.: Center for Applied Linguistics, 1972.

Zook, J., and Zook, J. *Hexology*. Paradise, Pa.: Zook, 1978.

Index

Aberglobin (*See* Evil eye)

Abortion, 66, 144–49.

Access, to health care:
barriers to, 60–61, 187–90, 209–10, 227–30
improvement of, 280–81
limits on, 47–48
poverty and, 166

Acculturation, 76

Acupuncture:
in Chinese culture, 203–4
figurine, 195, 213
treatment goal, 204

Afghanistan:
birth rituals, 127
death rituals, 132

African Americans (*See* Blacks)

Agape love, 122

Ageism, 78

Albania:
birth rituals, 127
death rituals, 132

Alcoholism, in American Indians, 185–86

Aleut Indians (*See* American Indians)

Alfalfa, 116

Algeria:
birth rituals, 127
death rituals, 132

Aliens, illegal, 74–75

Alka-Zone, 27, 44

Allopathy:
characteristics, 98
vs. curanderismo, 248
development of, 112
philosophy of, 110
systems, 111

Alternative therapies:
definition, 66
expenditures for, 67
trends in, 112
types of, 110–11
use of, 66–67

AMA (*See* American Medical Association)

American Folklife Center, Library of Congress, 43

American Folklore Society, 43

American Indians (*See also* specific tribes):
anecdotal health practices, 30
blood quantum level, 190
communication styles, 190–91

culture-based health events, 183–84
death rituals, 137
domestic violence among, 186–87
healers, 179–81
health and illness beliefs, 177
health care eligibility, 187–90
as health-care providers, 191–92
history, 175–77
land reclamation efforts, 176
mean age, 162
mental illness in, 185–86
mortality rates and causes, 184–85
natural remedies, 181–83
population characteristics, 160–61
tribal breakdown, 176

Americanization, of beliefs, 75–76

American Medical Association (AMA), 98

American Public Health Association:
Black Caucus, 235
Latino Caucus, 259

Amulets:
Chinese, 202
Hispanic, 242–43
Israeli, 104
Japanese, 1, 25, 195, 213
Palestinian, 1, 25
types of, 103–4

Ancestry (organization), 43

Ancient rituals, 123

Anemias:
alpha-thalassemia, 266
Cooley's (beta-thalassemia), 266
hemolytic, 266
sickle-cell, 225, 230
starch eating related to, 223

Angelou, Maya, 222

Anise, 116

Appalshop, 42

Archive of Folk Culture, Library of Congress, 43

Argo starch, eating, 222–23

Aromatherapy, 110

Asafetida, 218

Asian Americans:
Chinese (*See* Chinese Americans)
countries of origin, 195
as health-care providers, 211–12
health problems of, 208
household income, 163
language difficulties, 209–10

Taoism, 197–98
Teas, 249
Telotherapy, 122, 151
Terminology, preferred ethnic, 159–60
Territoriality, cultural influence on, 86–87
Texas:
    German Americans in, 267–68
    Polish Americans in, 271–72
Thailand:
    birth rituals, 130
    death rituals, 135
Thalassemia syndromes, 266
Therapeutic Touch, 121
The Spirit Catches You and You Fall Down, 71
Thousand-year-old eggs, 97, 106, 119
Thunderbird, 97, 119
Thyme, 118
Tienchi flowers, 195, 213
Tiger balm, 97, 119
Time orientation:
    cultural differences in, 87
    of Hispanic Americans, 257
Tomb of David (Israel), 121, 155
Tomb of Menachem Mendel Schneerson
        (Queens, NY), 121, 155
Traditional medicine (*See* Folk medicine)
Trajectory, illness (*See* Illness trajectory)
Transportation, as health care barrier, 166
Ts'ang viscera, 200–1
Tunisia:
    birth rituals, 130
    death rituals, 135
Turner, John Richard, 151
Turpentine preparations, 215, 219, 236
Turtle shells, 208

Unitarians:
    birth rituals, 126
    health beliefs, 148–49
Unlocking process, of defining health, 5–7
Urea, therapeutic value of, 208

Vaccination, smallpox:
    of African slaves, 218

    Chinese history of, 203
Vietnam:
    birth rituals, 130
    death rituals, 135
Virgin of Guadalupe, 108
Voodoo:
    in America, 221
    definition, 112
    forms, 221
    illness caused by, 102–3, 221–22
    modern, 220–21

Wandering souls, 103
War on Poverty, 58
We Believe in Niño Fidencio, 153
Welfare, 166
White Americans:
    countries of origin, 263
    culture-based health events, 262
    German (*See* German Americans)
    household income, 163
    immigration history, 261–62
    Italian (*See* Italian Americans)
    mean age, 162
    Polish (*See* Polish Americans)
    population characteristics, 161
    in poverty, 164
Witches:
    in Hispanic culture, 241
    illness caused by, 102–3, 140
World Health Organization (WHO), 3

Xenophobia, 78
X-ray machines, 45, 68

Yellow Emperor's Book of Internal Medicine
        (Huang-ti Nei Ching), 199–201
Yerberias, 242–43
Yin and yang:
    components, 199–200
    restoration, 204
Zitzow, Daryl, 78